ACSM's

CERTIFICATION REVIEW

SECOND EDITION

ACSM Certified Personal Trainersm
ACSM Health/Fitness Instructor®
ACSM Exercise Specialist®

SENIOR EDITORS

Jeffrey L. Roitman, EdD, FACSM
Director of Cardiac Rehabilitation
Research Medical Center
Kansas City, Missouri

Khalid W. Bibi, PhD
Professor, Sports Medicine, Health and Human Performance
Director, Health and Human Performance Center
Canisius College
Buffalo, New York

ASSOCIATE EDITOR

Walter R. Thompson, PhD, FACSM, FAACVPR
Professor of Kinesiology and Health (College of Education)
Professor of Nutrition (College of Health and Human Services)
Georgia State University
Atlanta, Georgia

ACSM's
CERTIFICATION REVIEW
SECOND EDITION

ACSM Certified Personal Trainer_{SM}
ACSM Health/Fitness Instructor®
ACSM Exercise Specialist®

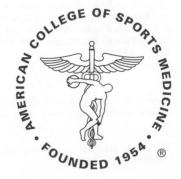

AMERICAN COLLEGE
OF SPORTS MEDICINE

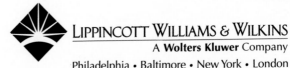

LIPPINCOTT WILLIAMS & WILKINS
A **Wolters Kluwer** Company

Philadelphia · Baltimore · New York · London
Buenos Aires · Hong Kong · Sydney · Tokyo

Executive Editor: Peter Darcy
Managing Editor: Rebecca Keifer
Marketing Manager: Christen Murphy
Production Editor: Jennifer Ajello
Designer: Risa Clow
ACSM Publications Committee Chair: Jeffrey L. Roitman, EdD, FACSM
ACSM Group Publisher: D. Mark Robertson
Compositor: Seven Worldwide
Printer: RR Donnelley

351 West Camden Street
Baltimore, MD 21201

530 Walnut Street
Philadelphia, PA 19106

Printed in China

Library of Congress Cataloging-in-Publication Data

ACSM's certification review: ACSM certified personal trainer, ACSM health/fitness instructor, ACSM registered clinical exercise specialist/American College of Sports Medicine; senior editors, Jeffrey L. Roitman, Khalid W. Bibi; associate editor, Walter R. Thompson.—2nd ed.
 p. ; cm.
 Rev. ed. of: ACSM's clinical certification review. c2001, and: ACSM's health & fitness certification review. c2001.
 Includes bibliographical references and index.
 ISBN 13: 978-0-7817-4592-5
 ISBN 10: 0-7817-4592-6
 1. Sports medicine—Outlines, syllabi, etc. 2. Sports medicine—Examinations, questions, etc. 3. Personal trainers—Outlines, syllabi, etc. 4. Personal trainers—Examinations, questions, etc. I. Roitman, Jeffrey L. II. Bibi, Khalid W. III. Thomspon, Walter R. IV. American College of Sports Medicine. V. Title: ACSM's clinical certification review. VII. Title: ACSM's health & fitness certification review. [DNLM: Examination Questions. 4. Exercise—Outlines. 5. Physical Fitness—Examination Questions. 6. Physical Fitness—Outlines. QT 18.2 A1866 2006]
 RC1213.A268 2006
 617.1′027′076—dc22

                                                                                    2005004037

To purchase additional copies of this book, call our customer service department at **(800) 638-3030** or fax orders to **(301) 824-7390**. International customers should call *(301) 714-2324.*

Visit Lippincott Williams & Wilkins on the Internet: *http://www.LWW.com.* Lippincott Williams & Wilkins customer service representatives are available from 8:30 am to 6:00 pm, EST.

08 09 10
9 10 11

Contributors

Theodore J. Angelopoulos, PhD, MPH, FACSM
Department of Child, Family, and Community Sciences
University of Central Florida
Orlando, Florida
Chapter 12, Electrocardiography

Elaine Filusch Betts, PhD, FACSM
Central Michigan University
Mount Pleasant, Michigan
Chapter 1, Anatomy and Biomechanics

Jeffery J. Betts, PhD
Central Michigan University
Mount Pleasant, Michigan
Chapter 1, Anatomy and Biomechanics

Khalid W. Bibi, PhD
The Health and Human Performance Center
Canisius College
Buffalo, New York
Chapter 11, Metabolic Calculations

Kathleen M. Cahill, MS, ATC, RCEP
Sugar Land, Texas
Chapter 8, Exercise Programming

David S. Criswell, PhD
Department of Exercise and Sport Sciences
University of Florida
Gainesville, Florida
Chapter 3, Human Development and Aging

Frederick S. Daniels, MS
CPTE Health Group
Nashua, New Hampshire
*Chapter 7, Safety, Injury Prevention, and
    Emergency Care*
Chapter 10, Program and Administration/Management

Brenda M. Davy
Virginia Tech University
Blacksburg, Virginia
Chapter 9, Nutrition and Weight Management

Michael R. Deschenes, PhD, FACSM
Department of Kinesiology
The College of William and Mary
Williamsburg, Virginia
Chapter 2, Exercise Physiology

Andrea L. Dunn, PhD, FACSM
Cooper Institute for Aerobics Research
Denver, Colorado
Chapter 5, Human Behavior and Psychology

Gregory B. Dwyer, PhD, FACSM
Department of Exercise Science
East Stroudsburg University
East Stroudsburg, Pennsylvania
Chapter 10, Program and Administration/Management

Stephen C. Glass, PhD, FACSM
Department of Movement Science
Grand Valley State University
Allendale, Michigan
Chapter 6, Health Appraisal and Fitness Testing

Chad Harris, PhD
Department of Kinesiology
Boise State University
Boise, Idaho
Chapter 1, Anatomy and Biomechanics

Mark J. Kasper, EdD
Department of Kinesiology and Physical Education
Valdosta State University
Valdosta, Georgia
Chapter 4, Pathophysiology and Risk Factors

Diana LaHue, RN, MSN
Electrophysiology Clinic
Research Medical Center
Kansas City, Missouri
Chapter 12, Electrocardiography

Bess H. Marcus, PhD
Department of Psychiatry and Human Behavior
Brown University
Providence, Rhode Island
Chapter 5, Human Behavior and Psychology

Robert S. Mazzeo, PhD, FACSM
Department of Integrative Physiology
University of Colorado
Boulder, Colorado
Chapter 3, Human Development and Aging

Susan M. Puhl, PhD
Associate Professor of Kinesiology
Department of Physical Education and Kinesiology
California Polytechnic State University
San Luis Obispo, California
Chapter 4, Pathophysiology/Risk Factors

Robert Tung, MD, FACC
Electrophysiology Clinic
Research Medical Center
Kansas City, Missouri
Chapter 12, Electrocardiography

Janet R. Wojcik, PhD
Department of Psychology
Virginia Tech University
Blacksburg, Virginia
Chapter 9, Nutrition and Weight Management

John W. Wygand, MA
Department of Health, Physical Education, and
    Human Performance Science
Adelphi University
Garden City, New York
Chapter 8, Exercise Programming

Reviewers

Amy Ables, PhD
University of Texas–Arlington
Arlington, Texas

Susan G. Beckham, PhD, FACSM
University of Texas at Arlington
Arlington, Texas

Lisa Colvin, PhD, FACSM
University of Louisiana–Monroe
Monroe, Louisiana

Dino G. Costanzo, MS
New Britain General Hospital
New Britain, Connecticut

Gregory B. Dwyer, PhD, FACSM
East Stroudsburg University
East Stroudsburg, Pennsylvania

Eric Hockstad, MD, FACC
Research Medical Center
Kansas City, Missouri

Fred Klinge
North Little Rock Athletic Club
North Little Rock, Arkansas

Dennis M. Koch
Canisius College
Buffalo, New York

Tom Lafontaine, PhD
PREVENT Consulting Services
Columbia, Missouri

Shel Levine, PhD
Eastern Michigan University
Ypsilanti, Michigan

Jacalyn McComb, PhD, FACSM
Texas Tech University
Lubbock, Texas

Claudio Nigg, PhD
University of Hawaii
Honolulu, Hawaii

Neal Pire, MA
Plus One Fitness
New York, New York

Brian Rieger, MS, RCEP
Research Medical Center
Kansas City, Missouri

Jeffrey Soukup
Appalachian State University
Boone, North Carolina

Foreword

What do you get when the hands of two expert editors blend the *American College of Sports Medicine's (ACSM) Health Fitness Certification Review* with the *ACSM's Clinical Certification Review*? You get the best of both resources, combined into one outstanding book called the *ACSM's Certification Review*. Drs. Jeffrey L. Roitman and Khalid W. Bibi and colleagues are to be highly commended for crafting what is the definitive review resource for health professionals preparing to take either the ACSM Health Fitness Instructor or Exercise Specialist certification examination.

For nearly 30 years, the ACSM has led the way in preparing professionals working in either the health and fitness or the clinical exercise setting. From university-based adult fitness programs and medical fitness centers to cardiac and pulmonary rehabilitation programs, ACSM-certified professionals deliver evidence-based health, exercise, and fitness programs throughout the United States and abroad.

This text represents the efforts of dozens of volunteer writers and reviewers who shared one common goal, to bring to life in a concise and understandable manner the knowledge, skills, and abilities (KSAs) at the heart of the ACSM certifications. These KSAs define the scope and depth of both the Health Fitness Instructor and the Exercise Specialist certifications and have themselves just undergone extensive revision. We are left with a contemporary resource for use by health fitness and rehabilitation professionals who are truly serious about being the best prepared to care for others interested in the primary and secondary prevention of disease.

Adopting a concise review format, the *ACSM's Certification Review* conveys the essential information that must reside "at the fingertips" of practicing fitness professionals and clinicians. This information is spelled out in more detail in *ACSM's Guidelines for Exercise Testing and Prescription*, 7th Edition and in *ACSM's Resource Manual for Guidelines for Exercise Testing and Prescription*, 5th Edition. Every person studying for the ACSM Health Fitness Instructor or Exercise Specialist certification will find that this single resource book both complements previously completed academic coursework and identifies areas that require additional study.

I encourage all health, fitness, and rehabilitation students as well as professionals to achieve an ACSM certification, contribute to their field, and advance the practice of your chosen profession regardless of whether you work in the community, a hospital, or an academic setting. And, in doing so, be sure to take your place in history as one of thousands of professionals who have been certified through the ACSM as being the best trained to help others in need of your services.

Best wishes as you expand your learning and extend your career.

Steven J. Keteyian, PhD, FACSM
Program Director
Preventive Cardiology
Henry Ford Heart and Vascular Institute
Henry Ford Health System
Detroit, Michigan

Preface

The *ACSM's Health & Fitness Certification Review* and *ACSM's Clinical Certification Review* have been revised to include both clinical and health/fitness information in a single volume. We made this change with intent that it will be positive for the certification candidate. First, candidates for ACSM certification can now find all the review material in a single resource, thus reducing the need for more than one review book because there is additional material in the this volume. It consolidates and simplifies resources and materials that accompany ACSM certification. Along with the seventh edition of the *ACSM's Guidelines for Exercise Testing and Prescription* and the fifth edition of the *ACSM's Resource Manual for Guidelines for Exercise Testing and Prescription*, this resource presents relevant information for ACSM certification candidates in an organized and user-friendly fashion. The information in the *ACSM's Certification Review* covers most of the knowledge, skills, and abilities (KSAs) for both ACSM Clinical and Health/Fitness certifications.

Features. The chapters in the *ACSM's Certification Review* coincide with the major categories of KSAs and are presented in **outline form** to allow quick, topical review of each area. **Tables and figures** supplement the outline text and allow easy access to supporting information. At the conclusion of each chapter is a **review test** consisting of multiple-choice study questions written in the same format and at a similar level of difficulty as the questions in the certification exam itself. Two **comprehensive examinations** that have been formulated using the same "blueprint" as the certification examination are presented as well. **Answers, with explanations,** are provided for the review test and comprehensive examination questions. A listing of **recommended readings** pertaining to each chapter also can be found at the end of the book, preceding the two comprehensive examinations; these references can be consulted for more-detailed information about the topics outlined in this review book.

How to Use This Book. The *ACSM's Certification Review* should be used by ACSM certification candidates who are ready (or nearly ready) for the certification examination and who want to review material associated with the KSAs. Those candidates who are just beginning the study process also may use this book as a study guide to

identify weaknesses and areas where more intense study may be necessary. This book is *not* meant to be a primary resource, because it is a "skeletal" outline of the critical material. The reader is further advised that the two recommended resources for all ACSM certification candidates are the seventh edition of the *ACSM's Guidelines for Exercise Testing and Prescription* and the fifth edition of the *ACSM's Resource Manual for Guidelines for Exercise Testing and Prescription*. These are invaluable primary resources for all certification candidates and professionals who need supplemental information about ACSM guidelines.

Finally, this book is intended primarily for those who are studying for the ACSM's Health/Fitness Instructor and Clinical Exercise Specialist certifications. Please note that we have not indexed the material to either the Clinical or HFI KSAs. All candidates for Clinical Certifications are held responsible for the HFI KSAs, so the entire book is useful for those studying for Clinical Certifications. HFI certification candidates should be aware of the KSAs that are pertinent to their certification and study accordingly. The clinical sections of this Review Book are not necessarily applicable to that certification.

In addition, it may be used for the ACSM Certified Personal Trainer, because those KSAs also are contained within the material covered here. However, that certification (Personal Trainer) was incomplete during the revision of this book, so not all those KSAs may be found within this material.

Summary. The features contained in the *ACSM's Certification Review*—the outline format, the tables and illustrations, the practice questions for each chapter, and the comprehensive examination at the end of the book—should make this study guide a valuable aid to ACSM certification candidates. Please be aware that questions about resources always arise. Sometimes, existing information is supplanted by new information. The seventh edition of the *ACSM's Guidelines for Exercise Testing and Prescription* is always the single, authoritative resource for examination-related questions. It is our hope that this type of presentation will assist all certification candidates to increase their level of knowledge and to prepare for the examination and certification process.

Acknowledgments. We would like to acknowledge the support and participation of our loved ones and thank them for their patience with our participation in this project and the hours we spent away from them. In addition, we thank Steven Keteyian, PhD, Chair of ACSM Committee on Certification and Registry Boards and those Committee members who provided oversight and review of this material.

Jeffrey L. Roitman, EdD, FACSM
Khalid W. Bibi, PhD
Senior Editors

Contents

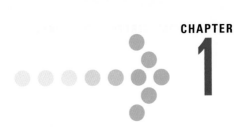

Anatomy and Biomechanics

JEFFREY J. BETTS, ELAINE FILUSCH BETTS, AND CHAD HARRIS

I. Introduction

A. GROSS ANATOMY
1. Can be learned as **regional or topographic anatomy** organized according to regions, parts, or divisions of the body (e.g., hand, mouth).
2. Can be learned as **systemic anatomy** organized according to organ systems (e.g., respiratory system, nervous system). **This chapter uses the systemic anatomy approach**, and it discusses the anatomy of the following systems only: skeletal, muscular (skeletal muscles), cardiovascular, and respiratory.

B. BIOMECHANICS
1. Is the field of study concerned with the principles of physics related to energy and force as they apply to the human body.
2. Is discussed in this chapter as it applies to specific movements or activities.

C. ORIENTATION *(FIGURE 1-1)*
1. **Proximal:** nearest to the body center, joint center, or reference point.
2. **Distal:** away from the body center, joint center, or reference point.
3. **Superior (cranial):** above, toward the head.
4. **Inferior (caudal):** lower than, toward the feet.
5. **Anterior (ventral):** toward the front.
6. **Posterior (dorsal):** toward the back.
7. **Medial:** closer to the midline.
8. **Lateral:** away from the midline.

D. BODY PLANES AND AXES
Segmental movements occur around an axis and in a plane. Each plane has an associated axis lying perpendicular to it.
1. The body has **three cardinal planes** *(Figure 1-2)*. Each plane is perpendicular to the others.
   a. The **sagittal plane** makes a division into right and left portions.
   b. The **frontal plane** makes a division into anterior (front) and posterior (back) portions.
   c. The **transverse plane** makes a division into upper (superior) and lower (inferior) portions.
2. These planes can be applied to the whole body or to parts of the body.
3. The body has three axes.
   a. The **mediolateral axis** lies perpendicular to the sagittal plane.
   b. The **anteroposterior axis** lies perpendicular to the frontal plane.
   c. The **longitudinal axis** lies perpendicular to the transverse plane.

II. Movement

Depending on the type of articulation between adjacent segments, one or more movements are possible at a joint *(Figure 1-3)*.

A. **FLEXION** is movement that decreases the joint angle. It occurs in a sagittal plane around a mediolateral axis.

B. **EXTENSION** is movement opposite to flexion and increases the joint angle. It occurs in a sagittal plane around a mediolateral axis.

C. **ADDUCTION** is movement toward the midline of the body in a frontal plane around an anteroposterior axis.

D. **ABDUCTION** is movement away from the midline of the body in a frontal plane around an anteroposterior axis.

E. **ROTATION** is movement around a longitudinal axis and in the transverse plane, either toward the midline (internal) or away from the midline (external).

F. **CIRCUMDUCTION** is a combination of flexion, extension, abduction, and adduction. The segment moving in circumduction describes a cone.

G. **PRONATION** is rotational movement at the radioulnar joint in a transverse plane about a longitudinal axis that results in the palm facing downward.

H. **SUPINATION** is rotational movement at the radioulnar joint in a transverse plane around a longitudinal axis that results in the palm facing upward.

I. **PLANTARFLEXION** is extension at the ankle joint.

J. **DORSIFLEXION** is flexion at the ankle joint.

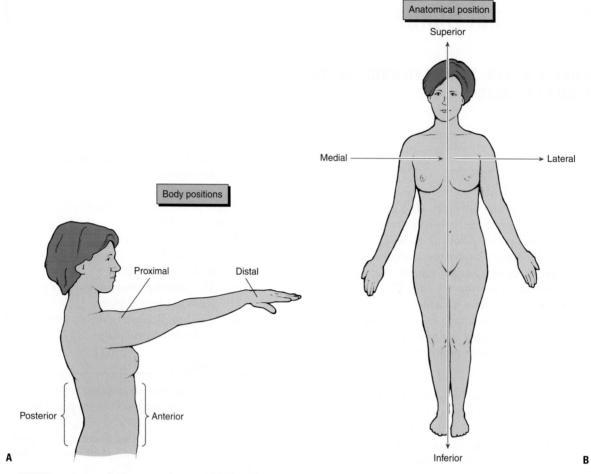

FIGURE 1-1. Terms of orientation. (Adapted from *ACSM's Resource Manual for Guidelines for Exercise Testing and Prescription,* 3rd ed. Baltimore, Williams & Wilkins, 1998, p 90.)

K. EVERSION is turning the sole of the foot away from the midline (outward).

L. INVERSION is turning the sole of the foot toward the midline (inward).

III. The Skeletal System

A. DIVISIONS (*FIGURE 1-4*)

1. Axial Skeleton

The axial skeleton includes the bones of the skull, vertebral column, ribs, and sternum. It forms the longitudinal axis of the body, supports and protects organ systems, and provides surface area for the attachment of muscles.

a. Skull

Of the 29 bones of the skull, the most significant in terms of exercise testing is the **mandible**, which may serve as an orienting landmark for palpating the carotid artery to assess pulse.

b. Spine

Also called the **vertebral column** (*Figure 1-5*), the spine serves as the main axial support for the body.

1) Vertebrae

The human spine commonly has 33 vertebrae: 7 cervical, 12 thoracic, 5 lumbar, 5 sacral (fused into one bone, the sacrum), and 4 coccygeal (fused into one bone, the coccyx).

2) Intervertebral Disks

Intervertebral disks are round, flat, or plate-like structures composed of fibrocartilaginous tissue.

a) The outer, fibrocartilaginous portion of the disk is the **annulus fibrosus**.

b) The inner gelatinous portion is **the nucleus pulposus**.

c) Disks unite the vertebral bodies and serve as **shock absorbers**.

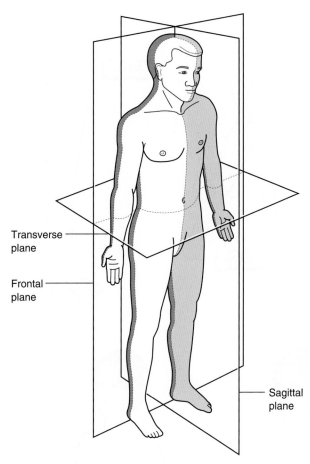

FIGURE 1-2. Planes of the human body.

Transverse plane

Frontal plane

Sagittal plane

(3)   Adult vertebral column
The adult vertebral column has **four major curvatures** *(Figure 1-5)*.
a)   **Normal spinal curves** are present in the major regions of the vertebral column when viewed sagittally.
(i)   The **thoracic curve** and **sacral curve** are posteriorly directed and termed **primary curves,** because they retain the same directional curvature as the spine in the fetus.
(ii)   The **cervical curve** and **lumbar curve** are anteriorly directed curves and are termed **secondary curves,** because they develop after birth as the infant progresses in weight bearing.

b)   **Commonly found abnormal curves** *(Figure 1-6)* include **scoliosis** (lateral deviation), **kyphosis** (exaggerated posterior thoracic curvature), and **lordosis** (exaggerated anterior lumbar curvature).
c.   Ribs
1)   The body has **12 pairs of ribs: 7 pairs of true ribs**, in which the costal cartilage articulates directly with the sternum, and 5 pairs that do not articulate directly with the sternum.
2)   The costal cartilage of ribs 8, 9, and 10 articulates with the costal cartilage of the adjacent superior rib. The cartilaginous ends of ribs 11 and 12 are free from articulation.
3)   The spaces between the ribs are called **intercostal spaces. Palpation of the intercostal spaces of the true ribs** is important for correct placement of **electrocardiography (ECG) electrodes** (in the fourth and fifth intercostal spaces).
d.   Sternum
The **sternum** lies in the midline of the chest and has three parts: the **manubrium** (superior), the **body** (middle), and the **xyphoid process** (inferior).
1)   The **sternal angle** is a slightly raised surface landmark where the manubrium meets the body of the sternum.
2)   The **xiphoid process** is also a surface landmark, situated at the bottom of the sternum and in the middle of the inferior border of the rib cage. **Palpation of the xiphoid** is necessary for cardiopulmonary resuscitation (CPR).
3)   **Palpation of the manubrium** helps to determine **proper paddle placement in defibrillation**.
2.   **Appendicular Skeleton**
a.   Includes the bones of the arms and legs and the pectoral and pelvic girdles.
b.   Functions to attach the limbs to the trunk.
1)   Clavicles
a)   Clavicles articulate with the sternal manubrium proximally and the scapulae distally and are positioned just superior to the first rib.

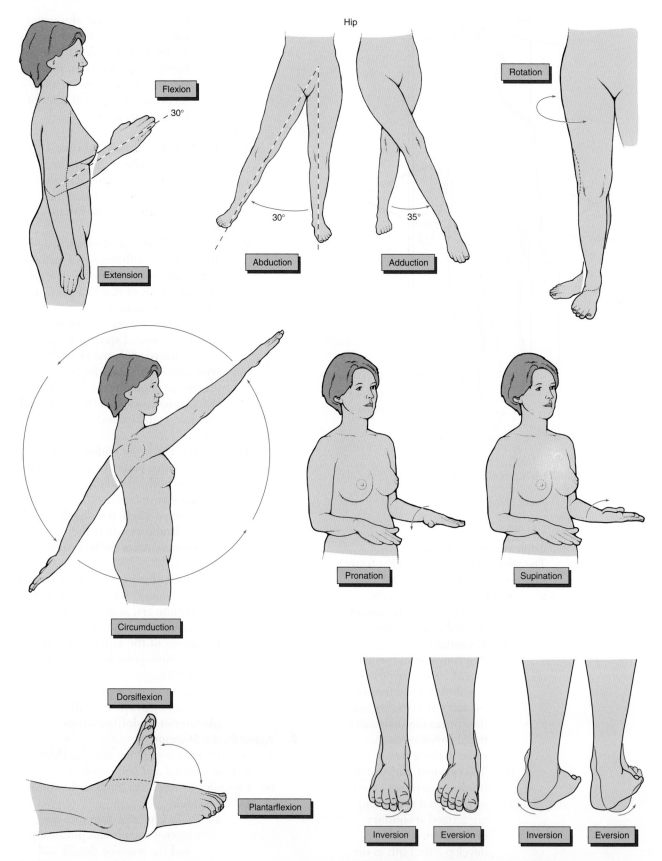

FIGURE 1-3. Body movements at joints. (Adapted in part from *ACSM's Resource Manual for Guidelines for Exercise Testing and Prescription*, 3rd ed. Baltimore, Williams & Wilkins, 1998, pp 83, 90, 91.)

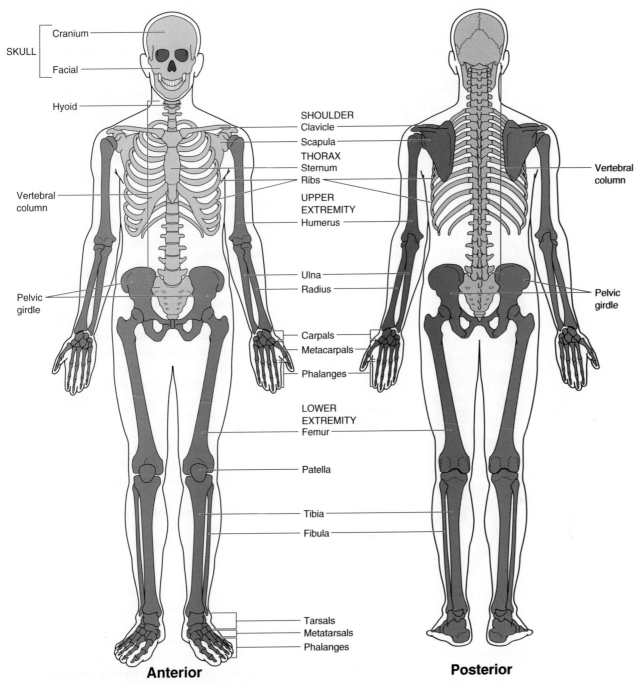

FIGURE 1-4. Divisions of the skeletal system.

b) Palpation of the clavicles helps to determine electrode placement for ECG and defibrillation.

2) Scapulae

a) Scapulae are situated on the posterior side of the body in the region of the first seven ribs.

b) Each scapula has two important landmarks:

(i) The **inferior angle** (used for skinfold site location)

at the bottom of the scapulae, forming the junction between the medial and lateral borders.

(ii) The **acromion process** (used for shoulder breadth measurement), the bony process at the most lateral part of the shoulder.

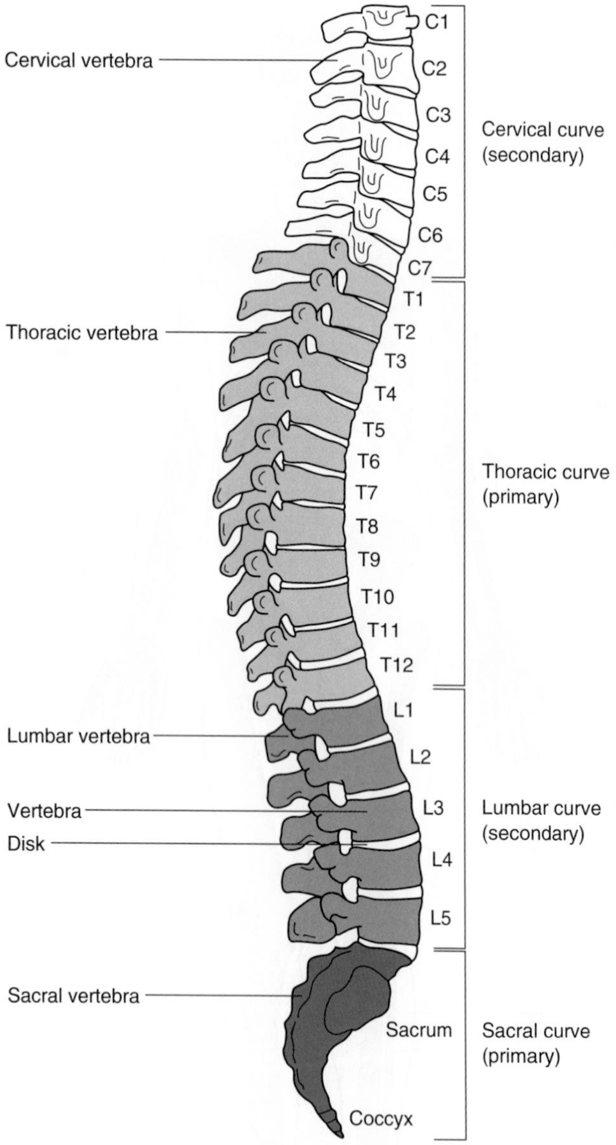

FIGURE 1-5. Lateral view of the spine, showing the vertebrae and disks.

3) Upper Arm
   a) The **humerus** proximally articulates with the glenoid fossa of the scapula and distally articulates with the ulna and radius.
   b) The most easily palpable aspects of the humerus are the **medial and lateral epicondyles** at its distal end. The epicondyles are located for elbow width measurement in estimating frame size.

4) Forearm
   The forearm includes two bones: the **ulna**, and the **radius**.

a) The most prominent bony landmark of the proximal forearm is the **olecranon process** on the posterior ulna.

b) At the distal end of the forearm are the **radial styloid process** laterally and the **ulnar styloid process** medially. These areas help to identify the proper location for assessing radial pulse.

B. LOWER BODY

The **appendicular skeleton** comprises the bones of the pelvic girdle, thigh, leg, and foot.

1. **Pelvic Girdle**
   a. The pelvic girdle is formed by the hip bones (**ilium**, **ischium**, and **pubis**), **sacrum**, and **coccyx**.
   b. The superiormost aspect of the **ilium** is the **iliac crest**, and the anteriormost structure is the **anterosuperior iliac spine**.
   c. These structures are easily palpated and serve as landmarks for skinfold measurements.

2. **Thigh**
   a. The thigh is formed by the **femur**. The most easily palpable landmark is the **greater trochanter** on the proximal lateral side.
   b. Distally, the **patella** is located anterior to the knee joint. It serves as a landmark for locating the thigh skinfold.

C. BONE

Bone is an **osseous tissue**. It is a supporting connective tissue composed of calcium salts and resistant to tensile and compressive forces. It is covered by a **periosteum** that isolates it from the surrounding tissues and provides for circulatory and nervous supply. Types include **compact** (cortical, dense) and **cancellous** (trabecular, spongy) bone.

1. **Functions**
   a. Provide structural support for the entire body.
   b. Protect organs and tissues of the body.
   c. Serve as levers that can change the magnitude and direction of forces generated by skeletal muscles.
   d. Provide storage for calcium salts to maintain concentrations of calcium and phosphate ions in body fluids.
   e. Produce blood cells.

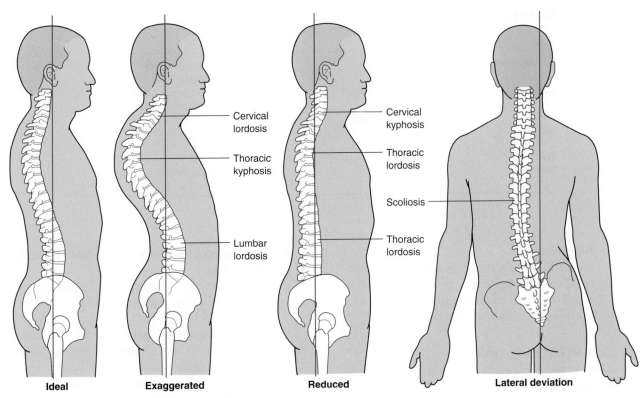

FIGURE 1-6. Ideal and abnormal spinal curvatures.

2. **General Bone Shapes**
   a. Long Bones
      1) Found in the appendicular skeleton.
      2) Consist of a central cylindrical shaft, or **diaphysis**, with an **epiphysis** at each end (e.g., femur).
          a) Diaphysis
              The diaphysis consists of compact bone surrounding a thin layer of cancellous bone, within which lies the medullary cavity, which is filled with **yellow bone marrow**.
          b) Epiphysis
              The epiphysis consists of cancellous bone surrounded by a layer of compact bone. **Red bone marrow** is contained in the porous chambers of spongy bone; **hematopoiesis** (production of red blood cells, white blood cells, and platelets) occurs within red bone marrow. Epiphyses articulate with adjoining bones and are covered with **articular (hyaline) cartilage**, which facilitates joint movement.

      3) Epiphyseal Plate
          In immature long bones, the junction between the epiphysis and the diaphysis is the location of the epiphyseal plate, where **growth** of long bone **occurs**.
   b. Short Bones
      1) Are almost cuboidal in shape (e.g., bones of the wrist and ankle).
      2) Are often covered with articular surfaces that interface with joints.
   c. Flat Bones
       Flat bones are thin and relatively broad (e.g., bones of the skull, ribs, and scapulae).
   d. Irregular Bones
       Irregular bones have mixed shapes that do not fit easily into other categories (e.g., vertebrae).

D. **CONNECTIVE TISSUES**
   Connective tissues are not generally exposed outside the body.
   1. **Basic Components**
      a. Specialized cells (e.g., in blood, bone, cartilage)
      b. Extracellular protein fibers (e.g., elastin, collagen, fibrin)
      c. Ground substance

TABLE 1-1. Types of Synovial Joints

Type	Example	Movements
Ball and socket	Hip, shoulder	Circumduction, rotation, and angular in all planes
Condyloid	Wrist (radiocarpal)	Circumduction, abduction, adduction, flexion, and extension
Gliding	Ankle (subtalar)	Inversion and eversion
Hinge	Knee, elbow	Flexion and extension in one (talocrural) plane
Pivot	Atlas/axis	Rotation around central axis
Saddle	Thumb	Flexion, extension, abduction, adduction, circumduction, and opposition

2. **Functions**
   a. Provide support and protection.
   b. Transport materials.
   c. Store mechanical energy reserves.
   d. Perform regulatory functions.

E. **JOINTS (ARTICULATIONS)**

A joint exists wherever two bones meet. The particular function and integrity of a joint depends on its anatomy and its requirement for strength or mobility.

1. **Classification**
   a. Structural Classes
      1) **Fibrous joints** (e.g., sutures of the skull)
      2) **Cartilaginous joints** (e.g., disk between vertebrae)
      3) **Synovial joints** (e.g., hip, elbow)
   b. Functional Classes
      1) **Immovable joints:** synarthroses
      2) **Slightly movable joints:** amphiarthroses
      3) **Freely movable joints:** diarthroses or synovial joints
2. **Types of Synovial Joints**
   See *Table 1-1.*
3. **Characteristics of Synovial Joints** *(Figure 1-7)*
   a. Bony surfaces are covered with **articular cartilage**.
   b. Surrounding the joint is a **fibrous joint capsule**.
   c. **Ligaments** join bone to bone.
   d. Inner surfaces of the **joint cavity** are lined with **synovial membranes**.
   e. Synovial fluid from the membrane provides lubrication to the joint.
   f. Some synovial joints, such as the knee, contain **fibrocartilaginous disks** (e.g., menisci).
   g. **Bursae** reduce friction and act as shock absorbers.

4. **Movements at Synovial Joints** (*Table 1-1* and *Figure 1-3*)
   Movements are determined by the structure of the joint and the arrangements of the associated muscles and bone.
   a. **Angular movements** (decrease or increase of the joint angle) include flexion, extension, hyperextension, abduction, and adduction.
   b. **Circular movements** include rotation (medial or lateral, supination or pronation) and circumduction. These movements occur at joints with a rounded surface articulating with the depression of another bone.
   c. **Special movements** include inversion, eversion, protraction, retraction, elevation, and depression.

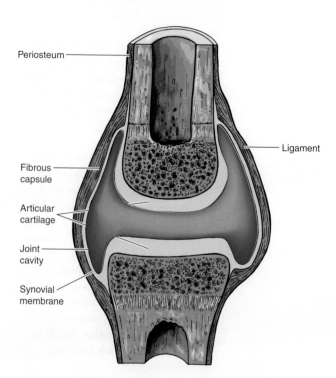

FIGURE 1-7. Synovial joint characteristics.

IV. The Muscular System

The muscular system includes skeletal, cardiac, and smooth muscle. Skeletal muscles can be controlled voluntarily.

A. GROSS ANATOMY OF SKELETAL MUSCLES

Skeletal muscle contains three layers of connective tissue.

1. The **epimysium** is the outer layer that separates the muscle from surrounding tissues and organs. The epimysium converges at the end of the muscle to form the tendon that attaches muscle to bone.
2. The **perimysium** is the central layer that divides the muscle into compartments called **fascicles** that contain skeletal muscle cells (muscle fibers).
3. The **endomysium** is the inner layer that surrounds each muscle fiber.

B. MUSCLE CONTROL

1. A **motor neuron** controls each skeletal muscle fiber.
2. The cell bodies of the motor neurons lie within the central nervous system.
3. A motor neuron and all the muscle fibers that it innervates comprise a **motor unit**.
4. Motor units are recruited separately for muscle contraction.
5. **Communication** between a motor neuron and a skeletal muscle fiber occurs at the **neuromuscular junction**.
6. Each axon of the motor neuron ends at a **synaptic knob** containing the neurotransmitter **acetylcholine (ACh)**.
7. The **synaptic cleft** separates the synaptic knob from the sarcolemma of the skeletal muscle fiber.
8. The **sarcolemma** of the motor end plate contains chemically gated sodium channels and membrane receptors that bind ACh.

C. MICROANATOMY OF THE MUSCLE CELL

1. The cytoplasm of the muscle cell is called **sarcoplasm**.
2. Extensions of the **sarcolemma** form a network of tubules called **transverse or T-tubules**.
3. The T-tubules extend into the sarcoplasm and communicate with the **sarcoplasmic reticulum**, which stores calcium in special sacs called **terminal cisternae**.
4. **Myofibrils** contain **myofilaments**, which consist of the contractile proteins **actin** and **myosin**.
5. Myofilaments are organized in repeating functional units called **sarcomeres**.
6. Actin and myosin form **cross-bridges** and slide past one another during muscle contraction, thus shortening the sarcomeres.
7. **Tropomyosin** covers the actin bridging site during resting condition. Tropomyosin is attached to **troponin**.
8. Tropomyosin and troponin regulate bridging of actin and myosin for **muscle contraction and relaxation**.

D. MUSCLE CLASSIFICATION

Each muscle begins at a proximal attachment (**origin**), ends at a distal attachment (**insertion**), and contracts to produce a specific **action**.

1. A prime mover, **or agonist,** is responsible for producing a particular movement. Prime movers and their associated joints and movements are outlined in *Table 1-2* and *Figures 1-8* and *1-9*.
2. An **antagonist** is a prime mover that opposes the agonist.
3. A **synergist** assists the prime mover but is not the primary muscle responsible for the action.

E. CLINICAL IMPORTANCE

1. Some muscles have importance for body composition testing, exercise testing, etc.
2. In the upper body, identification and palpation of the **sternocleidomastoid, pectoralis major, biceps brachii,** and **triceps brachii** are of particular importance to exercise testing.
3. In the lower body, identification and palpation of the **gluteus maximus, quadriceps femoris,** and **gastrocnemius** are of particular importance to exercise testing.
4. An important landmark for skinfold measurement is the **inguinal crease**, which is a natural, diagonal crease in the skin formed where the musculature of the thigh meets the pelvic girdle.

V. The Cardiovascular System

A. HEART

The heart receives blood from the veins and propels it into the arteries. It is located near the center of the thoracic cavity and is divided into four chambers: right and left atria, and right and left ventricles. It is enclosed by connective tissues of the pericardium in the mediastinum.

1. **Anatomy**
   a. The **atria** lie superior to the **ventricles**.
   b. The **coronary sulcus** marks the border between the atria and the ventricles.

TABLE 1-2. Muscles that Are Prime Movers

Joint	Movement	Muscle(s) [Portion]
Shoulder	Abduction	Deltoid [middle], supraspinatus
	Adduction	Latissimus dorsi, pectoralis major, teres major, posterior deltoid
	Extension	Latissimus dorsi, pectoralis major [sternal], teres major, deltoid [posterior]
	Horizontal extension	Deltoid [posterior], infraspinatus, latissimus dorsi, teres major, teres minor
	Hyperextension	Latissimus dorsi, teres major
	Flexion	Deltoid [anterior], pectoralis major [clavicular]
	Horizontal flexion	Deltoid [anterior], pectoralis major
	Lateral rotation	Infraspinatus, teres minor
	Medial rotation	Latissimus dorsi, pectoralis major, teres major, subscapularis
Shoulder girdle	Abduction (protraction)	Pectoralis minor, serratus anterior
	Adduction (retraction)	Rhomboids, trapezius [middle fibers]
	Depression	Pectoralis minor, subclavius, trapezius [lower fibers]
	Elevation	Levator scapulae, rhomboids, trapezius [upper fibers]
Scapula	Upward rotation	Serratus anterior, trapezius [upper and lower fibers]
	Downward rotation	Pectoralis minor, rhomboids
Elbow	Flexion	Biceps brachii, brachialis, brachioradialis
	Extension	Triceps brachii
Radioulnar joint	Supination	Supinator, biceps brachii
	Pronation	Pronator quadratus, pronator teres
Wrist	Abduction (radial flexion)	Flexor carpi radialis, extensor carpi radialis longus, extensor carpi radialis brevis
	Adduction (ulnar flexion)	Flexor carpi ulnaris, extensor carpi ulnaris
	Extension/hyperextension	Extensor carpi radialis longus, extensor carpi radialis brevis, extensor carpi ulnaris
	Flexion	Flexor carpi radialis, flexor carpi ulnaris, palmaris longus
Trunk	Flexion	Rectus abdominus, internal oblique, external oblique
	Extension/Hyperextension	Erector spinae group, semispinalis
	Lateral flexion	Internal oblique, external oblique, erector spinae group, multifidus, quadratus lumborum, rotatores
	Rotation	Internal oblique, external oblique, erector spinae group, multifidus, rotatores, semispinalis
Hip	Abductors	Gluteus medius, piriformis
	Adductors	Adductor brevis, adductor longus, adductor magnus, gracilis, pectineus
	Extensors	Biceps femoris, gluteus maximus, semimembranosus, semitendinosus
	Flexors	Iliacus, pectineus, psoas major, rectus femoris
	Lateral rotation	Gemelli, gluteus maximus, obturator externus, obturator internus
	Medial rotation	Gluteus medius, gluteus minimus
Knee	Extension	Rectus femoris, vastus intermedius, vastus lateralis, vastus medialis
	Flexion	Biceps femoris, semimembranosus, semitendinosus
Ankle	Extension (plantar flexion)	Gastrocnemius, soleus
	Flexion (dorsiflexion)	Extensor digitorum longus, peroneus tertius, tibialis anterior
Foot (intertarsal)	Eversion	Peroneus brevis, peroneus longus, peroneus tertius
	Inversion	Flexor digitorum longus, tibialis anterior, tibialis posterior

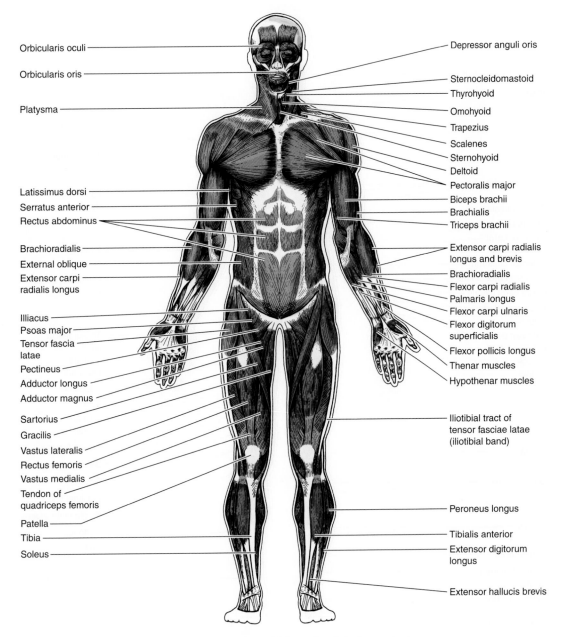

Orbicularis oculi

Orbicularis oris

Platysma

Latissimus dorsi
Serratus anterior
Rectus abdominus

Brachioradialis
External oblique
Extensor carpi
radialis longus

Illiacus
Psoas major
Tensor fascia
latae
Pectineus
Adductor longus
Adductor magnus

Sartorius
Gracilis
Vastus lateralis
Rectus femoris
Vastus medialis
Tendon of
quadriceps femoris

Patella
Tibia
Soleus

Depressor anguli oris

Sternocleidomastoid
Thyrohyoid
Omohyoid
Trapezius
Scalenes
Sternohyoid
Deltoid
Pectoralis major
Biceps brachii
Brachialis
Triceps brachii

Extensor carpi radialis
longus and brevis
Brachioradialis
Flexor carpi radialis
Palmaris longus
Flexor carpi ulnaris
Flexor digitorum
superficialis
Flexor pollicis longus
Thenar muscles
Hypothenar muscles

Iliotibial tract of
tensor fasciae latae
(iliotibial band)

Peroneus longus

Tibialis anterior
Extensor digitorum
longus

Extensor hallucis brevis

FIGURE 1-8. Anterior superficial muscles of the human body.

c. The atria have thin muscular walls and, when not filled with blood, are called **auricles**.

d. The ventricles have thicker muscular walls.

e. The **interventricular sulcus** marks the boundary between the left and right ventricles.

f. The great veins and arteries of the circulatory system are connected to the base of the heart.

g. The **apex** lies inferiorly at the tip of the heart.

2. **Internal Anatomy**

a. The right atrium receives blood from the systemic circulation through the **superior and inferior venae cavae**.

b. **Coronary veins** return venous blood from the myocardium to the **coronary sinus**, which opens into the right atrium.

c. Each atrium communicates with the ventricle on the same side by way of an **atrioventricular (AV) valve**. The right AV valve is a **tricuspid valve**; the **left AV valve** is a **bicuspid (mitral) valve**.

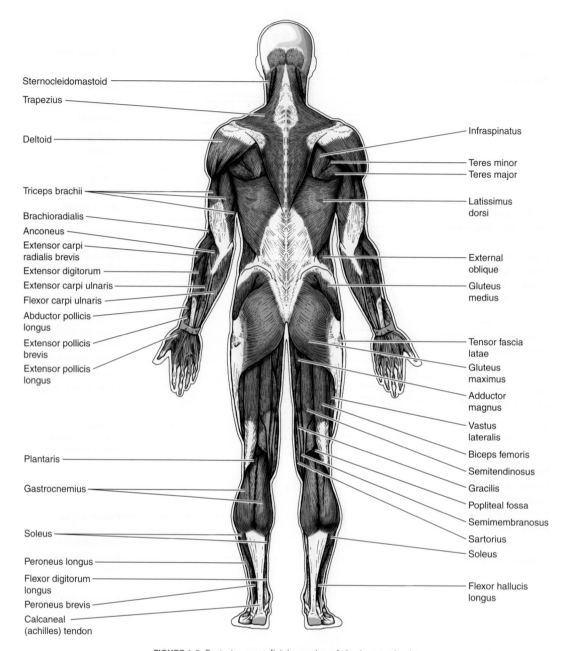

Sternocleidomastoid

Trapezius

Deltoid

Triceps brachii

Brachioradialis

Anconeus

Extensor carpi
radialis brevis

Extensor digitorum

Extensor carpi ulnaris

Flexor carpi ulnaris

Abductor pollicis
longus

Extensor pollicis
brevis

Extensor pollicis
longus

Plantaris

Gastrocnemius

Soleus

Peroneus longus

Flexor digitorum
longus

Peroneus brevis

Calcaneal
(achilles) tendon

Infraspinatus

Teres minor
Teres major

Latissimus
dorsi

External
oblique

Gluteus
medius

Tensor fascia
latae

Gluteus
maximus

Adductor
magnus

Vastus
lateralis

Biceps femoris

Semitendinosus

Gracilis

Popliteal fossa

Semimembranosus

Sartorius

Soleus

Flexor hallucis
longus

FIGURE 1-9. Posterior superficial muscles of the human body.

d. Each cusp is braced by **chordae tendinae, which are connected to papillary muscles**.

e. Unoxygenated blood leaving the right ventricle flows through the right semilunar (**pulmonic**) valve to the pulmonary artery.

f. Oxygenated blood leaving the left ventricle flows through the left semilunar (**aortic**) valve to the aorta.

3. **Circulation Through the Heart (Physiology)**

a. **Blood from the periphery** flows through the heart according to the following sequence: superior and inferior venae cavae, right atrium, tricuspid valve, right ventricle, pulmonic semilunar valve, pulmonary arteries, and lungs.

b. **Blood from the lungs** flows through the heart according to the following sequence: left pulmonary vein, left atrium, bicuspid valve, left ventricle, aortic semilunar valve, ascending aorta, and systemic circulation.

B. **CIRCULATORY SYSTEM**

1. **Blood Vessels**

a. Arteries

Arteries are muscular-walled vessels that carry blood away from the heart, decrease progressively in size to become **arterioles**, and then connect to capillaries.

b. Capillaries
Capillaries are vessels composed of one cell layer that functions to exchange nutrients and waste materials between the blood and tissues.

c. Veins
Veins are vessels that carry blood toward the heart, and they are classified according to size.
1) **Venules** are small veins that carry blood from the capillaries to medium-sized veins.
2) Medium-sized veins are larger in diameter and empty into large veins.
3) Large veins include the two **venae cavae**.

2. Blood flow
a. The heart circulates oxygenated blood through arteries to arterioles to capillaries.
b. At the capillaries, blood delivers oxygen and nutrients to the tissues and carries waste products away.
c. Unoxygenated blood returns to the capillaries and travels to venules and then to veins, which return blood to the heart.

VI. The Respiratory System

A. DIVISIONS
1. The **upper respiratory tract** consists of the **nose** (including the nasal cavity) and paranasal sinuses, the **pharynx**, and the **larynx**.
2. The **lower respiratory tract** consists of the **trachea** and the **lungs**, which include the **bronchi**, **bronchioles**, and **alveoli**.

B. LUNGS
Lungs are organs of respiration where oxygenation of blood occurs. They occupy the **pleural cavities** and are covered by a **pleural membrane**.
1. The **right lung** has three distinct lobes: superior, middle, and inferior.
2. The **left lung** has two lobes: superior, and inferior.
3. The **apex** of each lung extends into the base of the neck above the first rib.
4. The **base** of each lung rests on the **diaphragm**, which is the respiratory muscle that separates the thoracic from the abdominopelvic cavities.

C. AIR FLOW AND GAS EXCHANGE
1. Air enters the respiratory system through two external **nares** and proceeds through the **nasal cavity** and **sinuses**.
   a. Air is **warmed, filtered, and moistened** before entry into the nasopharynx at the internal nares.
   b. **Cilia** line the nasal cavity and function to sweep mucus and to trap microorganisms.
2. The incoming air then passes through the **pharynx**.
   a. The pharynx extends between the internal nares and the entrances to the **larynx and esophagus**.
   b. The pharynx is shared by the digestive and respiratory systems.
3. Incoming air leaving the pharynx passes through a narrow opening in the larynx called the **glottis**. Air movement causes the vocal cords to vibrate, generating sound.
4. From the larynx, incoming air enters the **trachea**.
   a. The trachea extends from the larynx into the lungs.
   b. **C-shaped cartilages** of the trachea perform several functions.
   1) To protect, support, and maintain an open airway.
   2) To prevent overexpansion of the respiratory system.
   3) To allow large masses of food to pass along the esophagus.
5. Air enters the **lungs** via the **tracheobronchial tree**, which consists of the **bronchi, bronchioles, and alveoli**.
   a. The trachea branches to form the right and left **primary bronchi**.
   b. Each primary bronchus enters a lung and branches into **secondary bronchi**.
   c. Further branching forms smaller, narrower passages that terminate in units called **bronchioles. Variation in the diameter of the bronchioles** controls the resistance to air flow and ventilation of the lungs.
   d. **Terminal bronchioles** are the smallest branches and supply air to the **lobules** of the lung.
   e. The lobules consist of **alveolar ducts and alveoli**, where actual **gas exchange** occurs. **Alveoli** are one-cell-layer thick and have an abundance of capillaries on the outer surface.

VII. Applied Anatomy

Knowledge of basic surface anatomy is essential in assessing pulse rate and blood pressure, obtaining anthropometric measurements, determining ECG lead placements, and performing CPR and emergency defibrillation.

A. ASSESSMENT OF PULSE RATE

Pulse is a measurement of heart rate. It can be palpated on any large- or medium-sized artery (most commonly the carotid, brachial, or radial) by using a fingertip to compress the vessel and sense the pulse (*Figure 1-10*).

1. The **carotid artery** runs along the trachea as the **common carotid**. At approximately the level of the mandible, the common carotid bifurcates to the **external and internal carotid arteries**. The carotid artery can be palpated inferior to the mandible and lateral to the larynx in the groove between the trachea and the sternocleidomastoid muscle.

2. The **brachial artery** runs along the medial side of the upper arm between the biceps brachii and triceps brachii muscles to a point just distal of the elbow joint. The artery can be palpated in the groove between the biceps and triceps or, more commonly, at the medial antecubital space on the frontal aspect of the elbow.

3. The **radial artery** divides from the brachial artery and continues distally along the forearm on the radial (thumb) side. The radial artery is easily palpable at the distal lateral wrist immediately superior to the thumb.

B. ASSESSMENT OF SYSTEMIC ARTERIAL BLOOD PRESSURE

1. Reflects hemodynamic factors (e.g., cardiac output, peripheral vascular resistance, blood flow).
2. **Is an indirect measurement of the pressure inside an artery** caused by the force exerted (by the blood) against the vessel wall.
3. Is usually measured in the arm over the brachial artery, medial to the biceps tendon, **using a sphygmomanometer and a stethoscope.**
4. In **blood pressure measurement**, the arterial reference indicator on the cuff is placed over the brachial artery. The bottom of the cuff is located approximately 1 inch above the antecubital space, and the stethoscope is positioned in the medial antecubital space (*Figure 1-11*).

C. ASSESSMENT OF ANTHROPOMETRIC MEASURES

1. **Skinfold Measurements**

   Because of the assumed relationship between subcutaneous fat and total body fat, skinfold measurements are a common method of **estimating body fat percentage**. Various skinfold sites may be measured using skinfold calipers (*Figure 1-12*).

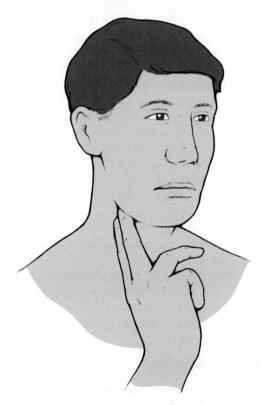

Assessing carotid pulse

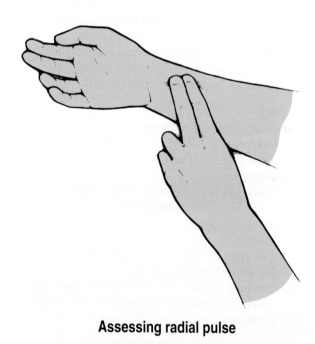

Assessing radial pulse

FIGURE 1-10. Assessing carotid and radial pulses. (Adapted from *ACSM's Resource Manual for Guidelines for Exercise Testing and Prescription,* 3rd ed. Baltimore, Williams & Wilkins, 1998, p 94.)

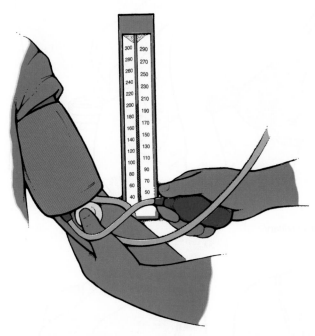

FIGURE 1-11. Measurement of blood pressure. (Adapted from *ACSM's Resource Manual for Guidelines for Exercise Testing and Prescription,* 3rd ed. Baltimore, Williams & Wilkins, 1998, p 93.)

a. **Chest/pectoral**: diagonal fold, half the distance between the anterior axillary line and the nipple in men or a third of this distance in women.

b. **Midaxillary**: vertical fold, on the midaxillary line at the level of the xiphoid process.

c. **Subscapular**: diagonal fold (45° angle), 1 to 2 cm inferior to and along the line of the inferior angle of the scapula.

d. **Triceps brachii**: vertical fold, on the posterior midline of the upper arm midway between the acromion and olecranon processes.

e. **Biceps brachii**: vertical fold, on the anterior arm over the belly of the muscle, 1 cm above the triceps brachii site.

f. **Abdominal**: vertical fold, 2 cm to the right of the umbilicus.

g. **Suprailiac**: diagonal fold, on the anterior axillary line immediately superior to the natural line of the iliac crest.

h. **Thigh**: vertical fold, on the anterior midline of the thigh midway between the inguinal crease and superior patellar border.

i. **Calf**: vertical fold, at the midline of the medial border of the calf at the greatest circumference.

2. **Body Circumferences or Girth Measurements (Table 1-3)**

a. Assess the **circumferential dimensions** of various body parts.

b. Provide an indication of **growth, nutritional status, and fat patterning**.

c. Are determined using a **tape measure**.

d. Involve the following common sites (*Figure 1-13*):

1) **Arm**: midway between the acromion and olecranon processes.

2) **Forearm**: at the maximum forearm circumference.

3) **Abdomen**: at the level of the umbilicus.

4) **Waist**: at the narrowest part of the torso, inferior to the xiphoid process and superior to the umbilicus.

5) **Hip**: at the maximum circumference of the hips/buttocks, above the gluteal fold.

6) **Thigh**: at the maximum circumference of the thigh, below the gluteal fold.

7) **Calf**: at the maximum circumference between the knee and ankle joint.

3. **Body Width Measurements**

a. Provide information for determining **frame size and body type**.

b. Can be used **to estimate desirable weight** based on stature.

c. Are measured using **spreading calipers, sliding calipers, or an anthropometer**.

d. Involve the following common sites:

1) **Elbow**: the distance between the lateral and medial epicondyles, with the elbow flexed to 90°.

2) **Biacromial**: the distance between the acromion processes.

3) **Knee**: the distance between the lateral and medial condyles, with the knee flexed to 90°.

4) **Bi-iliac**: distance between the iliac crests.

D. **ELECTROCARDIOGRAPHY**

1. ECG Lead Placement (*Figure 1-14*)

a. The **standard or Mason-Likar 12-lead system** uses 10 electrodes: 4 limb electrodes, and 6 precordial electrodes.

1) Limb Electrodes

a) **Right arm (RA) and left arm (LA) electrodes** are positioned just inferior to the distal ends of the right and left clavicle, respectively.

b) **Right leg (RL) and left leg (LL) electrodes** are positioned just superior to the iliac crest along the midclavicular line.

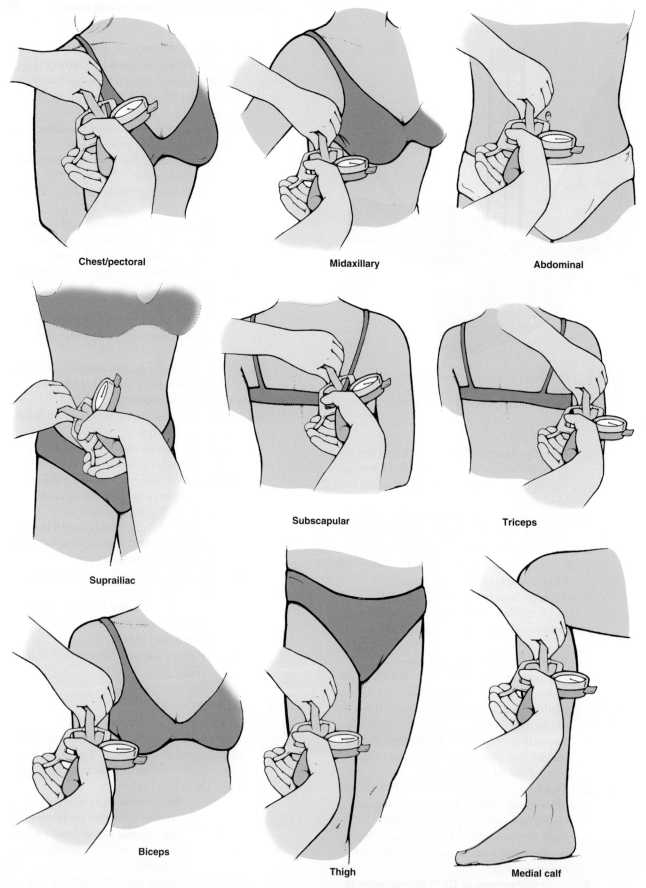

FIGURE 1-12. Obtaining skinfold measurements. (Adapted from *ACSM's Resource Manual for Guidelines for Exercise Testing and Prescription*, 3rd ed. Baltimore, Williams & Wilkins, 1998, pp 95–97.)

TABLE 1-3. Standardized Description of Circumference Measurement Sites and Procedures

Circumference site	Description
Abdomen	At the level of the umbilicus
Calf	Between the knee and the ankle, at the maximum circumference
Forearm	At the maximal forearm circumference, palms facing forward with the arms hanging downward, but slightly away from the trunk
Hips	Above the gluteal fold, at the maximal circumference of the hips or buttocks, whichever is larger
Arm	Midway between the acromion and olecranon processes, with the arm to the side of the body
Waist	At the narrowest part of the torso (superior to the umbilicus and inferior to the xiphoid process)
Thigh	With the legs slightly apart, at the maximal circumference of the thigh (below the gluteal fold)

Procedures
- All limb measurements should be taken on the right side of the body using a tension-regulated tape
- The subject should stand erect but relaxed
- Place the tape perpendicular to the long axis of the body part in each case
- Pull the tape to proper tension without pinching skin
- Take duplicate measures at each site and retest if duplicate measurements are not within 7 mm or 0.25 inch

From American College of Sports Medicine: *ACSM's Guidelines for Exercise Testing and Prescription,* 5th edition, Reference Cards. Baltimore, Williams & Wilkins, 1995, Table 4-3.

2) **Precordial (or "V") Electrodes**
   a) **V_1 and V_2** are positioned at the fourth intercostal space on the right and left sternal border, respectively.
   b) **V_4** is located on the midclavicular line at the fifth intercostal space.
   c) **V_3** is positioned at the midpoint between V_2 and V_4.
   d) **V_5 and V_6** are positioned on the anterior axillary line and midaxillary line, respectively, both at the level of V_4.

b. **Bipolar Electrodes**
   Electrode placement for the bipolar leads can take various configurations. Electrodes may be placed at the manubrium, the right fifth intercostal space at the anterior axillary line, and the standard electrode placements of RA, RL, LL, and V_5.

2. **CPR and Defibrillation**
   a. In **CPR**, chest compressions are done with the hand on the sternal body, at the

xyphoid. The middle finger is placed on the xyphoid notch with the index finger next to it. The heel of the opposite hand is then placed superior to the index finger *(Figure 1-15)*.
   b. The upper electrode for **defibrillation** is placed just inferior to the clavicle and to the right of the sternum. The lower electrode is located at the midaxillary line just lateral to the left nipple *(Figure 1-16)*.

VIII. Principles of Biomechanics

For movement to occur, a net force must be present. **Biomechanics** is the study of the forces and torques affecting movement and the description of the resulting movement.

A. FORCES
1. A **force** can be thought of as a push or a pull that either produces or has the capacity to produce a change in motion of a body.
2. Multiple forces from multiple directions may act on a body. The sum of these forces, or the **net force**, determines the resulting change in motion.

B. NEWTON'S LAWS
The relationships between forces, torques, and the resulting movements were described by Sir Isaac Newton (1642–1727). Three laws describe the interactions:
1. The **law of inertia** states that a body will maintain its state of rest or uniform motion in a straight line unless acted on by an external force.
2. The **law of acceleration** states that the acceleration of a body resulting from an applied force will be proportional to the magnitude of the applied force, in the direction of the applied force, and inversely proportional to the mass of the body. The formula for acceleration is

$a = F/m$

where

F = force
m = mass
a = acceleration

3. The **law of reaction** states that when two bodies interact, the force exerted by the first body on the second is met by an equal and opposite force exerted by the second body on the first. In other words, **for every action, there is an equal and opposite reaction.**

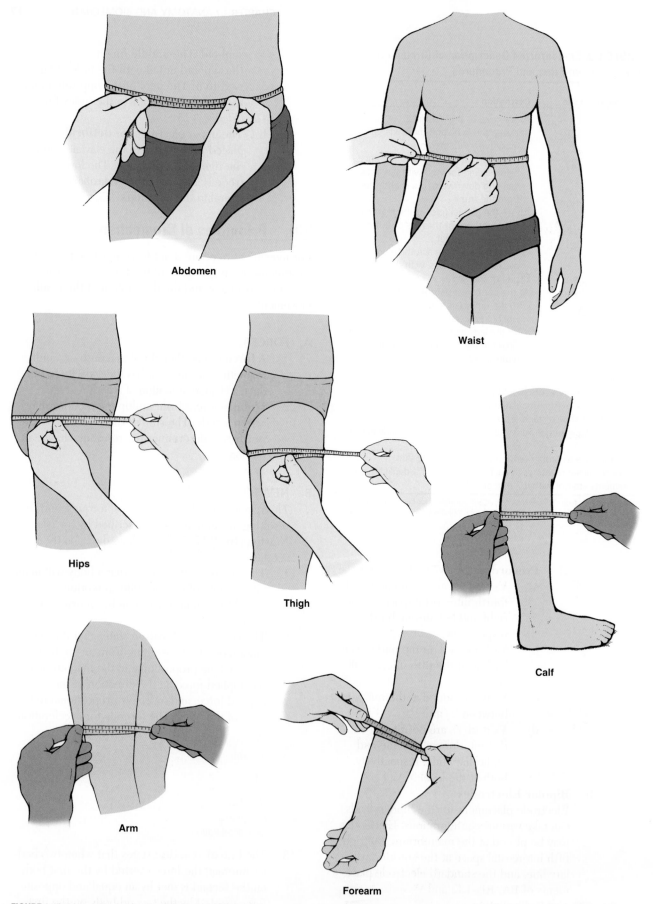

FIGURE 1-13. Measuring body circumferences. (Adapted from *ACSM's Resource Manual for Guidelines for Exercise Testing and Prescription,* 3rd ed. Baltimore, Williams & Wilkins, 1998, pp 97–99.)

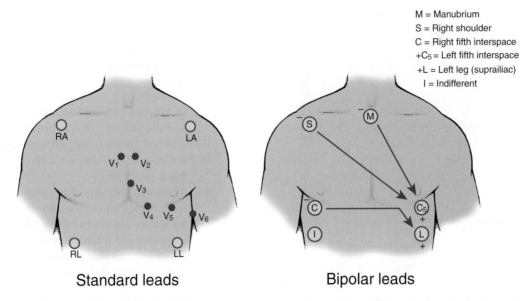

M = Manubrium
S = Right shoulder
C = Right fifth interspace
+C$_5$ = Left fifth interspace
+L = Left leg (suprailiac)
I = Indifferent

Standard leads   Bipolar leads

FIGURE 1-14. ECG lead placement. (Adapted from *ACSM's Resource Manual for Guidelines for Exercise Testing and Prescription,* 3rd ed. Baltimore, Williams & Wilkins, 1998, p 92.)

C. FORCES AFFECTING MOVEMENT

The forces influencing movement can be classified as reaction, friction, and muscular.

1. **Ground Reaction Force**
    a. In accordance with **Newton's law of reaction**, as a body applies a force to the ground, the ground applies an equal and opposite force to the body.
    b. Ground reaction forces are measured with a force plate in **three directions**: vertical, anteroposterior, and mediolateral. The net effect of the three-dimensional forces determines the resulting movement.
    c. **Typical patterns** of ground reaction force are seen in **walking and running** (*Figure 1-17*).
    d. **Abnormalities in gait** can be assessed by evaluating ground reaction force patterns.

2. **Frictional force**
    a. When two objects interact, **friction** acts parallel to the surface contact of the objects in a direction opposite the motion or impending motion (*Figure 1-18*).

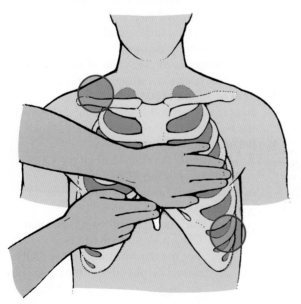

FIGURE 1-15. Hand positions for cardiac compression in CPR. (Adapted from *ACSM's Resource Manual for Guidelines for Exercise Testing and Prescription,* 3rd ed. Baltimore, Williams & Wilkins, 1998, p 99.)

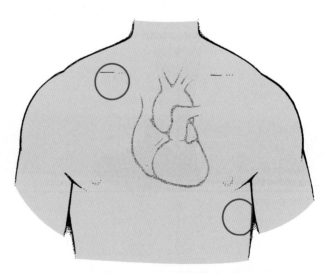

FIGURE 1-16. Standard placement for defibrillation electrodes. (Adapted from *ACSM's Resource Manual for Guidelines for Exercise Testing and Prescription,* 3rd ed. Baltimore, Williams & Wilkins, 1998, p 100.)

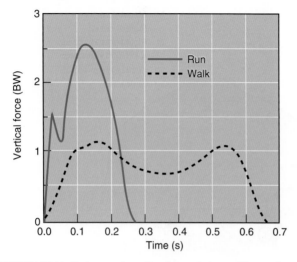

FIGURE 1-17. Vertical ground reaction forces during walking and running.

b. **Frictional force** (*Ff*) is influenced by the nature and interaction of the contacting surfaces (the coefficient of friction, *m*) and the force pressing the surfaces together (the normal force, *N*). The formula for frictional force is

$$Ff = mN$$

3. **Muscular Force**
   a. To move body segments, muscular forces must be present. Muscles provide a **pulling force on bone.** Across any joint, the net effect of individual muscle forces acting across the joint determines the joint movement.
   b. Because all segmental movement is rotational, not only the net muscular force but

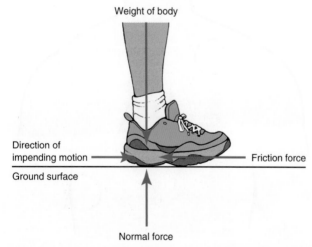

Weight of body

Direction of impending motion

Friction force

Ground surface

Normal force

FIGURE 1-18. Friction force during foot contact of a running stride. (Adapted from *ACSM's Resource Manual for Guidelines for Exercise Testing and Prescription,* 3rd ed. Baltimore, Williams & Wilkins, 1998, p 105.)

also **the distance the force acts from the rotational axis of the joint** influence movement. **Torque** is the rotary effect of force produced by a muscle or a group of muscles.
   c. Also affecting movement are the **length of the muscle at the time of contraction** and the **velocity of muscle shortening.**
   d. **Normal movement patterns** result from the coordinated actions of the muscles acting across a joint.
   e. **Abnormal movement patterns** result from disruptions in the coordinated muscular actions because of the application of inappropriate force, co-contraction of musculature, muscular weakness, or neurologic disorders affecting muscular recruitment.

D. **PRINCIPLES OF BALANCE AND STABILITY**
Each segment of the body is acted on by the **force of gravity** and has a **center of gravity.**
   1. **Line of Gravity (LOG)**
      Line of gravity is the downward direction of the force of gravity on an object (vertically, toward the center of the earth).
   2. **Center of Gravity (COG)**
      a. Is the **point of exact center around which the body freely rotates.**
      b. Is the **point around which the weight is equal on all sides.**
      c. Is the **point of intersection of the three cardinal body planes.**
      d. Lies approximately anterior to the second sacral vertebra when all segments of the body are combined and the body is considered to be a single, solid object (in **anatomic position**).
      e. Changes as the segments of the body move away from the anatomic position.
   3. **Base of Support (BOS)**
      Base of support is the area of contact between the body and the supporting surface.
   4. **Balance and Stability**
      a. **Balance** is maintained when the COG remains over the BOS.
      b. **Stability** is firmness of balance; the COG must fall within the BOS.
         1) **Increased stability** occurs when COG is closer to the BOS.
         2) For **maximum stability,** the COG should be placed over the center of the BOS.

E. **APPLIED WEIGHTS AND RESISTANCES**
   1. The ability of any force to cause rotation of a lever is known as **torque.**

2. **Rotation** of a segment of the body is dependent on:
   a. The magnitude of force exerted by the **effort force and the resistance force.**
   b. The **distance of these two forces from the axis of rotation.**
3. Moving the COG of segments alters resistive torque. **Changing the torque provides a method for altering the difficulty of an exercise when weight is applied** (*Figure 1-19*).
   a. Weight applied at the end of an extended arm changes the COG of the arm to a more distal position, requiring greater muscular support to maintain the arm in a horizontal position. Conversely, by shifting the mass of the weight proximally, less muscular effort is required.
   b. Some externally applied forces (e.g., exercise pulleys) do not act in a vertical direction, and those **forces exert effects that vary according to the angle of application**.
   c. Weights applied to the extremities frequently exert traction (**distractive force**) on joint structures. A distractive force is sometimes used to promote normal joint movement in rehabilitation exercise, but distractive force can also be injurious or undesirable.

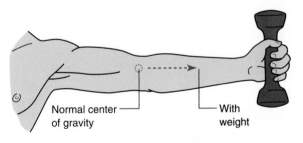

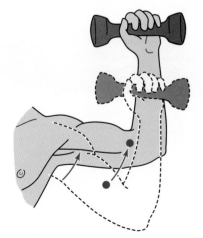

FIGURE 1-19. A change in center of gravity changes the torque.

F. **MOTION**
1. **Translatory Motion**
   a. Occurs when a freely movable object moves in a straight line when a force is applied on center of the object.
   b. Occurs when, regardless of where the force is applied, the object is free to move in a rectilinear or a curvilinear path.
2. **Rotary Motion**
   a. Occurs when a force is applied off-center to a freely movable object.
   b. Occurs when, regardless of where the force is applied, the object is free to move only in a rotary path.
3. **Velocity**
   a. Velocity represents the distance traveled in a period of time.
   b. **Acceleration** refers to increasing velocity.
   c. **Deceleration** refers to decreasing velocity.
4. **Momentum**
   Momentum is the mathematical product of the mass and velocity of a moving object.

G. **LEVERS**
A lever is a rigid bar that **revolves around a fixed point or axis (fulcrum).**
Levers are **used with force to overcome a resistance.**
1. **Parts of a Lever**
   a. The **axis** is the pivot point between the force and the resistance.
   b. The **force arm** is the distance from the axis to the point of application of force.
   c. The **resistance arm** is the distance from the axis to the resistance.
2. **Classes of Levers (*Figure 1-20*)**
   a. In a **first-class lever**, the axis is between the force and the resistance arm, and the force arm may be greater than, smaller than, or equal to the resistance arm.
   b. In a **second-class lever**, the resistance lies between the effort force and the axis of rotation, and the force arm is greater than the resistance arm.
   c. In a **third-class lever**, the effort force lies closer to the axis of the lever than the resistance, and the force arm is smaller than the resistance arm.
   d. When the principles of levers are actually applied in the body, the joint serves as the axis, the contraction of skeletal muscles around the joint serves to generate the force, and the moving segment (including anything supported by that segment) is the resistance.

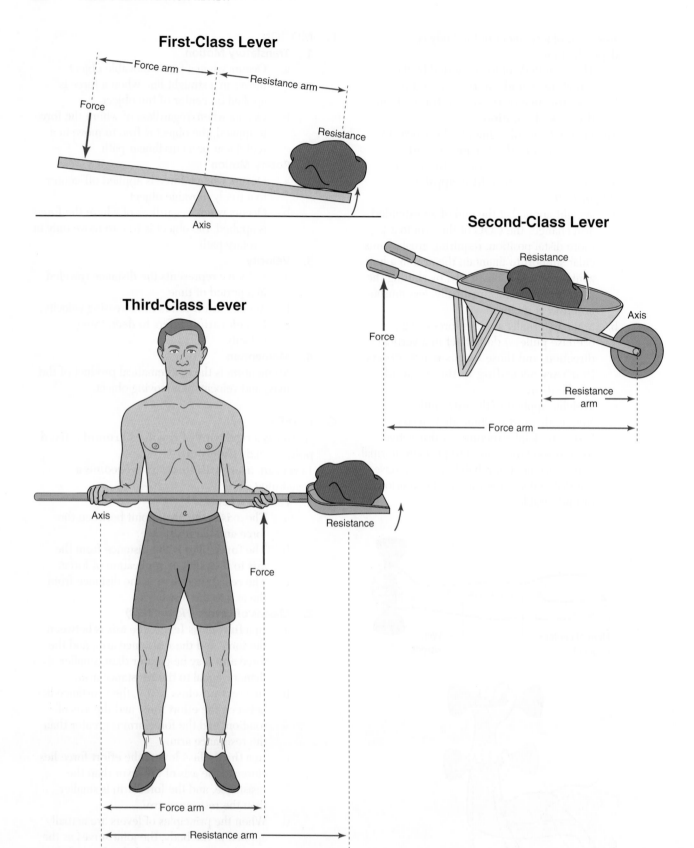

FIGURE 1-20. Lever systems.

IX. Application of Biomechanical Principles to Activity

A. WALKING

1. Normal Walking Gait

a. **Locomotion** occurs from repetition of the **gait cycle**, which is the time between successive ground contacts of the same foot (*Figure 1-21*).

   1) A **stride** is the time between ground contacts of the right heel. **Stride length** is therefore measured from initial contact of one lower extremity to the point at which the same extremity contacts the ground again.

   2) Half of a stride is a **step**, defined as the time from ground contact of one heel to ground contact of the other heel.

   3) Normally, 60% of the gait cycle is in **stance** (foot in contact with the ground), and 40% is in **swing** (foot not in contact with the ground).

b. Typical **walking speed** in adults is approximately 1.5 m/s. Decreases in walking speed occur with aging, injury, and disease.

c. A typical length of stride, or **cycle length (CL)**, is approximately 1.5 m, and a typical rate of stride, or **cycle rate (CR)**, is approximately 1 cycle/s. With increasing gait speed, CL and CR increase.

d. In the frontal plane, **pelvic movement** during walking is approximately 5 cm on each side, alternating as each leg assumes a support role. In the transverse plane, the pelvis rotates a total of 8°, half of it anteriorly and half of it posteriorly.

e. In a normal walking gait, the vertical **ground reaction force** pattern is bimodal in shape and of maximum magnitude on the order of 1- to 1.2-fold the body weight. The two peaks represent heel contact to midstance and midstance to push off.

2. Phases of the Gait Cycle

During a single gait cycle, each extremity passes through two phases.

a. Stance Phase

   1) Begins when one extremity contacts the ground (heel strike).

   2) Continues as long as some portion of the foot is in contact with the ground (toe off).

   3) Subdivisions of the Stance Phase

     a) **Heel strike**.

     b) **Foot flat**.

     c) **Midstance**.

     d) **Heel off**.

     e) **Toe off**.

b. Swing Phase

   1) Begins when the toe of one extremity leaves the ground.

   2) Ends just before heel strike or contact of the same extremity.

   3) Subdivisions of the Swing Phase

     a) **Initial swing (acceleration)**.

     b) **Midswing**.

     c) **Terminal swing (deceleration)**.

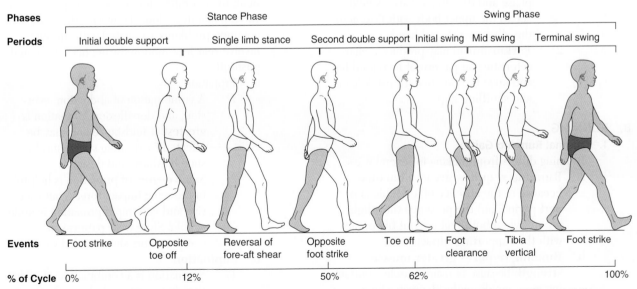

Phases	Stance Phase				Swing Phase		
Periods	Initial double support	Single limb stance	Second double support	Initial swing	Mid swing	Terminal swing	
Events	Foot strike	Opposite toe off	Reversal of fore-aft shear	Opposite foot strike	Toe off	Foot clearance	Tibia vertical	Foot strike
% of Cycle	0%	12%	50%	62%			100%

FIGURE 1-21. Normal walking gait cycle. (Adapted from Rose J, Gamble JG [eds]: *Human Walking*, 2nd ed. Baltimore, Williams & Wilkins, 1994, p 26.)

3. **Abnormal Walking Gait**

Deviations from a normal walking gait occur for various reasons (e.g., pain from injury, decreased flexibility or range of motion) and take many different forms. **Common causes of gait abnormalities** include muscular weakness and neurologic disorders.

a. Muscular Weakness

1) **Weakness in the gluteus maximus** may contribute to an anterior lean of the upper body at heel strike.

2) **Weakness in the gluteus medius and minimus** decreases their stabilizing function during the stance phase of gait, possibly leading to an increased lateral shift in the pelvis (increased frontal plane movement) and side-to-side movement during gait.

3) Severe **weakness in the plantarflexors** reduces push-off and thus step length on the affected side.

4) **Dorsiflexor insufficiency** results in slapping of the foot during heel contact (foot drop) and increased knee and hip flexion during the swing phase.

5) Because of the inability to adequately support loads or control knee extension, **weakness of the quadriceps femoris** may lead to forward lean of the trunk or hyperextension of the knee joint (genu recurvatum).

b. Neurologic Disorders

1) In **hemiplegia**, the affected leg is often circumducted during the swing phase and the affected arm is held across the upper body with flexion in the elbow, wrist, and hand.

2) **Parkinsonism** may produce a characteristic gait pattern of increased hip and knee flexion, forward trunk lean, and shuffling step.

B. **RUNNING**

1. **Normal Running Gait**

Running differs from walking in several ways.

a. **Running requires greater balance** because of the absence of a double support period and the presence the "flight phase" when both feet are out of contact with the supporting surface.

b. **Running requires greater muscle strength** because of many muscles contracting more rapidly and with greater force.

c. **Running requires greater range of motion** because of greater joint angles at the extremes of the movement.

d. The **direction of the driving force is more horizontal** and the **stride is longer**.

e. The body has a **greater forward incline.**

f. **Rotary actions** of the spine and pelvic regions **are increased**.

g. **Arm actions are higher and more vigorous.** (The arms should move in an anterior/posterior direction to improve efficiency.)

h. **Stride length and frequency are increased** with increasing speed.

i. The normal running gait is similar to the walking gait but with the addition of a **flight phase**, during which both feet are off the ground.

j. **Cycle length (CL)** and **cycle rate (CR)** are related to running speed:

$$\text{velocity} = CL \times CR$$

Up to approximately 5 m/s, CL increases with speed, and CR stays relatively constant or increases slightly. Increases in speed beyond 5 m/s generally result from increased CR.

k. At running speeds up to 6 m/s, vertical **ground reaction forces** are between two- and threefold the body weight. These forces are realized at heel strike as an impact peak and during push off as an active peak.

2. **Abnormal Running Gait**

As with walking, running gait disorders are difficult to generalize due to their complexity and varying manifestations. However, the most common problems associated with running involve rear foot motion during heel strike and push-off.

a. Pronation

1) A combination of abduction, eversion, and dorsiflexion, pronation is greatest at midstance and may be affected by running speed and by shoe hardness and design.

2) Some degree of pronation is helpful in reducing impact forces, but excessive and very rapid pronation is undesirable. Shoe wear patterns in overpronators show medial wear.

b. **Supination**

1) Supination is a combination of adduction, inversion, and plantarflexion.

2) Excessive supination (marked by excessive shoe wear on the lateral side) at take off may impair running performance because of misdirection of propulsive forces.

C. SWIMMING

1. **Buoyancy**
   a. Is the tendency of a body to float when submerged in a fluid.
   b. **Is dependent on the percentage of weight composed of bone and muscle,** because these tissues are more dense (and, therefore, less buoyant) than other body tissues.
   c. According to **Archimedes' principle**, a body immersed in fluid is buoyed up with a force equal to the weight of the displaced fluid.

2. **Propelling Forces**
   a. Result from the **stroke and kick.**
   b. Should contribute to **forward progress,** not to vertical or lateral movement.
   c. During the propelling phase, the arms, hands, and feet should present a large surface to the water and should push against the water.

3. **Resistive Forces**
   Resistive forces result from:
   a. Skin resistance (friction).
   b. Wave-making resistance caused by up-and-down body movement.
   c. Eddy current resistance.

D. LIFTING AND BODY MECHANICS

1. In applying the laws of motion to lifting, reaching, pushing, pulling, and carrying of objects, the effects of gravity, friction, muscular forces, and external resistance are important.

2. The **basic principles of good body mechanics** are:
   a. **Assume a position close to the object,** or move the position of the object closer to the COG, allowing the use of upper extremities in a shortened position (short lever arms). Lower torque is required, thus allowing muscles to function more efficiently.
   b. **Position COG as close to the object's COG as possible,** reducing torque and energy requirements.
   c. **Widen the BOS** by lowering the COG and maintaining the COG within the BOS.
   d. **Position the feet according to the direction of movement** required to perform the activity, thus increasing stability.
   e. **Avoid twisting** when lifting.
   f. When possible, **push, pull, roll, or slide an object** rather than lift it.
   g. **Use the "power position"** (*Figure 1-22*).
      1) Knees slightly bent.
      2) Body bent forward from the hips.
      3) Back straight.
      4) Chest and head upright.

E. LOW BACK PAIN: MECHANISMS, PREVENTION, AND TREATMENT

Back pain **occurs most commonly in the lumbar region** of the vertebral column. It may be caused by traumatic injury, history of poor posture, faulty body mechanics, stressful living and working habits, lack of flexibility or strength, or a general lack of physical fitness.

1. **Mechanism of Injury in Disk Herniation**
   a. The **lumbar vertebrae are the most massive but also the least mobile,** because they **support much of the body weight.**
   b. The **lumbar disks** are the thickest of the intervertebral disks and **are subject to the most pressure.**
   c. As loading on the vertebral column increases, the intervertebral disks become more important as **shock absorbers.**

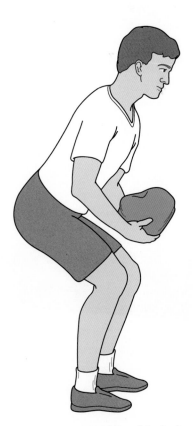

FIGURE 1-22. Power position of the body.

d. **Excessive or repetitive stresses** on the lumbar region because of slumped sitting, forward bending, lifting, or twisting may cause **herniation of the disk**.

1) The **inner nucleus pulposus of the disk** breaks through the surrounding fibrocartilaginous annulus fibrosus and **protrudes** beyond the intervertebral space.

2) The disk protrusion often occurs in a posterior direction. This causes **pressure on the nerves in the disk wall and nerve roots**, sending pain along the back and leg. This pain is referred to as **radiating symptoms** or **radiculopathy**.

2. **Prevention and Treatment of Low Back Pain**

a. Low back pain can occur because of various mechanisms of injury or overuse.

Therefore, **people with low back pain should be evaluated by a physician**.

b. Knowledge of **proper body mechanics, adequate physical conditioning, and flexibility** may help to prevent low back pain.

1) **Disk protrusion with radiculopathy**: Backward bending of the spine, with avoidance of forward bending and slumped sitting postures, is often recommended to relieve pressure on the nerve root.

2) **Pain caused by muscle guarding and spasm** in the absence of signs of disk herniation is often treated with **muscle stretching**. Maintaining flexibility in the back is also helpful as a preventive method.

Review Test

DIRECTIONS: Carefully read all questions, and select the BEST single answer.

1. The C-shaped cartilages of the trachea allow all of the following to occur EXCEPT
    A) Ciliated movement of mucus-secreting cells.
    B) Distention of the esophagus.
    C) Maintenance of open airway.
    D) Prevention of tracheal collapse during pressure changes.

2. Functions of bone include all of the following EXCEPT
    A) Support for the body.
    B) Protection of organs and tissues.
    C) Production of red blood cells.
    D) Production of force.

3. In the organization of skeletal muscle, the muscle cell contains the contractile proteins. Which of the following is a contractile protein?
    A) Myosin.
    B) Muscle fascicle.
    C) Myofibril.
    D) Muscle fiber.

4. A client in your exercise class has been complaining of back pain with no radicular symptoms. This person has been treated medically and is now joining the exercise program to improve flexibility in the low back. Which exercise would be most appropriate for this person to address the stated goal?
    A) Hip flexor stretch.
    B) Knee-to-chest stretch.
    C) Gastrocnemius stretch.
    D) Lateral trunk stretch.

5. All of the following statements are true regarding long bones EXCEPT
    A) The diaphysis is composed of compact bone.
    B) The epiphysis consists of spongy bone.
    C) Most bones of the axial skeleton are of this type.
    D) The central shaft encases the medullary canal.

6. The arm is capable of performing all of the following motions EXCEPT
    A) Flexion.
    B) Abduction.
    C) Inversion.
    D) Supination.

7. The prime movers for extension of the knee are the
    A) Biceps femoris.
    B) Biceps brachii.
    C) Quadriceps femoris.
    D) Gastrocnemius.

8. A baseball pitcher has been complaining of weakness in the lateral rotation motions of the shoulder. You have been asked to evaluate him for a strengthening program. Which of the following muscles would you have him concentrate on strengthening?
    A) Subscapularis.
    B) Teres major.
    C) Latissimus dorsi.
    D) Teres minor.

9. Cartilage is categorized as which of the following types of connective tissue?
    A) Loose.
    B) Dense.
    C) Fluid.
    D) Supporting.

10. Blood leaving the heart to be oxygenated in the lungs must first pass through the right atrium and ventricle. Through which valve does blood flow when moving from the right atrium to the right ventricle?
    A) Bicuspid valve.
    B) Tricuspid valve.
    C) Pulmonic valve.
    D) Aortic valve.

11. An abnormal curve of the spine with lateral deviation of the vertebral column is called
    A) Lordosis.
    B) Scoliosis.
    C) Kyphosis.
    D) Primary curve.

12. Which of the following is considered to be a "ball-and-socket" joint?
    A) Ankle.
    B) Elbow.
    C) Knee.
    D) Hip.

13. Which of the following is the ability of a force to cause rotation of a lever?
    A) Center of gravity.
    B) Base of support.
    C) Torque.
    D) Stability.

14. Standard sites for the measurement of skinfolds include the
    A) Medial thigh.
    B) Biceps.
    C) Infrailiac.
    D) Forearm.

15. A standard site for the measurement of circumferences is the
    A) Abdomen.
    B) Neck.
    C) Wrist.
    D) Ankle.

16. The most common site used for measurement of the pulse during exercise is the
    A) Popliteal.
    B) Femoral.
    C) Radial.
    D) Dorsalis pedis.

17. Blood from the peripheral anatomy flows to the heart through the superior and inferior venae cavae into the
    A) Right atrium.
    B) Left atrium.
    C) Right ventricle.
    D) Left ventricle.

18. Arteries are large-diameter vessels that carry blood away from the heart. As they course through the body, they progressively decrease in size until they become
    A) Arterioles.
    B) Anastomoses.
    C) Venules.
    D) Veins.

19. The law of inertia
    A) States that a body at rest tends to remain at rest, whereas a body in motion tends to continue to stay in motion with consistent speed and in the same direction unless acted on by an outside force
    B) States that the velocity of a body is changed only when acted on by an additional force
    C) States that the driving force of the body is doubled and that the rate of acceleration is also doubled.
    D) States that the production of any force will create another force that will be opposite and equal to the first force.

20. Running is a locomotor activity similar to walking but with some differences. In comparison to walking, running requires greater
    A) Balance.
    B) Muscle strength.
    C) Range of motion.
    D) All of the above.

21. Who first described that a body immersed in fluid is buoyed up with a force equal to the weight of the displaced fluid?
    A) Einstein.
    B) Freud.
    C) Whitehead.
    D) Archimedes.

22. Which of the following bones articulates proximally with the sternal manubrium and distally with the scapula and is helpful to palpate in electrode placement?
    A) Scapula.
    B) Sternum.
    C) Clavicle.
    D) Twelfth rib.

23. Which of the following is NOT a characteristic of the "power position" used for lifting with proper body mechanics?
    A) Shoulders slouched.
    B) Back straight.
    C) Body bent forward from the hips.
    D) Knees slightly bent.

24. The intervertebral disks have which of the following characteristics?
    A) Calcified outer ring.
    B) Gelatinous inner nucleus portion.
    C) Gray matter surrounding the neural cell bodies.
    D) All of the above.

25. Pain caused by low back muscle guarding and spasm in the absence of signs of disk herniation is often treated with muscle stretching. Which of the following is (are) helpful stretching activities for the low back?
    A) Knee to chest.
    B) Double-knee to chest.
    C) Lower trunk rotation.
    D) All of the above.

26. Which of the following will increase stability?
    A) Lowering the center of gravity.
    B) Raising the center of gravity.
    C) Decreasing the base of support.
    D) Moving the center of gravity farther from the edge of the base of support.

27. Which type of musculoskeletal lever is most common?
    A) First-class.
    B) Second-class.
    C) Third-class.
    D) Fourth-class.

28. Angular motion occurs when
    A) A force is applied off-center to a freely-moveable object.

B) A freely-movable object moves in a straight line when a force is applied on-center.

C) An object is free to move only in a linear path.

D) All of the above.

29. In a second-class lever, the
A) Axis is located between the effort force and the resistance.
B) The resistance is located between the effort force and the axis.
C) The effort force is located between the resistance and the axis.
D) None of the above.

30. Slapping of the foot during heel strike and increased knee and hip flexion during swing are characteristic of
A) Weakness in the gluteus medius and minimus.
B) Weakness in the quadriceps femoris.
C) Weakness in the plantarflexors.
D) Weakness in the dorsiflexors.

31. Which of the following is characteristic of running versus walking?
A) Less vigorous arm action.
B) Decreased stride length.
C) Period of nonsupport.
D) Period of double-support.

32. Low back pain occurs most commonly in the lumbar region, because
A) The lumbar vertebrae are the least mobile.
B) The lumbar disks are subject to the most pressure.
C) The lumbar vertebrae support much of the body weight.
D) All of the above.

33. The rear-foot motion called pronation results from a combination of
A) Abduction, eversion, and plantarflexion.
B) Adduction, inversion, and plantarflexion.
C) Abduction, eversion, and dorsiflexion.
D) Adduction, inversion, and dorsiflexion.

ANSWERS AND EXPLANATIONS

1–A. Cilia line the nasal cavity, not the trachea. The C-shaped cartilages of the trachea provide a certain rigidity to support the trachea and maintain an open airway so that collapse does not occur. In addition, the rigidity caused by these cartilages prevents overexpansion of the trachea when pressure changes occur in the respiratory system. The proximity of the trachea to the esophagus (the esophagus is posterior to the trachea) could cause obstruction to the airway if a large bolus of food is passed in the esophagus. This is remedied by the arrangement of the C-shaped cartilages of the trachea, with the open end of the C being posterior. Distention of the esophagus can occur without compromise to the airway.

2–D. The bones of the skeletal system act as levers for changing the magnitude and direction of forces that are generated by the skeletal muscles attaching to the bones. The bones of the skeletal system provide structural support for the body through their arrangement in the axial and appendicular skeletal divisions. The axial skeleton forms the longitudinal axis of the body, and it supports and protects organs as well as provides attachment for muscles. The appendicular skeleton provides for attachment of the limbs to the trunk. It is in the bone marrow that blood cells are formed.

3–A. The skeletal muscle consists of bundles of muscle fibers called muscle fascicles, or fasciculi. Each fasciculus contains muscle cells. Within the muscle cells are cylinders called myofibrils, which are responsible for the contraction of the muscle fiber. The myofibrils have this ability because they contain myofilaments, which are the contractile proteins actin and myosin. Actin is a thin filament that is twisted into a strand. Myosin is a thick filament that has a tail and a head. During activation of the muscle, actin and myosin interact, causing cross-bridging between the two filaments. The myosin pulls the actin, which shortens the muscle and causes tension development.

4–B. Treatment of a low back complaint depends on the mechanism of injury or overuse. In the case of disk herniation, which is often accompanied by radiating symptoms into the leg, positioning of the spine can often alleviate painful symptoms because of reduced pressure on the spinal nerves. In the case of the individual addressed in this question, flexibility of the lumbar spine is prescribed to reduce symptoms. Performance of the knee-to-chest stretch exercise would be the most appropriate in this case, because it allows sustained stretch of the lumbar spinal musculature to increase muscular length and to improve flexibility. The lateral trunk stretch is not sufficient to improve the flexibility of muscles supporting the lumbar spine.

5–C. The majority of bones of the appendicular (rather than the axial) skeleton are long bones. Long bones have a central shaft (called the diaphysis) that is made of compact (dense) bone. The shaft forms a cylinder around a central cavity of the bone, which is called the medullary canal.

6–C. Inversion is a specialized movement that can be performed by the sole of the foot but not by the arm. The arm is capable of angular and circular movements. Angular movements decrease or increase the joint angle and include flexion, extension, abduction, and adduction. Circular movements can occur at joints having a bone with a rounded surface that articulates with a cup or depression on another bone. Included in circular movements are circumduction and rotation, including the specialized rotational movements of supination and pronation.

7–C. The quadriceps femoris muscle is the major muscle responsible for knee extension, as dictated by its proximal and distal attachments. The muscle has four heads (quad), three of which originate from the anterior portion of the ilium and one of which originates on the shaft of the femur. All four heads converge and insert on the tibia via a common tendon (patellar). Contraction of the muscle causes the knee to extend. The biceps brachii is found in the upper body and is an elbow flexor. Although the biceps femoris and gastrocnemius muscles cross the knee joint, they do so posteriorly and are primarily active in knee flexion and ankle plantarflexion, respectively.

8–D. The subscapularis, teres major, and latissimus dorsi are all medial rotators of the arm. They function as antagonists to the teres minor, which is a lateral rotator of the arm.

9–D. Connective tissues of the body are categorized according to specific characteristics of their ground substance. Connective tissue has many types of cells and fibers in a somewhat syrupy ground substance. Loose and dense connective tissues are of this type. Fluid connective tissue cells are suspended in a watery ground substance; included in this category are blood and lymph. Supporting connective tissues have a dense ground substance, with very closely packed fibers. Cartilage and bone are found in the supporting connective tissue category.

10–B. Blood from the peripheral anatomy flows to the heart through the superior and inferior venae cavae into the right atrium. From the right atrium, the blood passes through the tricuspid valve to the right ventricle, then out through the pulmonary semilunar valve to the pulmonary arteries, and then to the lungs to be oxygenated. The tricuspid valve is so-named because of the three cusps, or flaps, of which it is made. The bicuspid valve is a similar valve, having only two cusps, that is found between the left atrium and left ventricle. Blood leaving the left ventricle will pass through the aortic semilunar valve to the ascending aorta and then out to the systemic circulation.

11–B. The vertebral column serves as the main axial support for the body. The adult vertebral column exhibits four major curvatures when viewed from the sagittal plane. Scoliosis is an abnormal lateral deviation of the vertebral column. Kyphosis is an abnormal increased posterior curvature, especially in the thoracic region. Lordosis is an abnormal, exaggerated anterior curvature in the lumbar region. A primary curve refers to the thoracic and sacral curvatures of the vertebral column that remain in the original fetal positions.

12–D. The ankle is a gliding joint and allows flexion, extension, inversion, and eversion. The shoulder and hip are both ball-and-socket joints, allowing circumduction, rotation, and angular motions. The knee is a hinge joint, allowing flexion and extension in only one plane.

13–C. The center of gravity is the point of exact center around which the body freely rotates, the point around which the weight is equal on all sides, and the point of intersection of the three cardinal planes of the body. Balance is maintained when the center of gravity stays over the base of support, and stability is the firmness of balance. Torque is the ability of any force to cause rotation of the lever and is calculated as the product of the force and the perpendicular distance from the axis of rotation at which the force is applied.

14–B. The standard sites for the measurement of skinfold thicknesses include the abdominal, triceps, biceps, chest, medial calf, midaxillary, subscapular, suprailiac, and thigh (a measurement taken on the anterior midline of the thigh).

15–A. The standard sites for the measurement of body circumferences are the abdomen, calf, forearm, hips, arm, waist, and thigh.

16–C. The most common sites for measurement of the peripheral pulse during exercise are the carotid and radial. These sites are more easily accessible during exercise than the femoral, popliteal, posterior tibial, or dorsalis pedis.

17–A. Blood from the peripheral anatomy flows to the heart through the superior and inferior venae cavae into the right atrium. From the right atrium, blood passes through the tricuspid valve to the right ventricle and then out through the pulmonary semilunar valve to the pulmonary arteries and to the lungs to be oxygenated.

18–A. Arteries are large-diameter vessels that carry blood away from the heart. As they course through the body, they progressively decrease in size until they become arterioles, the smallest vessels of the arterial system. From the arterioles, blood enters the capillaries, which are one layer thick. Venules and veins return blood back to the heart.

19–A. The law of inertia states that a body at rest tends to remain at rest whereas a body in motion tends to continue in motion, with consistent speed and in the same direction, unless acted on by an outside force. The law of acceleration states that the velocity of a body is changed only when acted on by an additional force, that the driving force of the body is doubled, and that the rate of acceleration is also doubled. The law of counterforce states that the production of any force will create another force that will be opposite and equal to the first force.

20–D. Running is a locomotor activity similar to walking, but with some differences. In comparison with walking, running requires greater balance, muscle strength, and range of motion. Balance is necessary because of the absence of the double-support period and the presence of the float periods, in which both feet are out of contact with the supporting surface. Muscle strength is necessary because many muscles are contracting more rapidly and with greater force during running as compared with walking. Joint angles are at greater extremes with the running gait.

21–D. Archimedes first described the principle of buoyancy. If a body displaces water weighing more than itself, the body will float. When the lungs are filled with air, most individuals float in water. However, the ability to float is dependent on the percentage of weight that is composed of bone and muscle, because these tissues are denser than other body tissues.

22–C. The clavicle articulates with the sternum and scapula, which the twelfth rib does not do. Also, the location of the clavicle is helpful in placing

electrodes for some ECG lead placements and defibrillation to avoid the large muscle mass in the area and to apply the shock in an appropriate location for effect.

23–A. The power position does not indicate a slouching of the shoulders; rather, it focuses on stabilization of the low back. The power position is to maintain a stable center of gravity and keep the load distributed effectively, which is why the head and neck are up, etc.

24–B. The intervertebral disk acts as a shock absorber for the spinal column and, therefore, has the gelatinous inner portion to absorb the forces experienced. It is often a herniation of this portion of the disk that occurs in back disk injury and must be repaired surgically.

25–D. Pain caused by muscle guarding and spasm in the absence of signs of disk herniation is often treated with muscle stretching. Maintaining flexibility in the back is helpful as a preventative measure as well. All three of these exercises are good for stretching the lower back.

26–A. Lowering the center of gravity will increase stability. Stability would also be increased by increasing the size of the base of support and/or by moving the center of gravity closer to the center of the base of support.

27–C. Third-class lever systems are the most common in the musculoskeletal system. An example would be the arrangement of the biceps brachii: The insertion of the biceps brachii, which provides the effort force, is between the elbow joint (the axis) and center of gravity of the forearm (the resistance). Examples of first- and second-class levers can be found in the musculoskeletal system, but they are not common. There is no such thing as a fourth-class lever.

28–A. Angular motion will occur with a freely movable object when a force is applied off-center; it will also result when a force is applied to an object that is free to move only in a rotary path. A force applied on-center to a freely movable object, or to an object that is free to move only on a linear path, will result in linear motion.

29–B. In a second-class lever system, the resistance is located between the effort force and the axis; thus, the effort force moment arm is greater than the resistance moment arm, providing an advantage for force. When the axis is between the effort force and the resistance, the result is a first-class lever. When the effort force is between the resistance and the axis, the result is third-class lever.

30–D. Dorsiflexor weakness leads to foot drop during heel strike and, to ensure that the toe does not catch the walking surface, increased knee and hip flexion during swing. Weakness in the plantarflexors reduces push off and, thereby, step length. Weakness in the gluteus medius and minimus decreases their stabilizing function during stance and can lead to increased lateral shift in the pelvis. Quadriceps weakness can lead to forward lean of the trunk or knee hyperextension.

31–C. Only running has a period of nonsupport, when both feet are off the ground. Walking has a period of double-support, when both feet are in contact with the ground. In addition, running has a more vigorous arm action and increased stride length compared to walking.

32–D. Because of their location, the lumbar vertebrae must support the weight of the trunk and upper extremities; therefore, they are the largest vertebrae and have the thickest intervertebral disks. For this reason, they are the least mobile of the vertebrae and are subject to the greatest amount of pressure.

33–C. Pronation is a type of rear-foot motion that occurs during heel strike and push off in running. Pronation results from a combination of abduction, eversion, and dorsiflexion. Although a certain amount of pronation is normal and helpful in reducing impact forces, excessive and very rapid pronation may lead to injury. The rear-foot motion called supination results from a combination of adduction, inversion, and plantarflexion.

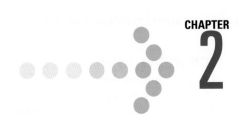

Exercise Physiology

MICHAEL R. DESCHENES

I. Bioenergetics

The term **bioenergetics** refers to the body's ability to acquire, convert, store, and utilize energy. The immediate source of energy for all cellular activities, including muscle contraction, is **adenosine triphosphate (ATP)**. In releasing its energy, ATP is cleaved to **adenosine diphosphate (ADP)**. Because only a limited amount of ATP is stored in the body, energy pathways (or systems) have been developed to replace ATP as it is utilized (e.g., exercise).

A. PHOSPHAGEN SYSTEM

1. This energy pathway is composed of the ATP and **phosphocreatine (PCr)** that are stored in muscle fibers.
2. Through the activity of the enzyme **creatine kinase**, PCr yields its phosphate group so that it can be added to ADP to synthesize ATP.
3. Although immediately available for use by the working muscle, the phosphagen system is limited in its capacity to supply energy. During exercise with all-out effort, for example, stored ATP and PCr can sustain activity for no more than 30 seconds.

B. NONOXIDATIVE SYSTEM

1. The nonoxidative system is sometimes referred to as the **anaerobic pathway**, because oxygen is not required for it to produce ATP.
2. In this system, only carbohydrates (e.g., glucose, glycogen) can be used to produce ATP. In the absence of oxygen, however, the breakdown of carbohydrates yields lactic acid (more accurately referred to as lactate), which can contribute to muscle fatigue as it accumulates.
3. The nonoxidative system is the main provider of energy to the working muscle in athletic events lasting from 30 seconds to 3 minutes.

C. OXIDATIVE SYSTEM

1. This ATP-producing pathway is also called the **aerobic system**, because oxygen is required for it to operate.
2. Both carbohydrates and lipids (fats)—and even, to a limited extent, proteins—can be used to synthesize ATP by this pathway.
3. The metabolic byproducts that result from **oxidative phosphorylation** are water and carbon dioxide, which have no fatiguing effects on working muscle.
4. In activities lasting more than 3 minutes in duration and in which intensity is limited, muscles primarily rely on oxidative metabolism to produce ATP.
5. Although a prolific producer of ATP, this system is disadvantaged by the fact that it is relatively slow in synthesizing the ATP demanded by exercising muscle. Moreover, should inadequate oxygen be delivered to the working muscle, it will also depend on the nonoxidative system to produce energy, resulting in lactate accumulation. The exercise intensity at which this occurs is referred to as the **anaerobic threshold** or the **lactate threshold**.

II. Skeletal Muscle

Skeletal muscle is tissue that has been specialized to move the bony levers of the skeletal system, thus enabling mobility (or movement) of the body. Other types of muscle in the body include cardiac muscle (discussed later) and smooth muscle, which among other things assists in the regulation of blood flow to various parts of the body. Among these three types of tissue, however, skeletal muscle is the most abundant, accounting for nearly 50% of the human body's mass. Like all types of tissue, skeletal muscle is comprised of individual cells. Skeletal muscle cells are typically termed **myocytes** or **myofibers**. The structure of these cells and the manner in which they are arranged yield insight regarding the mechanism of muscle function.

A. CONNECTIVE TISSUE

1. The **endomysium** is a layer of connective tissue that is wrapped around each myofiber.
2. A group of as many as 150 myofibers lying in parallel are bundled together to form a **fasciculus**, which is encased by a layer of tissue called the **perimysium**.
3. The layer of connective tissue that surrounds the entire muscle is referred to as the **epimysium** (*Figure 2-1*).

B. MAJOR ORGANELLES

1. Unlike most cells, each individual myofiber contains more than one nucleus. Indeed, these multinucleated cells may possess 200 to 300 nuclei per millimeter of fiber length.
2. The endoplasmic reticulum, which is termed the **sarcoplasmic reticulum**, is richly developed in the myofiber, because the **calcium** ions that it stores are needed to stimulate muscle contraction.

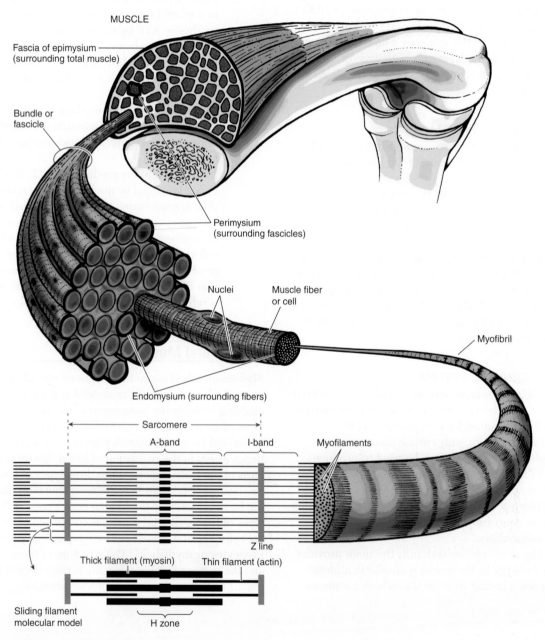

FIGURE 2-1. Cross-section of skeletal muscle. (With permission from *ACSM's Resource Manual for Guidelines for Exercise Testing and Prescription*, 3rd ed. Baltimore, Williams & Wilkins, 1998, p 80.)

3. The plasma membrane of the myofiber is referred to as the **sarcolemma**.
4. The voltage-gated sodium channels that are regularly distributed along the sarcolemma allow electrical stimulation of the myofiber via the generation of **action potentials**. As a result, myofibers are considered to be "excitable" cells.
5. Because muscle tissue demonstrates a high degree of metabolic activity, mitochondrial content is substantial in myofibers, providing much ATP via the oxidative pathway.

C. PROTEIN FILAMENTS
1. The contractile filaments myosin and actin account for roughly 60% of the protein content of the myofiber. **Myosin** is the larger protein and is sometimes called **the thick filament; actin** is the smaller of the contractile proteins and is termed the **thin filament**.
2. Regulatory filaments are essential for triggering the contractile event. These regulatory filaments are **troponin** and **tropomyosin**.

D. TYPES OF MUSCLE FIBERS
1. Myofibers can be classified using several different methods. The most common is based on the isoform of myosin expressed by the cell.
2. Humans have three myosin isoforms (types I, IIa, and IIx, corresponding to the fiber types of I, IIA, and IIB, respectively).
   a. **Type I** fibers have slow-twitch properties but high oxidative capacity.
   b. **Type IIB** myofibers are fast twitch with low oxidative potential.
   c. **Type IIA** myofibers are intermediate in both twitch velocity and oxidative capacity.
3. Exercise of high intensity and short duration (e.g., sprinting) is principally powered by type II myofibers, whereas activities featuring low intensity and long duration (e.g., marathon running) are almost exclusively dependent on type I myofibers.

E. MECHANISM OF THE MYOFIBER TWITCH
1. Both regulatory and contractile filaments are essential to the generation of myofiber twitch. In turn, the force generated by the whole muscle is a function both of the number of myofibers within that muscle that are twitching and of the rate at which these twitches occur.
2. The **sliding filament theory** of muscle contraction explains how these protein filaments interact to produce a twitch of the fiber. The sequence of events is as follows:
   a. As the nervous system excites the myofiber's sarcolemma and its **T-tubules**, calcium stored within the sarcoplasmic reticulum is released into the cell's cytosol.
   b. Calcium binds to troponin, causing the associated tropomyosin to undergo a conformational shift.
   c. As a result of this shift, **active sites** on the actin filament are exposed.
   d. **Cross-bridge** heads located on the myosin molecule bind to the exposed, active sites of actin.
   e. The enzyme ATPase, which is found on the cross-bridge head, cleaves ATP, resulting in the **power stroke** that pulls actin toward the center of the myosin molecule. This sliding action of the actin over the myosin results in shortening of the fiber and generation of force.
   f. When a new ATP molecular binds to the myosin cross-bridge head, the link between myosin and actin is broken, allowing the entire process to repeat itself so long as the cytosolic calcium levels remain elevated. **The calcium pump** is responsible for delivering cytosolic calcium back into the sarcoplasmic reticulum, thus returning the myofiber to a state of relaxation.

III. The Pulmonary System
The pulmonary system allows the body to breathe and, thus, exchanges gases with the environment. During inspiration (inhalation), air is taken into the lungs, and during expiration (exhalation), air leaves the lungs to reenter the environment. The purpose of inspiration is to bring needed oxygen into the body; the purpose of expiration is to eliminate carbon dioxide, a byproduct of metabolism, from the body.

A. ANATOMY
1. Air enters the pulmonary system through the mouth and nose.
   a. Inhaling through the nose has the advantages of warming the air and removing many airborne particles that may cause irritation or even infection.
   b. During exercise, breathing through the mouth is generally required to accommodate the increased rate and depth of ventilation.
2. Passageways through the nose and mouth join together at the **pharynx** (throat).

3. Inhaled air then passes through the **larynx** before entering the cartilage-lined **trachea** (windpipe).
4. The trachea then branches to form two **bronchi**, each leading into one of the two lungs within the thoracic cavity.
5. Within the lungs, the bronchi divide to form numerous **bronchioles**.
6. At the end of each bronchiole is a cluster of **alveoli**. It is within these tiny air sacs that gases are exchanged between the lungs and the blood traveling through the capillaries surrounding each alveolus.

B. **MECHANISM OF BREATHING**
   1. **Inhalation**
      a. During inhalation, the inspiratory muscles contract to expand the size (or volume) of the thoracic cavity.
      b. To achieve this, the **diaphragm** contracts, moving downward toward the abdomen, whereas the external **intercostal muscles** pull the rib cage outward.
      c. During exercise, when the depth of breathing increases, accessory inspiratory muscles (e.g., sternocleidomastoid, scalenus) also contribute to expansion of the rib cage by lifting upward.
   2. **Exhalation**
      a. Under resting conditions, expiration is a passive process that involves relaxation of the inspiratory muscles and consequent recoiling of the thoracic cavity, returning the lungs back to their original dimensions. This increases the pressure inside the lungs, forcing air out of the body through the nose and the mouth.
      b. During exercise, exhalation becomes an active process in which the abdominal and internal intercostal muscles contract to more forcefully collapse the size of the thoracic cavity and drive air out of the lungs.

C. **RESPONSES TO EXERCISE AND TRAINING**
   1. **Minute Ventilation ($\dot{V}_E$)**
      a. $\dot{V}_E$ is the volume of air either inspired or expired (the amount will be the same) over the course of 1 minute.
      b. At rest, $\dot{V}_E$ is approximately 6 L.
      c. Exercise results in an elevation of $\dot{V}_E$, and exercise intensity determines the degree of this increase. This enhancement of $\dot{V}_E$ occurs in two phases.
         1) Initially, a sharp increase in the depth of breathing occurs.
         2) As the exercise stimulus becomes more intense, the rate of breathing substantially increases, and a secondary, less pronounced increase in the depth of breathing becomes apparent.
      d. During maximal intensity exercise, $\dot{V}_E$ may be 20- to 25-fold higher than the typical 6 L/min that is observed under resting conditions.
         1) This response is a consequence of both an increment in **tidal volume**, which is the amount of air entering or leaving the lungs in a single breath, from 0.5 to approximately 4 L, as well as an increase in **respiratory rate** from 12 to almost 50 breaths per minute.
         2) Despite this, the work of breathing remains fairly constant. At rest, 3% of the body's energy expenditure is accounted for by breathing, and even during maximal effort exercise, the energy used to power ventilation represents only 5% of the body's energy needs.
      e. In healthy individuals, exercise capacity is not limited by ventilation, nor does long-term exercise training induce adaptations in ventilatory capacity.
   2. **Maximal Aerobic Capacity ($\dot{V}O_2$max)**
      a. Training adaptations are evident, in the exercise intensity at which the anaerobic threshold occurs.
      b. In untrained individuals, anaerobic threshold occurs at approximately 55% of one's $\dot{V}O_2$max.
      c. The anaerobic threshold of well-trained endurance athletes occurs at a much greater exercise intensity, perhaps 80% to 85% of their $\dot{V}O_2$max.

IV. The Cardiovascular System

The cardiovascular system is comprised of the heart and the blood vessels that carry blood throughout the body. The heart is actually a powerful, fatigue-resistant muscle that acts as a pump to drive blood returning from all parts of the body to the lungs, where it can be oxygenated, and the newly oxygenated blood out to the rest of the body. Blood vessels are responsible for delivering the nutrient rich blood ejected from the heart to all the needy tissues of the body and for returning blood carrying metabolic byproducts from those tissues back to the heart. For clarity, the two components of this system will be addressed individually.

A. THE HEART

1. **Anatomy**

    a. The human heart is comprised of four separate chambers.

       1) The two upper chambers are referred to as the **atria** (singular, atrium).

       2) The two lower chambers are called **ventricles**.

    b. The right atrium receives blood from all parts of the body through the vena cava and the left atrium from the lungs.

    c. The atria pump blood into the ventricles, and the right and left ventricles, respectively, drive blood to the lungs and the rest of the body.

    d. The right and left sides of the heart (the pulmonary and systemic pumps, respectively), are separated by the **septum**, a thick wall of connective tissue.

    e. The right and left atria contract in unison, as do the right and left ventricles. The contractions of the atria and of the ventricles, however, are staggered. In this way, while blood is being delivered to the ventricles, those chambers are in their resting phase, and during contraction of the ventricles, the atria are at rest.

2. **Physiology**

    a. The heart's pumping action is described as the **cardiac cycle**.

    b. **Systole** refers to the contractile phase of the **myocardium**, when blood is forced out of the atria and ventricles.

    c. **Diastole** is the relaxation phase between contractions of the ventricles (systole); this phase occurs when the chambers fill with blood for the next cycle.

    d. Several terms are important in understanding the function of the cardiac cycle.

       1) **Stroke Volume (SV)**
          The SV is the volume of blood ejected by each ventricle per contraction (or beat) of the heart. At rest, SV is typically 70 mL.

       2) **Heart Rate (HR)**
          The HR is the number of times the heart contracts per minute. Under resting conditions, HR is approximately 72 bpm.

       3) **Cardiac Output ($\dot{Q}$)**
          Cardiac output is the amount of blood pumped from the heart by each ventricle per minute. (In most clinical situations, these and the following ventricular volumes are referenced to the left ventricle, primarily because of the importance of left ventricular function in end-organ perfusion.) In turn, cardiac output is a function of SV and HR, where

          $$\text{cardiac output} = HR \times SV$$

          Using normal resting values of HR (72 bpm) and SV (70 mL/beat), cardiac output at rest is approximately 5 L/min.

       4) **End-Diastolic Volume (EDV)**
          The EDV is the amount of blood in each ventricle at the end of the resting phase (diastole) of the cardiac cycle. According to the **Frank-Starling law**, EDV will significantly affect SV, because the greater the volume of blood in the ventricle, the greater the stretch imparted on the myocardium. As stretch increases, so does contractile force, both by elastic recoil of the muscle and by optimizing the length of the fibers composing the myocardium. At rest, normal EDV would be approximately 125 mL.

       5) **End-Systolic Volume (ESV)**
          The ESV is the volume of blood remaining in each ventricle following its contraction. At rest, ESV equals approximately 55 mL.

       6) **Ejection Fraction**
          The ejection fraction is the percentage of the blood in the ventricle during diastole that is actually pumped out during systole. Sometimes, it is defined as the ratio of SV to EDV, or

          $$\text{ejection fraction} = SV/EDV$$

          Under resting conditions, the ejection fraction is roughly 56%, although it can be as high as 67%.

3. **Acute Effects of Exercise on Cardiac Function**

    a. The greater demand for blood that occurs when exercise begins results in an increase in cardiac output.

       1) This acute response in cardiac function is directly linked to the intensity of exercise, and at maximal effort, cardiac output can be five- to sixfold higher (25–30 L/min) than that at rest (5 L/min). This elevated pumping capacity is brought about by increases in both HR and SV.

       2) The SV increases until the exercise intensity reaches approximately 50%

of $\dot{V}O_2$max, at which point it levels off. Consequently, further elevations in cardiac output are accounted for primarily by increased HR.

3) A linear relationship exists between HR and exercise intensity. As a result, monitoring HR is a common method of assessing exercise intensity.

b. As greater amounts of blood are pumped to the working muscle, the amount of blood returning to the heart is similarly enhanced.

1) This leads to elevations in EDV, which can be as high as 160 mL when SV is at its peak value.

2) The relationship between SV and EDV is as follows:

a) As EDV increases during exercise, so does SV.

b) In young, untrained men, SV may increase from 70 mL at rest to 100 mL during exercise.

3) Another method used by the heart to amplify its pumping ability during exercise is to increase its contractility. This increased force of contraction results in a change in ejection fraction from approximately 56% at rest to as high as 70%.

4. Long-Term Effects of Training on Cardiac Function

a. Chronic aerobic training has little or no impact on **maximal HR**.

b. In contrast, **resting HR** may be significantly decreased following a prolonged training program.

1) Because resting cardiac output remains 5 L/min in those who are trained, SV increases to counter this reduction in HR. At rest, SV may increase to 85 mL following long-term exercise training. During high-intensity exercise, SV of aerobically trained athletes may be as high as 170 mL, contributing to the elevated maximal cardiac output (35–40 L/min) observed in those athletes.

2) During exercise of any submaximal intensity, cardiac output remains essentially unaltered with exercise training. However, among trained individuals, this cardiac output is sustained with lower HR and higher SV values than are noted in untrained individuals.

5. Effects of Posture

a. During normal upright posture, gravity affects the return of blood to the heart.

b. In the supine or prone positions, the return of blood from the legs is more efficient. As a result of these postural influences, SV during exercise (e.g., swimming) is greater at any given intensity than it is during upright exercise (e.g., running, cycling).

c. Because cardiac output is unaffected by posture, the greater SV that occurs during supine exercise is accompanied by a lower HR than would be seen during exercise of the same intensity in the upright position.

1) This lowering of HR during exercise in the supine position must be borne in mind when monitoring exercise intensity with HR response.

2) Specifically, HR may underestimate exercise intensity during exercise performed in a lying position.

B. VASCULATURE

1. Anatomy

Five types of vessels make up the vascular system.

a. **Arteries** are thick-walled, large-diameter vessels that carry blood away from the heart. The largest artery is the **aorta**, which directly receives blood from the left ventricle. Because of their proximity to the heart, the blood pressure, or the force exerted by the blood on the walls of the vessels, is highest in the arteries.

b. Each artery then branches off to form several **arterioles**, which are smaller in size and demonstrate a lower blood pressure than their feeder vessels.

c. Each arteriole then gives rise to between two and five **capillaries**. The diameter of a capillary is very small, barely larger than the size of a red blood cell. Similarly, the walls of a capillary are very thin—only a single cell in thickness—thus allowing the exchange of nutrients and gases with the tissue.

d. Several capillaries then join together to form a **venule**, and it is these venules that begin the return of blood to the heart.

e. A number of venules form a single, larger **vein**, and it is these low-pressure, large-diameter vessels that ultimately return blood to the heart.

2.   **Physiology**

a.   The main function of the vascular system is to satisfy the demand of active tissue for blood, both to provide nutrients and oxygen and to remove metabolic byproducts and carbon dioxide.

b.   One-way valves located at regular intervals throughout the vasculature ensure unidirectional blood flow through this network and allow the circulation of blood within the entire body.

c.   Proper function of the vasculature entails not only providing direction for the delivery of blood but also regulating flow rates that are appropriate for the needs of the tissue. In effect, the greater the metabolic activity displayed, the greater the flow rate of blood to the specific tissue.

d.   The blood supply required by skeletal muscle can vary dramatically, thus challenging the vascular system.

   1)   To meet the increased demand for blood that occurs in exercising muscle, arterioles **vasodilate**. However, to satisfy working muscle, blood flow to other tissue, especially the viscera, is reduced as a result of **vasoconstriction** within arterioles in those internal organs (e.g., kidneys, liver, spleen).

   2)   Vasodilation is elicited by a relaxation of the smooth muscle that is layered around the walls of the arterioles, whereas contraction of the smooth muscle causes vasoconstriction and restriction of blood flow.

3.   **Blood Pressure**

a.   The force exerted by the blood on the vessel walls as it flows through that vessel is referred to as blood pressure.

   1)   Because the heart pumps blood in a pulsatile rather than a constant fashion, blood pressure oscillates.

   2)   The degree of this pulsatility differs throughout the vascular network.

      a)   It is most pronounced at the arteries, where blood exits the heart.

      b)   It is greatly muted as blood travels within the capillaries, however, and it is no longer evident as the blood moves through the venules and veins on its return to the heart.

b.   As blood is pumped from the heart, the resistance imposed by the vessels to its flow is termed **afterload**.

   1)   Along with **preload**, or the amount of blood in the ventricle immediately before contraction, afterload greatly affects SV.

   2)   Enhanced preload facilitates increased SV, whereas increased afterload may decrease SV. That is, significant afterload creates greater resistance to the ejection of blood from the left ventricle; as a result, SV is reduced.

   3)   Afterload is directly related to the **compliance** of the arterial system.

      a)   The greater the compliance, the more easily the arterial walls can be stretched to accommodate the surge of blood during systole, allowing for greater SV.

      b)   A healthy arterial system demonstrates adequate compliance, allowing the heart to overcome vascular resistance.

      c)   Atherosclerosis decreases arterial compliance and increases blood pressure.

c.   Typically, blood pressure is assessed at arterial vessels, and several measurements are important.

   1)   **Systolic Blood Pressure** (SBP) The SBP is the pressure exerted on arterial walls during contraction of the left ventricle. This value can be used to estimate the contractile force generated by the heart. In healthy individuals, SBP under resting conditions is approximately 120 mm Hg. **Resting values greater than 140 mm Hg indicate hypertension.**

   2)   **Diastolic Blood Pressure** (DBP) The DBP is the pressure exerted on the arterial walls during the resting phase between ventricular beats. This value reflects the peripheral resistance or health of the vasculature. In healthy adults, resting DBP is approximately 80 mm Hg. **Values greater than 90 mm Hg are considered to be hypertensive.**

   3)   **Pulse Pressure** The pulse pressure is the difference between the SBP and the DBP. Assuming a healthy person at rest, this value is roughly 40 mm Hg.

4)   **Mean Arterial Pressure** (MAP)
The MAP is the average pressure exerted throughout the entire cardiac cycle, and it reflects the average force driving blood into the tissue. This value can be calculated as

MAP = DBP + 1/3(SBP − DBP)

Therefore, in a healthy person, resting MAP is approximately 93 mm Hg.

5)   **Rate-Pressure Product** (RPP)
The RPP, also called the **double product**, is a rough correlate of the myocardial oxygen uptake and, thus, of the workload of the left ventricle. Alterations in HR and blood pressure contribute to changes in RPP, because RPP is a function of SBP multiplied by HR, or

RPP = SBP × HR

At rest, a healthy individual displays a double product of approximately 8,640 (120 mm Hg × 72 bpm).

4. **Acute Effects of Exercise on Vascular Function**
The vascular system undergoes two major modifications during exercise.

a.   The first modification is to redistribute blood flow to meet the increased demand of the working muscles.

1)   This **shunting** of blood away from the visceral organs to the active skeletal muscles occurs via vasoconstriction of arterioles within the viscera and vasodilation of arterioles in the muscle tissue.

2)   Shunting has a dramatic effect on the distribution of blood. For example, at rest, only approximately 20% of cardiac output is directed toward muscle, but during high-intensity exercise, as much as 85% of the blood ejected from the heart may be delivered to skeletal muscle.

b.   The second modification is a general vasodilation that results in decreased (to a third of the resting values) total peripheral resistance, which accommodates the rise in cardiac output that occurs during exercise. In fact, vasodilation enables the exercise-induced increase in pumping capacity of the heart.

1)   Despite this vasodilation, the several-fold increase in cardiac output during exercise still results in elevated systolic pressure.

2)   Also, like cardiac output, increases in systolic pressure are dependent on the exercise intensity.

a)   During maximal effort rhythmic exercise (e.g., running), systolic pressure may exceed 200 mm Hg.

b)   During sustained submaximal exercise, systolic pressure is generally maintained at 140 to 160 mm Hg.

3)   Diastolic pressure either remains steady or decreases slightly, even during maximal effort exercise.

4)   A sudden, significant drop in systolic pressure (>10 mm Hg from baseline BP) with increased workload when accompanied by other symptoms of ischemia or an increase in diastolic pressure (>115 mm Hg) or systolic pressures (>250 mm Hg) are criteria for termination of exercise testing.

5. **Long-Term Effects of Training on Vascular Function**

a.   A prolonged endurance training program results in several beneficial vascular adaptations.

1)   Under resting conditions, trained individuals display reduced SBP, DBP, and MAP.

2)   As a therapeutic measure in treating hypertension, however, exercise appears to be effective among those people who are mildly hypertensive.

b.   During submaximal exercise at any given intensity, those who are trained demonstrate lower SBP, DBP, and MAP. Maximal SBP is typically higher among well-conditioned individuals, whereas maximal DBP and MAP are attenuated compared with those of untrained individuals.

c.   Endurance training also improves the ability of the vascular system to redistribute blood flow during the onset of exercise so that shunting of blood to working muscles occurs more quickly.

d.   Another well-documented adaptation to endurance training is an improved capillarity within the muscle. As a result of this (along with increased mitochondrial density of myofibers), trained muscle shows an enhanced capacity to extract oxygen from the blood delivered to it.

6. **Effects of Mode of Exercise**
   a. At any given submaximal intensity, rhythmic upper body endurance exercise (e.g., arm cranking) elicits higher SBP and DBP than those values evident during more conventional endurance exercise (e.g., running, cycling).
      1) This probably results from the smaller muscle mass involved and the greater resistance to blood flow that occurs during arm-cranking exercise.
      2) The additional cardiovascular strain associated with upper body exercise should be considered when making exercise recommendations, particularly for those who may have cardiovascular disease.
   b. Resistance exercise (e.g., weight lifting) features forceful contractions of myofibers that impede blood flow through the muscle, thus elevating blood pressure. The degree of this increased peripheral resistance and concomitant pressure elevations is proportionate to the force exerted by the muscle and the total muscle mass that is contracting.
      1) The amplification of blood pressure during resistance exercise is even more pronounced when **isometric** (no movement) contractions are performed. Systolic pressures greater than 450 mm Hg have been recorded during maximal intensity isometric contractions.
      2) These blood pressure responses should be accounted for when prescribing exercise programs for those with cardiovascular disease or who are unfit. Moderate intensity resistance exercise featuring repetitions with full range of motion (concentric and eccentric contractions) should be recommended to those who may have cardiovascular limitations.

V. Blood

The blood performs a host of functions, only one of which is to carry oxygen throughout the body. Because of the many tasks performed by the blood, both at rest and during exercise, numerous cellular and noncellular constituents can be identified.

A. COMPOSITION

Blood, which accounts for approximately 8% of a person's body weight, is composed of fluid (**plasma**) along with several types of cells (**erythrocytes, leukocytes, platelets**).

1. **Plasma**
   a. Plasma comprises approximately 55% of the blood's volume in men and 58% in women.
   b. The main component of plasma is water (90–93%); however, it also contains dissolved substances, such as proteins (e.g., albumins, globulins, fibrinogen), electrolytes (e.g., sodium, potassium, calcium.), gases (e.g., oxygen, carbon dioxide, nitrogen), nutrients (e.g., glucose, lipids, amino acids, vitamins), waste products (e.g., urea, creatinine, uric acid, bilirubin), and various hormones.

2. **Cells**
   a. Erythrocytes (Red Blood Cells)
      Only small amounts of oxygen are dissolved in the plasma, but the vast majority (98.5%) of the oxygen transported in the blood is bound to hemoglobin, a protein found only in the erythrocytes. Hemoglobin also carries some (30%) of the carbon dioxide transported by the blood. By far, erythrocytes are the most abundant of the cell types in the blood, accounting for more than 99% of the blood's cells. **Hematocrit** is the percentage of blood volume that is composed of erythrocytes. In men, the average hematocrit is 40% to 50%; in women, it is usually 35% to 45%. This gender difference exists because the male hormone testosterone affects production of erythrocytes. Because of lower hematocrit levels, women have a reduced hemoglobin content: men are normally approximately 14–17 g/100 mL of blood compared to 12–15 g/100 mL of blood in women.
   b. Leukocytes (White Blood Cells)
      Leukocytes are components of the immune system. Their primary function is to destroy potentially infectious agents that enter the body.
   c. Platelets
      Platelets are the smallest component of the blood. Their main function is to accumulate and form a plug where damage has occurred to the wall of the blood vessel and, thus, to prevent the loss of blood.

B. ACUTE EFFECTS OF EXERCISE

1. The most obvious effect of exercise is to induce **hyperemia**, or an increase in the volume of blood delivered to the working muscles. This

allows a greater delivery of oxygen and nutrients as well as a more efficient removal of carbon dioxide and metabolic byproducts (e.g., lactate).

2. Another response that is commonly observed during prolonged endurance exercise is the movement of plasma out of the blood vessels and into the surrounding tissue. This **cardiovascular drift** serves to prevent overheating of the body by having more water available for sweating and is more pronounced during exercise in hot environments. However, this drift decreases the total volume of blood in the vasculature, resulting in decreased SV and increased HR even though exercise intensity remains constant.

3. The movement of plasma out of the blood also leads to **hemoconcentration,** which is apparent in elevations in hematocrit and hemoglobin values.

C. LONG-TERM EFFECTS OF TRAINING

Endurance training is associated with several favorable adaptations of the blood.

1. Production of erythrocytes significantly increases, leading to a greater oxygen-carrying capacity.

2. Plasma volume increases to an even greater extent, and as a result, relative measures of hemoglobin and hematocrit (per unit volume of blood) are actually decreased in well-conditioned athletes. This has been termed **runner's anemia**, but it is not considered to be a pathologic adaptation.

3. Because the total amount of red blood cells and hemoglobin are enhanced by training, the oxygen-carrying capacity of the blood is also enhanced.

4. Increased plasma volume in trained individuals has several advantageous effects.

   a. At rest, it results in a higher SV and lower HR.

   b. During exercise, increased plasma volume enhances the capacity for thermoregulation; recall the effect of cardiovascular drift.

   c. Similar to resting conditions, a trained person's SV is higher and HR lower during submaximal exercise than those of an untrained individual.

   d. Maximal SV and cardiac output are also more impressive in a trained individual, in large part because of their greater plasma volumes.

Review Test

DIRECTIONS: Carefully read all questions, and select the BEST single answer.

1. Which of the following is NOT a major food fuel during exercise?
   A) Glucose.
   B) Fatty acids.
   C) Protein.
   D) Glycogen.

2. The chemical energy that is directly converted to do work is
   A) ATP.
   B) Creatine phosphate.
   C) Beta oxidation of fatty acids.
   D) All of the above.

3. Which of the following is true when two people of different weights (80 and 70 kg) are exercising at 5 mph/5% grade on a treadmill?
   A) $\dot{V}o_2$ will be different if expressed in mL/kg/min.
   B) $\dot{V}o_2$ will be the same if expressed in L/min.
   C) Cardiac output will be the same in L/min.
   D) None of the above.

4. Which of the following would provide the SMALLEST potential energy source in the body?
   A) Fat.
   B) Protein.
   C) PCr.
   D) ATP.

5. Before and after 10 weeks of endurance training, an individual performs a submaximal exercise test at a constant work rate. Which of the following changes would most likely occur as a result of the endurance training?
   A) A lower cardiac output.
   B) An increase in oxygen consumption.
   C) An increase in the blood flow to the exercising muscle.
   D) Lower blood lactate levels.

6. When compared with leg exercise, arm exercise results in a relatively
   A) Increased HR at all intensities.
   B) Lower SBP at all intensities.
   C) Increased venous return at all intensities.
   D) Increased $\dot{V}o_2$max.

7. During exercise of increasing intensity, the SV of normal adults
   A) Continues to increase throughout the duration of exercise up to $\dot{V}o_2$max.
   B) Remains relatively stable during submaximal exercise of greater than approximately 50% of $\dot{V}o_2$max.
   C) Will continue to increase and then level off just before the achievement of $\dot{V}o_2$max.
   D) None of the above.

8. The simplest and most rapid method to produce ATP during exercise is through
   A) Glycolysis.
   B) The ATP-PCr system.
   C) Aerobic metabolism.
   D) Glycogenolysis.

9. In general, the higher the intensity of the activity, the greater the contribution of
   A) Aerobic energy production.
   B) Anaerobic energy production.
   C) The Krebs cycle to the production of ATP.
   D) The electron-transport chain to the production of ATP.

10. The energy to perform long-term exercise (≥15 min) comes primarily from
    A) Aerobic metabolism.
    B) A combination of aerobic and anaerobic metabolism, with anaerobic metabolism producing the bulk of the ATP.
    C) Anaerobic metabolism.
    D) None of the above.

11. In a rested, well-fed athlete, most of the carbohydrate used as a substrate during exercise comes from
    A) Muscle glycogen stores.
    B) Blood glucose.
    C) Liver glycogen stores.
    D) Glycogen stored in fat cells.

12. Fast-twitch muscle fibers have which of the following characteristics compared with slow-twitch muscle fibers?
    A) Easily fatigued and well-developed aerobic system.
    B) High force production and well-developed blood supply.
    C) High PCr stores and high ATPase stores.
    D) None of the above.

13. The motor neuron and all the muscle fibers it innervates are called a
    A) Motor junction.
    B) Motor unit.
    C) Motor end plate.
    D) None of the above.

14. The three principal mechanisms for increasing venous return during dynamic exercise are
    A) A decrease in SV, HR, and compliance of the vascular system.
    B) Venoconstriction, pumping action of muscle, and the pumping action of the respiratory system.
    C) An increase in vascular resistance, increase in HR, and decrease in blood pressure.
    D) None of the above.

15. Any physical activity with a performance time of approximately 30 seconds or less relies on which of the following energy systems?
    A) ATP.
    B) PCr.
    C) ATP-PCr.
    D) Aerobic glycolysis.

16. Which of the following is NOT a muscle type?
    A) Skeletal.
    B) Smooth.
    C) Cardiac.
    D) Generic.

17. When a motor unit is stimulated by a single nerve impulse, it responds by contracting one time and then relaxing. This is called a
    A) Twitch.
    B) Summation.
    C) Tetanus.
    D) Summary.

18. Which muscle protein contains many cross-bridges?
    A) Myofibril.
    B) Sarcomere.
    C) Troponin.
    D) Myosin.

19. Cardiac muscle action potentials are longer in duration than those of skeletal muscle. The longer action potential does not allow the muscle to
    A) Twitch.
    B) Undergo summation.
    C) Have tetanus.
    D) Summarize.

20. Which of the following cardiovascular variables does NOT increase as a result of chronic exercise while performing a single bout of maximal exercise?
    A) Maximal HR.
    B) Maximal cardiac output.

C) Maximal SV.
D) Maximal oxygen consumption.

21. Myocardial oxygen consumption is best estimated from
    A) Maximal oxygen consumption.
    B) RPP.
    C) Cardiac output.
    D) HR.

22. During mild to moderate exercise, pulmonary ventilation increases primarily as a result of increased
    A) Tidal volume.
    B) Breathing frequency.
    C) Vital capacity.
    D) Total lung volume.

23. The anaerobic threshold occurs at the onset of
    A) Oxidative phosphorylation.
    B) Maximal oxygen consumption.
    C) Metabolic acidosis.
    D) Aerobic metabolism.

24. Which of the following statements about static exercise is accurate?
    A) It results in reduced pressure on the heart.
    B) It is inappropriate for any client with heart disease.
    C) It involves rhythmic, continuous activity.
    D) It results in increased HR and SBP.

25. Which of the following statements regarding arm versus leg exercise is correct?
    A) Target HR should not be used as a guide for arm exercise.
    B) Target HR for leg exercise should be decreased by 10 bpm for arm exercise.
    C) Target HR for leg exercise should be increased by 10 bpm for arm exercise.
    D) Higher maximal oxygen consumption should be expected in arm exercise.

26. End-diastolic volume is highest when measured with the client in which position?
    A) Recumbent.
    B) Sitting.
    C) Standing.
    D) Supine.

27. Which of the following are byproducts of aerobic metabolism?
    A) Carbon dioxide and water.
    B) Oxygen and water.
    C) ATP and oxygen.
    D) Hydrogen and oxygen.

28. Cardiac output is a function of
    A) HR, preload, afterload, and contractility.
    B) HR and SBP.

C) SV and EDV.

D) Maximal oxygen consumption and arteriovenous oxygenation difference.

29. Which of the following describes a normal postexercise blood pressure (BP) response?
    A) Elevated systolic and diastolic values compared to preparticipation values.
    B) Progressive decline in SBP.
    C) Progressive increase in SBP.
    D) Exaggerated decrease in DBP.

30. Stroke volume is defined as
    A) The product of cardiac output and total peripheral resistance.
    B) The difference between EDV and ESV.

C) The product of preload and HR.

D) The product of cardiac output and arteriovenous oxygen difference.

31. As a result of exercise training, cardiac output becomes
    A) Higher at any given workload.
    B) Lower at any given workload.
    C) Essentially unchanged at any given workload.
    D) Diminished because of reduced SV.

32. During exercise, SV increases as a result of
    A) The Frank-Starling law.
    B) Increased HR.
    C) Increased ejection fraction.
    D) Increased pulmonary artery pressure.

ANSWERS AND EXPLANATIONS

1–C. Glucose (and its storage form, glycogen) and fat are the primary sources of energy. For example, middle distance runners typically use carbohydrates and fats, whereas sprinters use ATP-PCr as the energy substrate. Most aerobic exercise activities are fueled by a mixture of carbohydrate and fat. If the intensity is high, more ATP energy will come from carbohydrates. Protein (amino acids) are used only in severe energy deficit.

2–A. All energy for muscular contraction must come from the breakdown of ATP. The energy is stored in the bonds between the last two phosphates; when work is performed, the last phosphate is split, forming ADP and releasing heat. This release of heat contributes to the necessary mechanical energy.

3–D. During weight-bearing exercise, when performing the same absolute workload, persons of different weights have the same relative $\dot{V}O_2$ (mL/kg/min), different absolute $\dot{V}O_2$ (L/min), and different cardiac output (because of different body mass).

4–D. The smallest potential energy source is ATP. The oxygen system is capable of using all three fuels: carbohydrate, fat, and protein. Significant amounts of protein are not used as a source of ATP energy during most types of exercise. Although all three can be used, the two most important are carbohydrates and fat. The carbohydrate, fat, and small amount of protein used by this energy system during exercise are completely metabolized, leaving only carbon dioxide and water (with small amounts of urea from protein).

5–D. Changes induced by training during submaximal work (defined as a workload at which the individual can achieve a steady state) include a reduction in submaximal HR, an increase in SV, and no change in cardiac output. Because the amount of work is less (expressed as a percentage of maximal work), the amount of accumulated blood lactate will be less at the same relative submaximal amount of work.

6–A. The upper extremity is approximately two-thirds the muscle mass of the lower extremity. At the same relative workload, the upper extremity requires an increased HR to meet the metabolic demand. Systolic blood pressure is actually increased and venous return decreased because of an increase in intrathoracic pressure as a result of the upper extremity work.

7–B. During dynamic upright exercise of increasing intensity, SV will increase with each increase in intensity until approximately 40% to 50% of $\dot{V}O_2$max. Beyond this intensity, SV will not increase, because the time available for ventricular filling during diastole has become too short.

8–B. Because the number of reactions is very small (two), the ATP-PCr system provides a very rapid source of energy, followed by glycolysis.

9–B. Most aerobic exercise activities are fueled by a mixture of carbohydrate and fat. If the intensity of exercise is high, more ATP energy will come from carbohydrates (anaerobic energy production). If the intensity of exercise is lower (and the duration long enough), less ATP energy comes from carbohydrates, because some ATP energy can be derived from fat under these conditions.

10–A. Activities lasting longer than 2 or 3 minutes rely on aerobic metabolism to generate ATP.

11–A. The storage form of carbohydrates and those that are easily accessible for use as an energy substrate are muscle glycogen stores. Glycogen is the storage form of glucose and is found in the muscle and in the liver. Once the ATP-PCr system has supplied energy within the first few seconds of physical activity, the glycogen stored in the muscle is next used to supply energy by breaking down to glucose and then creating ATP.

12–C. Fast-twitch muscle fibers are designed to deliver high power in a short period of time, as opposed to slow-twitch muscle fibers, which help to deliver sustained power over a longer period of time. The fast-twitch muscle fiber, then, has a relatively small number of mitochondria but a high activity level of ATPase, the enzyme that splits ATP and produces energy.

13–B. A motor unit consists of the efferent (motor) nerve and all the muscle fibers that are supplied (or innervated) by that nerve. The total number of fibers in each motor unit varies both among and within muscles.

14–B. Stroke volume and HR increase in a healthy person with dynamic exercise. Vascular resistance also decreases with dynamic exercise. The primary mechanisms responsible for increasing venous return during dynamic exercise are the pumping action of the muscles on the deep veins, the increased ventilation that helps to draw blood into the thorax from the abdominal cavity, and venoconstriction, which helps to maintain cardiac filling pressure or flow back to the heart on the venous side.

15–C. Enough PCr is stored in skeletal muscle for approximately 25 seconds of high-intensity work. Therefore, the ATP-PCr system has a capacity for approximately 30 seconds (5 seconds for stored ATP, 25 seconds for stored PC).

16–D. The human body has three types of muscle: skeletal, smooth (found in some blood vessels and in the digestive system), and cardiac (heart).

17–A. When a motor unit is stimulated by a single nerve impulse, it responds by contracting one time and then relaxing. This is called a twitch.

18–D. Myosin is also known as the thick filament and contains cross-bridges, which are very important during contraction.

19–C. The action potential in cardiac muscle is much longer in duration compared with that in skeletal muscle. This prevents the cardiac muscle from being tetanized. If cardiac muscle were tetanized, no relaxation (called diastole) of heart muscle would occur. This would prevent ventricular filling from occurring for the next contraction.

20–A. Maximal HR does not change significantly with exercise training. Maximal HR does, however, decline with age.

21–B. Determinants of myocardial oxygen consumption ($M\dot{V}O_2$) include HR, myocardial contractility, and the tension or stress in the ventricular wall. Ventricular wall tension reflects a combination of SBP and ventricular volume and is inversely related to myocardial wall thickness. During exercise, HR is the major contributor to myocardial oxygen demand, and oxygen supply is facilitated by increased coronary blood flow, which is enabled by decreased vascular resistance. Investigators have reported an excellent correlation between measured $M\dot{V}O_2$ and the RPP (HR $\times$ SBP). The HR alone has limited ability to assess $M\dot{V}O_2$, especially when SBP is elevated.

22–A. Pulmonary ventilation ($\dot{V}_E$), the volume of air exchanged per minute, generally approximates 6 L/min at rest in the average, sedentary adult male. At maximal exercise, however, $\dot{V}_E$ often increases 15- to 25-fold over resting values. The $\dot{V}_E$ is a function of tidal volume and respiratory rate. During mild to moderate exercise, $\dot{V}_E$ increases, primarily because of increasing tidal volume, whereas increases in respiratory rate are more important to augment $\dot{V}_E$ during vigorous exercise.

23–C. The anaerobic threshold represents the onset of metabolic acidosis. The anaerobic threshold can be determined by serial measurements of blood lactate or noninvasively assessed by expired gases during exercise testing, specifically pulmonary ventilation and carbon dioxide (CO_2). The anaerobic threshold indicates the peak work rate or oxygen consumption at which the body's energy demands can be met by aerobic metabolism. Metabolic acidosis can be attributed to the buffering of lactate by sodium bicarbonate so that CO_2 is released in excess of muscle metabolism, providing an additional stimulus for ventilation. Accordingly, values for $\dot{V}_E$ and CO_2 increase out of proportion to the exercise performed.

24–D. During static (or isometric) exercise, HR increases in relation to the tension exerted, and an abrupt and precipitous increase in SBP occurs. The increased HR and SBP (RPP) result in increased myocardial oxygen demand. Static exercise involves sustained muscle contraction against a fixed load or resistance with no change in the length of the involved muscle group or joint motion. Because static exertion is present in normal activities, it is not contraindicated in all cardiac clients, but it must be performed in a safe and controlled setting.

25–B. Maximal oxygen consumption during arm exercise in men and women is 64% to 80% of that during leg exercise. Similarly, maximal cardiac output is lower during arm exercise than during leg exercise, whereas maximal HR, SBP, and RPP are comparable or slightly lower during arm exercise. The latter have relevance to arm exercise training recommendations, particularly training intensity. Accordingly, an arm exercise prescription based on the assumption of a maximal HR equivalent to that of leg exercise testing may result in overestimation of the training HR. As a general guideline, the prescribed HR for leg training should be reduced by approximately 10 bpm for arm training.

26–A. End-diastolic volume depends on HR, filling pressure, and ventricular compliance. Posture affects venous return and preload, particularly during brief bouts of physical exertion. At rest, EDV is highest in the recumbent position and decreases progressively with movement to sitting and then to standing.

27–A. Aerobic production of ATP combines two complex metabolic processes: the Krebs cycle, and the electron-transport chain. During the Krebs cycle, hydrogen is produced, and carbon dioxide (CO_2) is removed. Oxidative phosphorylation uses oxygen as the final hydrogen acceptor to form CO_2 and water. The final products of cellular respiration, as measured by direct calorimetry, are heat, CO_2, and water.

28–A. The product of HR and SV determines the cardiac output. The SV is equal to the difference between EDV and ESV. The EDV is determined by HR, filling pressure, and ventricular compliance (preload). The ESV is determined by contractility and afterload.

29–B. During graded exercise, SBP increases with increased workload, resulting from increased cardiac output. On completion of exercise, SBP declines gradually because of decreasing demand by skeletal tissue for increased cardiac output and oxygen delivery.

30–B. Stroke volume is the amount of blood ejected from the left ventricle during cardiac systole. This volume is a fraction of the EDV (the amount of blood originally in the left ventricle just before ventricular systole). The remaining blood not ejected by the left ventricle is the ESV.

31–C. The product of HR and SV determines the cardiac output. Cardiac output in healthy adults increases linearly with increased work rate, from a resting value of approximately 5 L to a maximum of 20 L during upright exercise. At exercise intensities of up to 50% of maximal oxygen consumption, the increase in cardiac output is facilitated by increases in HR and SV. At higher intensities, the increase in cardiac output results almost solely from a continued increase in HR. Cardiac output remains essentially unchanged at any given workload.

32-A. In healthy adults, SV at rest in the upright position generally varies between 60 and 100 mL/beat, with a maximum SV of 100 to 200 mL/beat. During exercise, SV increases curvilinearly with the work rate until it reaches near maximum at a level equivalent to approximately 50% of aerobic capacity, increasing only slightly thereafter. Within physiological limits, enhanced venous return increases EDV, stretching cardiac muscle fibers and increasing the force of contraction (Frank-Starling law).

Human Development and Aging

ROBERT S. MAZZEO AND DAVID S. CRISWELL

I. Overview of Human Growth and Development

A. **AGE GROUPS** are typically defined as follows:
1. **Neonatal**: birth to 3 weeks.
2. **Infancy**: 3 weeks to 1 year.
3. **Early childhood**: 1 to 6 years.
4. **Middle childhood**: 7 to 10 years.
5. **Late childhood/prepuberty**: girls, 9 to 15 years; boys, 12 to 16 years.
6. **Adolescence**: the 6 years following puberty.
7. Adulthood
   a. **Early adulthood**: 20 to 29 years.
   b. **Middle adulthood**: 30 to 44 years.
   c. **Later adulthood**: 45 to 64 years.
   d. **Older adulthood**
      1) Old: 65 to 74 years.
      2) Older: 75 to 84 years.
      3) Very old/frail: 85 years and older.

B. **SIGNIFICANT VARIABILITY EXISTS IN GROWTH AND DEVELOPMENT** for a given chronological age group.

C. **AGING IS A COMPLEX PROCESS** that involves the interaction of many factors, including genetics, lifestyle, and disease *(Figure 3-1).*

D. **THE AGING POPULATION** in the United States is increasing. The number of those older than age 65 will reach 70 million by the year 2030, with those older than age 85 being the fastest-growing population segment *(Figure 3-2).*

E. **AGE AND EXERCISE**
1. A client's age must be considered when designing an exercise program. **Children, adolescents, and older adults have special physiological and behavioral characteristics that must be considered in program design to ensure safety and effectiveness.** A medical history and proper screening are recommended and, in some cases, are required by ACSM Guidelines.

2. **Both aerobic and resistance training are recommended for older adults** to improve health, functional capacity, and overall quality of life.

II. Age-Related Physiologic Changes

A. **CARDIOPULMONARY FUNCTION**
1. **Changes in Heart Rate, Stroke Volume, and Cardiac Output**
   a. Heart Rate
      1) Both **resting heart rate and exercise heart rate** are higher in children, most likely as compensation for the lower stroke volume and cardiac output relative to body mass. Additionally, hemoglobin concentration is lower in children than in adults.
      2) **Maximal heart rate** decreases by approximately 6 to 10 bpm per decade with advancing age.
   b. Stroke Volume
      1) **Resting stroke volume** remains relatively unchanged with advancing age.
      2) **Maximal stroke volume** decreases with advancing age.
   c. Cardiac Output
      1) Decreases in both maximal heart rate and stroke volume cause a significant decline in **maximal cardiac output** with age. Maximal heart rate and stroke volume are probably decreased because of increased stiffness of the left ventricle, causing decreased diastolic filling.
      2) **Cardiac output at any given submaximal oxygen consumption** is lower in adults than in children. Children compensate for this by increased oxygen extraction, which is achieved by increased blood flow through skeletal muscle.

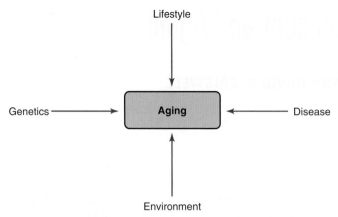

FIGURE 3-1. Factors that influence how we age. Genetics plays an important role, but other factors, such as lifestyle (e.g., exercise patterns, diet, stress), environment, and disease states, also contribute to the aging process.

d. Other Changes
   1) **Decreased arterial compliance and increased arterial stiffness** with age can result in elevated systolic and elevated diastolic blood pressures both at rest and during exercise.
   2) **Skeletal muscle capillary density** decreases with age, resulting in decreased muscle blood flow and oxygen extraction.
   3) **Left ventricular hypertrophy** increases with aging, apparently related to increased afterload associated with increased peripheral resistance.

   4) **Early left ventricular diastolic function** both at rest and during exercise decreases with age.

e. Maximal Oxygen Consumption ($\dot{V}O_2$max)
   1) The $\dot{V}O_2$max is determined by the capacity of the cardiovascular system to **deliver oxygen** to the working muscles and the capacity of the muscles to **extract oxygen** for oxidative metabolism.
   2) The $\dot{V}O_2$max is a function of maximal cardiac output and maximal arteriovenous oxygen difference.
   3) The $\dot{V}O_2$max may be expressed as an absolute value (L of oxygen per min), or it may be standardized to an index of body size (e.g., mass).
   4) The $\dot{V}O_2$max remains relatively unchanged throughout childhood and adolescence.
   5) The $\dot{V}O_2$max typically declines by 5% to 15% per decade after age 25; this decline is related to decreases in both maximal cardiac output and maximal arteriovenous oxygen difference. The rate of decline can be slowed by regular physical activity *(Figure 3-3)*

f. Changes in Pulmonary Function
   1) **Residual volume increases** and **vital capacity decreases** with aging.
   2) **Lung compliance increases** with aging, as the lungs lose elastin fibers and elastic recoil.
   3) Aging brings a **20% increase in the work of respiratory muscles** but a **decrease in the strength** of these muscles.

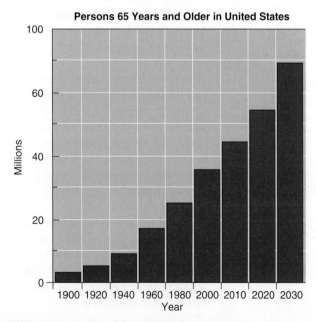

FIGURE 3-2. Estimation of the number of individuals who will be 65 years and older by the year 2000 and beyond. Note the exponential growth rate in this age group, making them the fastest-growing population segment in the United States.

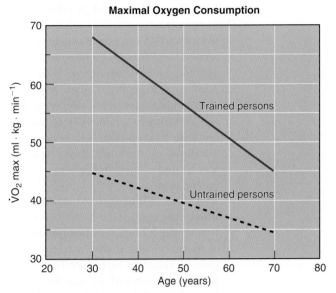

FIGURE 3-3. Changes in maximal oxygen consumption ($\dot{V}O_2$max) as a function of age in both conditioned and unconditioned individuals.

2. Changes During Growth and Development
   a. **A general increase in exercise capacity and absolute $\dot{V}O_2$ max (L/min) occurs during childhood.** This increase is dramatically accelerated during puberty, especially in boys, before leveling off after maturity.
   b. The large increase in absolute $\dot{V}O_2$max in adolescent boys corresponding to the growth spurt, which results from androgen-induced hypertrophy of the heart and stimulation of red blood cell and hemoglobin production, facilitates oxygen delivery. Furthermore, increased skeletal muscle mass associated with male adolescence increases the capacity for oxygen extraction.
   c. Despite the large increase in absolute $\dot{V}O_2$max, **relative $\dot{V}O_2$ max (mL/kg/min) plateaus in boys, and shows a slight decline in girls, during puberty.** Whether this represents inadequate physical conditioning of this age group or some other physiologic factor is unclear.
3. The $\dot{V}O_2$max is not related to endurance fitness in children and preadolescents.

B. MUSCULOSKELETAL FUNCTION
1. Changes in Muscle Mass
   a. An individual's **total number of muscle fibers** becomes fixed before adolescence; however, large changes in muscle mass remain possible via the mechanisms of **muscle fiber hypertrophy**.

b. At **adolescence**, males exhibit more rapid muscle growth **(hypertrophy)** than females do. Females do not exhibit disproportionate muscle growth during adolescence. Adolescent and postadolescent females have approximately 30% to 60% less muscle mass compared with males, both because of smaller stature and because of a smaller average muscle fiber size.
   c. A decline in muscle mass **(atrophy)** occurs with advancing age because of a progressive decrease in the number and size of muscle fibers *(Figure 3-4)*. This sarcopenia directly contributes to an **age-related decline in muscle strength.** Fast-twitch fibers (especially type IIb fibers) are particularly susceptible to atrophy in aging humans.
2. Changes in Muscle Strength
   a. **Muscle strength typically peaks in the mid-twenties** for both sexes and remains fairly stable through the mid-thirties.

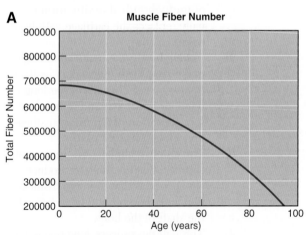

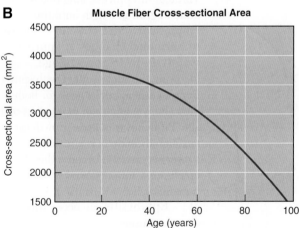

FIGURE 3-4. Alterations in muscle fiber number (A) and cross-sectional area (B) as a function of aging. A significant loss both in the number of fibers and fiber area begins around 50 to 55 years of age.

b. **Muscle strength declines** by approximately 15% per decade in the fifth, sixth, and seventh decades and by approximately 30% per decade thereafter.

3. Bone

a. **Bone is specialized connective tissue** composed of cells embedded in an extracellular organic matrix impregnated with an inorganic component. This inorganic component, primarily calcium phosphate crystals called hydroxyapatite, makes up approximately 65% of the dry weight of bone. Mature bone continuously undergoes a process called **bone remodeling**, in which bone matrix is reabsorbed and replaced by new matrix. **This process becomes unbalanced with advancing age such that bone formation does not keep pace with reabsorption.**

b. Bone Formation During Growth and Development

1) The human skeleton begins to develop in the embryo as the process of **endochondral ossification** gradually replaces the cartilage with bone tissue.

2) In long bones, the ossification begins in the **diaphysis**. Secondary ossification occurs at the ends of the long bone, or **epiphysis** and remains separated from the primary ossification by **epiphyseal plates**.

3) The epiphyseal plates are regions of cartilage that continue to produce chondrocytes that undergo ossification and, thereby, add bone tissue to the shaft of the bone.

4) Through this process, long bones continue to grow in length until **the epiphyseal plates close in response to hormonal changes at approximately 16 to 18 years of age**, following the adolescent growth spurt. Bone mass reaches its peak for both men and women by 25 to 30 years of age. Problems with bone growth can develop in children as a result of strenuous exercise, because the epiphysis is not yet united with the bone shaft.

a) **Epiphysitis** can occur with overuse.

b) **Fractures** can pass through the epiphyseal plate, disrupting normal bone growth.

c. Bone Loss During Aging and Development of Osteoporosis

1) **Osteoporosis** is a condition characterized by a decrease in bone mass and bone density, producing bone porosity and fragility. The efficiency of osteoblasts appears to decline with age, resulting in the inability of bone synthesis to keep pace with bone reabsorption. In women, this loss is accelerated immediately after menopause.

2) As a result, **older individuals are more susceptible to bone fractures**, which are a significant cause of morbidity and mortality in the elderly. **Hip fractures are the most common** and account for a large share of the disability, death, and medical costs associated with falls. Additionally, both wrist and vertebral fractures are not uncommon among those with osteoporosis.

3) Sex-Related Differences in Bone Loss

a) The age at which bone loss begins and the rate at which it occurs vary greatly between men and women.

b) Normally, **men** begin to lose bone mass by age 65; overall bone mineral content is approximately 10% lower than the peak value.

c) Bone loss in **women** may begin as early as age 30 to 35, and the rate of bone loss is greatly accelerated following menopause. By age 65, overall bone mineral content in women is approximately 15% to 20% lower than the peak value.

d) Some studies suggest that the **overall age-related loss of bone** mineral content in men is proportional to the loss of lean body tissue with aging. Women, however, exhibit a disproportionate loss of bone tissue after menopause. **Estrogen replacement** has been shown to be effective in attenuating this bone loss in postmenopausal women.

4) Classification of Osteoporosis
   a) With osteoporosis, susceptibility to fracture from minor trauma increases. Osteoporotic conditions affecting older adults are classified as type I or type II osteoporosis.
   b) **Type I** or **postmenopausal osteoporosis** is the most common and is associated with fractures of the vertebrae and distal radius. Approximately 90% of the cases of type I osteoporosis occur in women.
   c) **Type II** or **senile osteoporosis** is seen mostly in individuals older than 70 years of age and is manifested primarily by vertebral and hip fractures. The incidence of type II osteoporosis is also higher in women, with a female:male ratio of approximately 2:1.

5) Risk Factors
   Many of the risk factors for age-related bone loss and, hence, the risk for developing osteoporosis can be modified. The risk factors are:
   a) Being a **white** or **Asian female**.
   b) Being **thin-boned** or petite.
   c) Having a **low peak bone mass at maturity**.
   d) **A family history of** osteoporosis.
   e) Premature or surgically induced **menopause**.
   f) **Alcohol abuse**.
   g) **Cigarette smoking**.
   h) **Sedentary lifestyle**.
   i) Inadequate **dietary calcium intake**.
   j) **Chronic steroid use** (especially for males under the age of 70 years).
   k) **Vitamin D deficiency**

B. MUSCULOSKELETAL FUNCTION

1. Changes in Joints, Flexibility, and Balance
   a. **Connective tissue** (fascia, ligaments, tendons) **becomes less extensible** with age. Aging is associated with **degradation and increased cross-linkage of collagen fibers**, which comprise much of the connective tissue in the joints of the body. This increases the stiffness and decreases the tensile strength of collagen fibers.
   b. **Degeneration of joints**, especially in the spine, occurs with advancing age, perhaps largely because of **trauma to joint cartilage** causing the formation of scar tissue, which makes the connective tissue stiff and less responsive to stress, thus facilitating the loss of flexibility that is seen with aging.
   c. **Range of motion** (active as well as passive) **decreases** with age. (See **a** and **b** above for the reasons for this loss of range of motion.)
   d. **A progressive loss of flexibility begins** during young adulthood that relates to disuse, deterioration of joints, and degeneration of collagen fibers. **Osteoarthritis** can severely restrict range of motion. This disease occurs primarily in areas of the body that receive the greatest mechanical stress, thereby suggesting that **it may be caused by repeated trauma** rather than by aging.
   e. Balance and Postural Stability
      1) Balance and postural stability are **affected** by sensory and motor system changes.
      2) **Poor balance is one risk factor for falling.** (Other risk factors include medication use, diminished cognitive status, postural hypotension, and impaired vision.)
      3) **Age-related changes in the vestibular, visual, and somatosensory systems** result in diminished feedback to the postural centers.
      4) **The muscle effectors** may lack the capacity to respond appropriately to disturbances in postural stability.

D. FLEXIBILITY

1. Joint stiffness and loss of flexibility are common in the elderly. It is difficult to separate the effects of aging on joint flexibility from those of injury and wear-and-tear that occur over the life span.
   a. Aging is associated with **degradation and increased cross-linkage of collagen fibers**, which comprise much of the connective tissue in the joints. This increases the stiffness and decreases the tensile strength of collagen fibers.
   b. **Trauma to joint cartilage** causes the formation of scar tissue, which makes the connective tissue stiff and less responsive to stress.

1) **Range-of-motion exercises and static stretching** may increase flexibility in subjects of all ages.

2) It is unlikely, however, that any exercise could undo the extensive degenerative damage that is sometimes seen with osteoarthritis in the elderly.

2. Reaction Time, Movement Time, and Coordination

a. Childhood and Adolescence

1) Performance of tasks requiring **motor skills** improves consistently throughout the preadolescent and adolescent years. This improvement results from growth, the associated increases in strength and endurance, the progress of motor learning, and the development of greater coordination.

2) **Reaction time** decreases (improves) with maturational development. An abrupt decrease in reaction time occurs around 8 years of age, followed by a more progressive improvement throughout the remainder of childhood and adolescence.

3) **Speed of movement** also improves with age.

4) **Improvement of skill following a practice session** increases with age during childhood, indicating an increase in the capacity to integrate feedback during learning.

5) Gender Differences in Skill Performance

a) Gender differences in skill performance are minimal before adolescence.

b) During **adolescence**, the gap widens. The performance of girls in skills requiring strength and gross motor patterns (e.g., running, jumping) plateaus, whereas that of boys continue to improve.

c) Girls often outperform boys in skills requiring fine motor patterns.

d) Wide individual variations in quantitative skill performances are found at all ages in both genders.

b. Adulthood and Changes with Aging

1) Many **neurophysiologic changes** occur with aging that **affect motor performance**.

a) Decreased **visual acuity**.

b) **Hearing loss**.

c) Deterioration of **short-term memory**.

d) Inability to handle several pieces of information simultaneously.

e) Decreased **reaction time**.

2) The ability to maintain performance of a motor skill at a given level throughout middle and older adulthood depends on the type of skill in question.

3) **Skills requiring accuracy of movement** may be maintained at the level attained as a young adult.

4) Performance of **skills requiring speed and/or strength of movement** declines with age.

5) **Movement patterns** of older adults are generally well maintained from younger adulthood. **Decreases in performance** during adulthood result from decreases in range of motion, reaction time, movement time, and coordination.

6) It is often difficult to separate the effects of aging from those of disease and/or deconditioning resulting from inactivity. Nevertheless, **individuals who remain active and continue to practice motor skills can minimize the decline in performance** that occurs with aging.

E. **BODY COMPOSITION**

1. **Body fat percentage** generally increases from childhood to early adulthood, to between 15% and 20% in males and between 20% and 25% in females. Thereafter, body fat percentage gradually **increases with age** (*Figure 3-5*) because of increasing fat mass and decreasing muscle mass.

2. **In females, relative body fat increases during puberty** to approximately 20% to 25% of body mass because of hormonally induced accumulation of fat in the breasts and around the hips.

3. **Abdominal obesity** has reached epidemic proportions and plays a significant role in many diseases, including heart disease, cancer, and diabetes.

4. **Physiological changes associated with aging contribute to unfavorable changes in body composition**

a. **Inactivity is a primary factor in the increase of fat mass with age.** Energy expenditure from physical activity declines with age, and body fat mass increases when

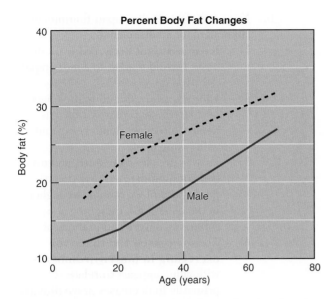

FIGURE 3-5. Changes in percentage body fat as a function of age in males and females.

an imbalance occurs between caloric intake and energy expenditure. However, **fat-free mass remains relatively constant**.

b. **A progressive decline in skeletal muscle mass begins around age 50.**

   1) **A gradual decrease in basal metabolic rate is associated with aging.** Coupled with a more sedentary lifestyle, this typically results in a loss of lean (metabolically active) muscle mass and a concurrent increase in the less metabolically active fat mass.

   2) During the **developmental years,** a positive nitrogen balance exists, with deposition of protein into skeletal muscle and increasing muscle mass.

   3) **After age 50,** individuals may enter into a state of negative nitrogen balance, contributing to a gradual loss of muscle mass.

   4) **After 70 years of age,** body mass begins to decline, typically by 1 to 2 kg in the eighth decade and accelerating thereafter.

   5) This decline in body mass represents a **loss of fat-free mass,** which exceeds the continued rise in fat mass.

   6) The average change in percentage body fat is linear between ages 25 and 75 for both men and women.

   7) The **age-related increase in fat mass** accumulates primarily in central areas **(abdominal areas)** as opposed to peripheral areas.

   8) **Increased** measurements of **central-to-peripheral adiposity,** such as the ratio of waist to hip circumference, have been linked to an **increased risk for cardiovascular disease**.

5. Application to Exercise Training in Older Adults

   a. Regular **aerobic exercise** has an obvious impact on energy balance by increasing energy expenditure.

   b. Regular **resistance training** has positive anabolic effects in older individuals, leading to the preservation of skeletal muscle mass, which can help to slow the age-related decline in basal metabolic rate.

   c. **Exercise training** can reduce the percentage body fat at any age. However, longitudinal studies of highly competitive athletes suggest that exercise does not prevent an age-related increase in body fat.

F. THERMOREGULATION

1. Children

   a. Children are less efficient than adults are at temperature regulation because of the **anthropometric and functional differences** of their immature thermoregulatory system.

   b. Children consistently sweat less than adults. Thus, children may have difficulty making thermoregulatory adaptations during extreme temperature conditions.

   c. The **surface area** of a child, relative to body mass, is greater than that of an adult, allowing a **greater rate of heat exchange** between the skin and the environment.

   d. In neutral or warm climates, the increased surface area may facilitate heat dissipation.

   e. In **climatic extremes,** this increased surface area becomes a major handicap by increasing unwanted heat transfer from the body to the environment during cold exposure (e.g., swimming in an unheated pool) and vice versa during exposure to heat (e.g., exercising when the ambient temperature exceeds the body temperature).

   f. **Sweating rate** for children is much lower than that for adults.

   g. Although the number of **sweat glands** in children equals the number in the adult, the rate of **sweat production** for each gland is half that of the adult glands.

   h. The threshold for sweating is higher in children than in adults.

   i. Children **acclimatize** to hot environments less efficiently and **at a slower rate** than adults. Children therefore require a **longer and more gradual program** of exposure to a hot environment for acclimatization.

   j. **Hypohydrated children** are at increased risk for heat-related illness, because the rise in core temperature in proportion to the degree of dehydration occurs at a greater rate.

2. Heat Disorders in Children

   a. **Children at highest risk for heat-related illness** include:

     1) Children with **diseases affecting the sweating mechanism** (e.g., cystic fibrosis, diabetes mellitus).

     2) Children with **diseases affecting the cardiovascular system** (e.g., congenital heart diseases, diabetes mellitus).

     3) Children with **obesity.**

     4) Children with a **history of heat stroke.**

   b. **Prevention** of heat-related illness can be achieved by ensuring that children who participate in physical activities, especially in hot, humid environments, are properly hydrated, acclimatized, and conditioned for the exercise.

3. Cold Injuries in Children

   a. Cold injuries are much less common than heat-related injuries.

   b. Cold injuries may be superficial (e.g., frostbite) or systemic (e.g., hypothermia).

   c. Little acclimatization occurs following repeated exposure to cold.

   d. Physical fitness does not appear to decrease the risk of cold injury.

   e. **Prevention** of cold-related injuries during exercise **is dependent on proper clothing and limitation of exposure to cold.**

   f. The greater ratio of body surface area to mass in children results in **greater heat loss in the cold, especially during swimming.** For this reason, children exercising in cool water should exit and warm up at least every 15 minutes.

4. Older Adults

   a. The **primary determinants of sweating rate are acclimation, fitness, hydration, and genetics.** Subtle age differences in sweat gland function exist, but age per se is a minor influence compared to the other factors in changes of sweating rate with aging. The same number of sweat glands are activated, but with less sweat output per gland, when stimulated pharmacologically.

   b. Numerous factors can impair thermoregulation in older adults, including:

     1) **Reduced total body water** predisposes the older adult to a more rapid dehydration.

     2) **Elderly men** exposed to prolonged heat stress exhibit lower subcutaneous blood flow values compared with young men.

     3) Heart rate, blood pressure, and oxygen consumption, expressed as a percentage of maximum, are higher in the older adult exercising at a submaximal workload in the heat.

     4) The **decreased tolerance for exercising in hot environments** with aging appears to relate primarily to decreases in **cardiovascular responses** to the heat stress and to a **compromised aerobic capacity.**

   c. Application to exercise training in older adults

     1) Initial studies suggest that regular aerobic exercise may attenuate the decrease of peripheral sweat production known to occur with aging.

G. HORMONES

1. Growth hormone

Loss in circulating growth hormone levels begins in the early thirties and continues throughout life. This contributes to the loss of muscle mass and strength associated with aging.

2. Testosterone

In men, **loss in circulating testosterone** levels begins in the early thirties and continues throughout life. This also contributes to the loss of muscle mass and strength associated with aging.

3. Ovarian Hormones

In women, during perimenopausal and postmenopausal conditions, a dramatic **drop in circulating levels of estrogen and progesterone** occurs. This contributes to the increased risk for heart disease and osteoporosis.

III. Special Consideration for Exercise Training in Children and Adolescents

A. BENEFITS AND RISKS

1. Children and adolescents tend to be more active than adults, but many fail to meet health-related standards for physical fitness.

2. Exercise programs for youths should increase physical fitness in the short term and lead to adoption of a physically active lifestyle in the long term.

B. STRENGTH TRAINING

1. Strength training in preadolescents, as compared to that in adolescents and adults, probably results in smaller absolute strength gains but equal relative increases in strength.
2. If proper instruction, exercise prescription, and supervision are provided, strength training in children and adolescents carries **no greater risk of injury** than comparable strength training programs in adults.
3. **No detrimental cardiorespiratory effects** of strength training in children and adolescents have been reported.

C. CARDIOVASCULAR CONSIDERATIONS

Most children with cardiovascular disorders may participate in physical activities. Each child with known or suspected heart disease should be carefully evaluated and his or her limits of physical activity set by the health-care provider or exercise professional.

1. Heart Murmurs
   a. Heart murmurs are commonly heard in children.
   b. Usually, these murmurs are **functional murmurs** and do not impair normal cardiovascular function.
   c. A diagnosis of heart murmurs caused by **anatomic defects** does not necessarily exclude children from physical activity. Such exclusion should be considered individually and an exercise prescription designed according to the primary physician's recommendations.
2. Dysrhythmias
   a. **Suspected dysrhythmias should be referred to a physician**.
   b. **Common symptoms** associated with dysrhythmias include:
      1) Sensation of "skipped beats."
      2) Headache
      3) Vomiting
      4) Loss of vision
      5) Syncope
      6) Near-syncope.
   c. Different types of dysrhythmias exist. **Some are benign**, whereas **others may preclude participation in physical activity**. The appropriate level of activity should be determined by a physician.

1) **Syncope** is the loss of muscle tone and consciousness caused by diminished cerebral blood flow. **Types of syncope include:**
   a) **Vasopressor syncope**, which is caused by external stimuli (e.g., anxiety or emotion).
   b) **Orthostatic syncope**, which is caused by pooling of blood in the lower extremities of the body.
   c) **Cardiovascular syncope**, which is caused by some form of heart disease.
2) **Symptoms of presyncope** include:
   a) Dizziness.
   b) Cold and clammy appearance.
   c) Diaphoresis.
   d) Significantly decreased blood pressure.
3) Following an episode of syncope or presyncope, children should be referred to a physician before participating in vigorous physical activity.

D. ORTHOPEDIC CONSIDERATIONS

1. **Bone Mass**
   During growth, overall **bone mass and bone mineral density increase** significantly. Weight-bearing physical activity during this time augments this process.
   a. Humans have increased capacity to add bone in response to exercise.
   b. **Weight lifting and compressive exercises** (e.g., gymnastics) have the greatest effect for enhancing bone mass in children.
   c. The beneficial effects of exercise on bone mass do not appear to occur if **dietary calcium intake** is inadequate.
2. **Orthopedic Injuries (Overuse Injuries)**
   Orthopedic injuries (overuse injuries) result from repetitive microtrauma of articular cartilage, bone, muscle, and/or tendon. They are commonly seen in children and adolescent athletes, particularly those specializing in one organized sport that involves cyclic forces applied to an anatomic structure.
   a. **Overuse injuries of bone (stress fractures)** commonly occur in the:
      1) Tibia, fibula, or foot in running sports.
      2) Femur, pelvis, or patella in jumping sports.
      3) Humerus, first rib, or elbow in overhand-throwing and racquet sports.

b. Risk Factors
  1) Training Error
    a) **Increased total volume** of training.
    b) **Increased rate of progression** of training intensity beyond approximately 10% per week.
  2) Muscle-Tendon Imbalance
    Growth may cause changes in relative strength and flexibility across major joints, especially during the adolescent growth spurt. Repetitive techniques at this age may result in asymmetric stresses on bones and joints.
  3) Anatomic Malalignments
    Malalignments (e.g., discrepancies of leg length, abnormalities of hip rotation) may result in excessive stress on skeletal units during repetitive exercise.
  4) High-Impact Forces During Running and/or Jumping Sports
    These high-impact forces can be reduced by the use of proper footwear but are exacerbated by hard playing surfaces.
  5) Growth
    Cartilage in growing children is more susceptible to repetitive trauma.

E. **ONSET OF PUBERTY IN GIRLS AND AMENORRHEA**
The age at which puberty begins in American girls varies from 9 to 14 years.
1. **Delayed onset of puberty and the abnormal absence or suppression of menses (amenorrhea) have been associated with chronic endurance training.**
  a. No single underlying cause has been identified.
  b. **Young competitive athletes** have a higher incidence of amenorrhea than either their nonathletic counterparts or older athletic women.
  c. Blood levels of estradiol, progesterone, and follicle-stimulating hormone are lower in adolescent and **young adult women** involved in intense exercise training.
  d. Recent evidence suggests that **excessive training may interfere with the normal menstrual cycle** in some women by inhibiting the release of gonadotropin-releasing hormone.
2. The **hormonal imbalances associated with long-term secondary amenorrhea** in young female athletes may have deleterious effects on the normal accumulation of bone tissue during growth, which in turn **may increase the risk of both skeletal fragility and osteoporosis later in life**.

F. **EXERCISE-INDUCED ASTHMA (EIA)**
1. Asthma is the most common chronic illness in childhood, affecting between 5% and 15% of children in the United States.
2. EIA consists of **cough, wheeze, chest tightness, chest pain, breathlessness,** or any combination of these during or, more often, immediately after exercise.
3. EIA has been reported to occur in approximately 80% of patients with asthma and in as many as 10% to 15% of apparently healthy children and adolescents.
4. The type of exercise affects the likelihood and severity of EIA episodes. Typically, **short and intense bouts of exercise are more likely to elicit EIA**.
5. **Ambient conditions** (e.g., cold, low humidity, polluted air) **can also exacerbate EIA**.
6. Children suffering from EIA are often physically unfit because of restriction of activity, either self-imposed or imposed by parents or physicians.
7. **Control of EIA** may be accomplished through pharmacologic intervention or nonpharmacologic approaches (e.g., use of a mask or scarf during exercise in cold weather). Once EIA symptoms are controlled, most children can safely engage in normal physical activity.
8. **Increasing the duration of warm-up** may help to prevent EIA by mitigating the mechanism causing bronchoconstriction within the airways at the onset of exercise that promotes EIA.

G. **UNIQUE RESPONSES OF CHILDREN DURING EXERCISE AND RECOVERY**
The basic physiologic responses to exercise are similar in healthy individuals of any age. However, age-related quantitative differences are seen during exercise and recovery.
1. **Metabolic Responses**
  a. **Submaximal, relative oxygen consumption** at a given workload in children is similar to that in adults for cycling exercise, but is 10% to 20% higher for running or walking.
  b. **Anaerobic capacity is lower in children** than in adults because of the lower concentration and rate of utilization of muscle glycogen as well as the low levels of phosphofructokinase in children.
  c. On initiation of exercise, **children reach metabolic steady state more quickly** than adults resulting in lower oxygen deficit.

2. **Cardiovascular Responses**
   a. **Cardiac output** at a given oxygen consumption **is slightly lower** in children than in adults.
   b. **Heart rate** at a submaximal load **is higher** in children than in adults because of the smaller heart size and stroke volume in children.
   c. **Maximal heart rate is higher in children** than in adults, but this does not fully compensate for the smaller heart size, **causing decreased maximal cardiac output**, in children.
   d. **Arterial blood pressure**, especially systolic blood pressure, at submaximal and maximal workloads **is lower** in exercising children than in adults.

3. **Pulmonary Responses**
   a. **Absolute maximal minute ventilation** is lower in children than in adults because of body size.
   b. **Relative minute ventilation during maximal exercise** in children is similar to that in adults, but is considerably higher than that in adults during submaximal exercise at a fixed $\dot{V}O_2$.
   c. Typically, children breathe at a higher frequency than adults do and have decreased ventilatory volume compared with adults during exercise.

4. Exercise at a given relative intensity (i.e., percentage of $\dot{V}O_2$max or maximum heart rate) is perceived to be easier by children.

H. TRAINABILITY OF CHILDREN AND ADOLESCENTS

1. **Skeletal Muscle Strength**
   a. **Resistance training** during preadolescence and adolescence **causes relative strength gains** (percentage improvements) similar to those found in young adults with adequate intensity and volume of training.
   b. **Strength gains** associated with resistance training are consistently associated with **muscle hypertrophy in adolescents and young adults.** However, muscle hypertrophy is rarely reported following resistance training in preadolescent children despite the increases in strength.
   c. **Neurologic adaptations** resulting in an **increase in motor unit activation** have been measured following strength training in preadolescents and adolescents. Increased motor unit activation has been inferred to mediate strength gains in young children.

   d. Resistance training in **prepubescent children** should focus on proper mechanics and form to help prevent injury.

2. **Functional Capacity**
   a. Children and adolescents respond to endurance training in a manner similar to that of adults.
   b. For preadolescents, the **magnitude of change in relative $\dot{V}O_2$max** is lower than would be expected from changes in endurance performance. It appears that the cardiovascular system of preadolescents is trainable, but to a lesser extent than that of adolescents and adults. Improvements in performance by endurance-trained children may result, in part, from increases in biomechanical efficiency.

IV. Exercise in Older Adults

A. GENERAL CONSIDERATIONS

1. Older adults who are inactive can greatly benefit from regular participation in a well-designed exercise program.
2. Benefits of regular exercise include:
   a. Enhanced fitness.
   b. Improved health status (because of reduction in risk factors associated with various diseases).
   c. Increased independence.
   d. An overall improvement in the quality of life.
3. Because of the age-related alterations in cardiovascular capacity, muscle mass and strength, flexibility, and balance, **a well-rounded program should incorporate aerobic, resistance, balance, and flexibility training.**
4. **Older individuals** with age-related limitations in range of motion, orthopedic problems, restricted mobility, arthritis, or other diseases may need an exercise program focusing on **minimal or nonweight-bearing, low-impact activities** (e.g., swimming).
5. Older adults may have a fear of falling. **Strength training and balance training can ameliorate the frequency of falls in older adults.**

B. MEDICAL SCREENING

1. The ACSM recommends screening for adults who are initiating exercise programs based on age and risk status.
   a. Screening requirements for initiating an exercise program are specified in the seventh edition of *ACSM's Guidelines for Exercise Testing and Prescriptions.*

b.   Refer to the seventh edition of *ACSM's Guidelines for Exercise Testing and Prescriptions* for methods and procedures associated with the screening process. Clients with **preexisting medical problems** (e.g., heart disease, arthritis, diabetes) or who take medications that can affect response to exercise **should be referred to their physician** for guidance before initiating an exercise program.

2.   **Evaluation by an exercise professional is beneficial** to document initial measurements of muscle strength, aerobic fitness capacity, flexibility, and range of motion. Any impairment in cardiopulmonary, musculoskeletal, or sensory function should be identified.

C. EXERCISE PRESCRIPTION

1.   Guidelines for exercise prescription are found in the seventh edition of *ACSM's Guidelines for Exercise Testing and Prescription.* Initiating exercise programs in older adults at the lower end of the recommended guidelines for exercise prescription (see above) may be a prudent course of action in newly exercising older adults.

2.   **Frequency** of exercise can be increased in deconditioned older adults. Frequencies of 5 to 7 days per week are appropriate if adjustments in duration and intensity are also prescribed.

3.   **Duration** of exercise sessions may range from 20 to 60 minutes of continuous or intermittent aerobic activity.

4.   Duration and intensity of exercise are interdependent and should be modified and adapted to individual functional capacity and interest.

5.   **Intensity** should be prescribed according to ACSM guidelines.

a.   **High-intensity activity** should be limited to shorter periods. In deconditioned older adults, high-intensity exercise should be discouraged.

b.   Generally, **light- to moderate-intensity exercise** of extended duration is recommended for older adults engaging in aerobic training programs.

c.   **For resistance training, higher relative intensity is recommended** to produce optimal training adaptations in muscle mass and strength.

D. BENEFITS AND PRECAUTIONS

1.   **Cardiovascular Endurance Benefits and Precautions**

a.   Cardiovascular Function

1)   Numerous studies have documented similar **increases in the $\dot{V}O_2$ max** of older (>60 years) compared to younger subjects following programs of endurance training.

2)   Depending on initial fitness levels, high-intensity exercise training **increases functional capacity** in the older adult as much as or more than that observed in young adults.

3)   **Improvements in $\dot{V}O_2$max and endurance in men** result from central cardiovascular adaptations (e.g., increased cardiac output) and increased arteriovenous oxygen difference. **In older women,** the increased $\dot{V}O_2$max appears to result primarily from increased arteriovenous oxygen difference.

4)   Moderate physical activity in older adults augments tolerance for daily activities and is associated with **less fatigue and dyspnea** (shortness of breath) and with **lower ratings of perceived exertion.**

b.   Coronary Artery Disease and Hypertension

1)   The prevalence of hypertension and coronary artery disease increases with advancing age. The **incidence** of these conditions and the **morbidity and mortality** associated with heart disease are **greatly reduced in physically active individuals.**

2)   Low-Intensity Endurance Training

a)   Effectively **lowers systolic and diastolic blood pressure** by 8 to 10 mm Hg in normotensive and moderately hypertensive older adults.

b)   **Reduces myocardial oxygen demand** as a result of peripheral adaptations (e.g., increased oxygen extraction, increased vagal tone, decreased catecholamine release) and central changes (e.g., decreased myocardial ischemia, improved left ventricular function) at similar levels of submaximal exercise.

c.   Cardiovascular Events

1)   **Appropriate screening** of exercise program participants (according to ACSM guidelines) is important, because the incidence of cardiovascular disease (both diagnosed and undiagnosed) increases with aging.

2)   The **incidence of cardiac events** during supervised adult fitness programs for apparently healthy older

programs for apparently healthy older adults **is very low**, with nonfatal cardiac events reported to occur at a rate of approximately 1 per 800,000 hours of supervised exercise and fatal events at a rate of approximately 1 per 1.1 million hours of supervised exercise.

(3) **High-intensity exercise** training increases the risk for cardiac events.

2. Strength Training

a. Muscle strength, power, and endurance begin to decline in middle adulthood.

b. This decline accelerates after 50 to 60 years of age and is attributable to a number of changes. These changes include:

   1) Decreased muscle fiber size.

   2) Decreased muscle fiber number.

   3) Decreased mitochondrial proteins and glycolytic, anaerobic, and oxidative enzyme activities.

   4) Decreased impulse conduction velocity.

c. **Regular physical activity seems to slow this decline.** One exception, however, is the loss of muscle fibers, which results from age-related loss of motoneurons and appears to be unaffected by exercise.

d. Men and women in the sixth decade of life gain strength, but at a slower rate, in response to resistance exercise.

e. **Older adults exhibit strength gains from resistance training** that are similar to or even greater than those seen in younger adults (because of lower initial strength levels). These strength gains are related to improved neurologic function and, to a lesser extent, increased muscle mass.

f. Regular **aerobic exercise enhances bone health**, particularly in postmenopausal women.

g. **Resistance training** can offset the normal, age-related declines in **bone health** by maintaining and, sometimes, even improving bone mineral density.

h. **Flexibility and balance can be improved** and the risk of falling reduced in older adults through an exercise program that incorporates resistance exercise, balance training, and stretching.

3. Balance

a. **Decreased balance** and an associated **increased occurrence of falls** in the elderly can be attributed to many factors. These factors include:

   1) Muscle weakness.

   2) Inflexibility.

   3) Degradation of neuromotor function.

   4) Obesity.

   5) Visual and vestibular deterioration.

b. Substantial evidence suggests that **physically active individuals maintain better balance during old age**.

   1) Regular exercise **improves muscle strength and flexibility**, which has a positive influence on speed and agility of walking as well as on **static balance.**

   2) Regular exercise also appears to have **positive effects on central nervous system functions**, such as attention, short-term memory, and information processing speed, all of which commonly deteriorate with age and greatly impact balance and coordination.

4. Preservation of Bone Mass

a. Bone mass **peaks in early adulthood** and declines slowly thereafter.

b. **Regular weight-bearing exercise** can slow the loss of bone mass with aging.

   1) The stimulation of osteoblastic bone formation on the periosteal surface of long bones following a given load is greater in the young than in the old, but it does occur in older adults if the stimulus is sufficient.

   2) The type of loading placed on the bone affects the degree of osteogenic stimulation. The **magnitude of the load during an exercise session seems to be of greater importance than the number of loading cycles.**

5. Immune Function

a. The **immune system deteriorates significantly with advancing age.** This is evidenced by the increased incidence of malignancy, infectious disease, and autoimmune disorders in the elderly.

b. Numerous studies have indicated that **lack of physical fitness and/or improper nutrition is also associated with compromised immune function.** It remains unclear how much of the age-related loss of immune function is directly caused physical inactivity; however, **available data suggest that immune function is better in the elderly who are compared with those who are sedentary.**

6. Obesity

a. Longitudinal and cross-sectional studies have indicated that **weight gain** during adulthood is not caused by aging but, rather, by an increasingly **sedentary lifestyle** in older adults. Secondarily, older adults who continue caloric consumption of their more active years also gain weight.

b. **Physical activity plays an important role in the prevention and treatment of obesity as age progresses.** Programs of physical activity must be continued for months or even years to effectively reduce and control body mass.

7. Insulin Resistance

a. **Insulin resistance**, a condition leading to **adult-onset diabetes**, is characterized by high levels of circulating insulin and reduced ability to maintain blood glucose concentration at a constant value.

b. Well-controlled studies have indicated that physical inactivity and obesity, but not aging, are related to increased risk for insulin resistance.

c. **Regular exercise can decrease abdominal fat and increase insulin sensitivity, which may normalize glucose tolerance.**

8. Psychological Benefits

a. Life Satisfaction
Older adults who exercise regularly have a more positive attitude toward work and are **generally healthier** than sedentary individuals.

b. Happiness
Strong correlations have been reported between the activity level of older adults and their self-reported happiness.

c. Self-Efficacy
1) Self-efficacy refers to the concept of or capability to perform a variety of tasks.
2) Older adults taking part in exercise programs commonly report that they are **able to do daily tasks more easily** than before they began the exercise program.

d. Self-Concept
Older adults improve their scores on self-concept questionnaires following participation in an exercise program.

e. Psychological Stress
Exercise is effective in reducing psychological stress.

9. Orthopedic Injury

a. The **incidence of musculoskeletal injury among regularly exercising older adults is considerably higher** than that in younger populations.

b. **Factors related to orthopedic injuries in older adults include**:
1) Inadequate warm-up.
2) Muscle weakness.
3) Sudden violent movements.
4) Rapid increases in exercise prescription.

10. Thermoregulatory Concerns

a. Older adults have **lower maximal cardiac output and compromised subcutaneous blood flow** during exercise. Furthermore, total body water is reduced, which decreases maximal capacity for sweating.

b. **Exercise training improves thermoregulation** in older adults. Nevertheless, leaders of exercise programs involving older adults should ensure the **availability of fluids** for the participants, and they should **avoid exercising outdoors in hot and humid conditions**.

E. UNIQUE RESPONSES OF OLDER ADULTS DURING EXERCISE AND RECOVERY (TABLE 3-1)

1. Cardiovascular and Hemodynamic Responses to Exercise

a. The **increase in heart rate** in response to a given increase in relative exercise intensity **is blunted** in older adults.

b. It appears that stroke volume and cardiac output at a fixed submaximal workload are similar in healthy young and old adults. However, **maximal stroke volume and cardiac output are decreased** in older adults because of decreased blood volume and maximal heart rate.

c. Age-related **reductions in arterial compliance and left ventricular contractile reserve** combine to increase blood pressure and attenuate the increase in ejection fraction during exercise in the older adult.

d. The response of arterial blood pressure to submaximal exercise appears unchanged with advancing age. Because blood volume is reduced, the **maintenance of blood pressure response** in the older subject **requires systemic vascular resistance to be elevated** above that found in young adults.

2. Pulmonary Regulation During Exercise

a. **Expiratory flow limitation occurs at lower exercise intensities** with aging because of a loss of lung elastic recoil. This

TABLE 3-1. Exercise Responses Commonly Observed in Older Adults and Suggested Testing Modifications

Characteristic	Suggested Modification
1. Low aerobic capacity	Begin test at a low intensity (2–3 metabolic equivalents [METs]).
2. More time required to reach metabolic steady state	Increase length of warm-up (3+ min) and stages (2–3 min).
3. Poor balance	Bike preferred over treadmill or step test.
4. Poor leg strength	Treadmill preferred over bike or step test.
5. Difficulty holding mouthpiece with dentures	Add support or use face mask to measure $\dot{V}o_2$.
6. Impaired vision	Bike preferred over treadmill or step test.
7. Impaired hearing	Use electronic bike or treadmill to avoid the necessity of following a cadence.
8. Senile gait patterns or foot problems	Bike preferred; if treadmill is used, increase grade rather than speed.

Adapted with permission from Skinner JS. Chapter 5: Importance of aging for exercise testing and exercise prescription. In JS Skinner, Ed: *Exercise Testing and Exercise Prescription for Special Cases.* Malvern, PA: Lea & Febiger, 1993, p. 79.

change can compromise inspiratory muscle function and increase ventilatory work. Older adults reach expiratory limitation at lower exercise intensities than younger adults do.

b. **Dead space is increased** in the older adult from approximately 30% of tidal volume in the young to 40% to 45% in the aged. This requires that total ventilatory response be elevated during exercise in the older adult to maintain alveolar ventilation and arterial P_{CO_2}.

c. The reduction in pulmonary arteriolar compliance with aging **elevates blood pressures in the pulmonary artery and capillaries during exercise.** This may contribute to a **diffusion limitation of gas exchange** in the older adult during moderate-to-intense exercise.

F. **TRAINABILITY OF OLDER ADULTS**

1. The precise decrements in trainability of older adults remain controversial, because training programs for the elderly rarely employ the same absolute workloads as programs for young adults.

2. **Older adults can adapt to exercise training** and sizgnificantly improve health and mobility.

3. When planning an exercise program for older adults, keep in mind the following:

   a. Aging is associated with a **reduced adaptability to physiologic stimuli**.

   b. Exercise programs for older adults require **more time to produce improvements** in variables such as muscle strength, $\dot{V}o_2max$, and muscle oxidative capacity.

   c. The **goal** of most exercise programs for older adults should be to **increase self-sufficiency and the ability to move with relative ease** and to perform activities of daily living.

Review Test

DIRECTIONS: Carefully read all questions, and select the BEST single answer.

1. In terms of chronological age, early childhood is usually described as
   A) Birth to 3 weeks.
   B) 3 weeks to 1 year.
   C) 1 to 6 years.
   D) 7 to 10 years.

2. Which age group is the fastest-growing segment of the U.S. population?
   A) Preadolescents.
   B) Adolescents.
   C) Adults aged 65 to 85 years.
   D) Adults older than 85 years.

3. Increased afterload associated with increased peripheral resistance as a result of aging causes
   A) Left ventricular hypertrophy.
   B) Kidney failure.
   C) Liver damage.
   D) Liver failure.

4. An increase in both systolic and diastolic blood pressure at rest and during exercise often accompanies aging. Blood pressure usually increases because of
   A) Increased arterial compliance and decreased arterial stiffness.
   B) Decreased arterial compliance and increased arterial stiffness.
   C) Decrease in both arterial compliance and arterial stiffness.
   D) Increase in both arterial compliance and arterial stiffness.

5. The $\dot{V}O_2$max remains relatively unchanged throughout childhood. However, after age 25, it typically decreases by
   A) 0% to 5% each decade.
   B) 5% to 15% each decade.
   C) 15% to 20% each decade.
   D) 15% to 20% each year.

6. Cardiac output is a function of heart rate and stroke volume. In children, why is heart rate higher at rest and during exercise?
   A) Because in children, stroke volume is directly related to how much left ventricular stiffness reduces diastolic filling
   B) Because in children, cardiac output is regulated more by peripheral resistance than by any other variable

   C) Because children typically have a lower stroke volume compared to adults.
   D) Because children typically have a more elevated peripheral resistance compared to adults.

7. The $\dot{V}O_2$max increases as a result of physical training in elderly persons. This occurs for all of the following reasons EXCEPT
   A) In men, the increase is a function of improved central and peripheral adaptations.
   B) In women, the increase is a function of improved peripheral adaptations.
   C) In both men and women, regular aerobic exercise slows the decline with aging.
   D) In both men and women, regular aerobic exercise speeds the decline with aging.

8. The total number of muscle fibers is fixed at an early age, but
   A) At adolescence, males exhibit rapid hypertrophy of muscle.
   B) In comparison to males, females exhibit a more rapid hypertrophy of muscle.
   C) Males lose muscle mass faster at an early age when they remain sedentary.
   D) Males tend to exhibit muscle hypertrophy at a later age than females.

9. Strenuous exercise can predispose children to which of the following?
   A) Osteoporosis.
   B) Osteoarthritis.
   C) Malignant tumors.
   D) Epiphysitis.

10. Advancing age brings a progressive decline in bone mineral density and calcium content; this process is accelerated in women immediately following menopause. Which condition is commonly associated with this condition?
    A) Osteoarthritis.
    B) Osteoporosis.
    C) Arthritis.
    D) Epiphysitis.

11. All of the following musculoskeletal changes typically occur with advancing age EXCEPT
    A) Decreased flexibility.
    B) Impaired balance.
    C) Inhibited range of motion.
    D) Skeletal muscle hypertrophy.

12. Body fat generally increases with advancing age, particularly between childhood and early adulthood, because of
    A) An exponential increase in caloric consumption.
    B) A great increase in caloric consumption and a small decline in fat production.
    C) Body fat accumulation as a result of an imbalance between caloric intake and energy expenditure.
    D) Alterations in resting metabolic rate.

13. Which of the following factors does NOT impair an older individual's ability to thermoregulate?
    A) Reduced total body water.
    B) Decreased renal function.
    C) Decreased vascular peripheral responsiveness.
    D) Enhanced sweat response.

14. A medical history as well as risk factor screening are important before prescribing an exercise program for older adults. Individuals with one or more risk factors for exercise participation should be referred
    A) Directly to the hospital and admitted for further evaluation.
    B) In 1 month to the nearest exercise facility.
    C) For diagnostic exercise tolerance testing.
    D) Immediately to a hospital emergency room.

15. Which of the following can an older person expect as a result of participation in an exercise program?
    A) Overall improvement in the quality of life and increased independence.
    B) No changes in the quality of life but an increase in longevity.

C) Increased longevity but a loss of bone mass.
D) Loss of bone mass with a concomitant increase in bone density.

16. Which of the following would generally be the preferred mode of exercise for an elderly person?
    A) Jogging.
    B) Calisthenics.
    C) Swimming.
    D) Archery.

17. An exercise program for elderly persons generally should emphasize increased
    A) Frequency.
    B) Intensity.
    C) Duration.
    D) Intensity and frequency.

18. For optimal cardiovascular as well as balance and flexibility adaptations, an elderly person generally should exercise how many days per week?
    A) 1.
    B) 2.
    C) 3.
    D) 5 to 7.

19. In response to regular resistance training,
    A) Older men and women demonstrate similar or even greater strength gains when compared to younger individuals.
    B) Younger men have greater gains in strength than older men.
    C) Younger women have greater gains in strength than older women.
    D) Younger men and women demonstrate similar or greater strength gains compared to older persons.

ANSWERS AND EXPLANATIONS

1–C. Typical age groupings/distinctions are as follows: neonatal, birth to 3 weeks; infancy, 3 weeks to 1 year; early childhood, 1 to 6 years; middle childhood, 7 to 10 years; late childhood/prepuberty, 9 to 15 years in females and 12 to 16 years in males; adolescence, the 6 years following puberty; adulthood, 20 to 64 years; older adulthood, 65 and older.

2–C. The number of individuals in the United States older than 65 years will reach 70 million by the year 2030, with people older than 85 years then being the fastest-growing segment of the population.

3–A. Left ventricular hypertrophy increases with age, apparently related to increased afterload associated with increased peripheral vascular resistance.

4–B. A decrease in arterial compliance and an increase in arterial stiffness with age can result in elevated systolic and diastolic blood pressure both at rest and during exercise.

5–B. A function of cardiac output and arteriovenous oxygen difference, $\dot{V}O_2max$ can remain relatively unchanged throughout adulthood. Without any exercise intervention, however it decreases 5% to 15% each decade after age 25. Both cardiac output and arteriovenous oxygen difference decline with age; regular physical activity will help reduce these effects.

6–C. At rest and during exercise, heart rate is higher in children because of compensation for a lower stroke volume. Maximal heart rate and maximal stroke volume both decrease with age, causing a significant decline in maximal cardiac output.

7–D. Regular aerobic training produces similar increases in $\dot{V}O_2$max in younger and older adults. In men, this increase seems to be both central and peripheral, whereas in women, the changes seem to be peripheral. Men and women who participate in regular endurance exercise programs reduce the loss in $\dot{V}O_2$max with aging.

8–A. At adolescence, males exhibit a rapid hypertrophy of muscle that is disproportionately greater than that observed in females. The total number of muscle fibers seems to be fixed at an early age in both genders. Muscle mass declines (atrophy) with advancing age because of a progressive decrease in the number and size of fibers, with a greater selective loss of type II fibers.

9–D. Because in children the epiphysis is not yet united with the bone shaft, strenuous exercise can cause problems with bone growth. Epiphysitis can occur with overuse. Also, fractures can pass through the epiphyseal plate, leading to disruption in normal bone growth.

10–B. Advancing age brings a progressive decline in bone mineral density and calcium content. This loss is accelerated in women immediately after menopause. As a result, older adults are more susceptible to osteoporosis and bone fractures.

11–D. Connective tissue (fascia, ligaments, tendons) become less extensible with age. Degeneration of joints, especially the spine, occurs with advancing age, causing decreased range of motion along with a progressive loss of flexibility. Balance and postural stability are also affected because of age-related changes in both sensory and motor systems.

12–C. The energy expenditure related to physical activity declines with age, making inactivity a primary factor responsible for the increase in fat mass with age. Body fat accumulates because of an imbalance between caloric intake and energy expenditure.

13–D. A number of factors can impair an older individual's ability to thermoregulate, including reduced total body water, decreased renal function, decreased vascular peripheral responsiveness, rapid dehydration, and blunted sweat response.

14–C. Awareness of preexisting medical problems and current medication use (gained through a medical history and risk factor screening) is necessary before an exercise program is prescribed. Persons with one or more risk factors should be referred for diagnostic exercise tolerance testing.

15–A. Most older adults are not sufficiently active. This population can benefit greatly from regular participation in a well-designed exercise program. Benefits of such a program include increased fitness, improved health status (reduction in risk factors associated with various diseases), increased independence, and overall improvement in the quality of life.

16–C. For older adults, who often suffer from limited range of motion, orthopedic problems, restricted mobility, arthritis, and other disorders, an emphasis on minimal or nonweight-bearing, low-impact activities (e.g., swimming) is generally most appropriate.

17–A. Increased frequency of exercise is generally recommended for older adults to optimize cardiovascular as well as balance and flexibility adaptations. The recommended duration of exercise depends on the intensity of the activity; higher-intensity activity should be conducted over a shorter period of time.

18–D. An older person will benefit more from increased frequency of exercise than from increased intensity or duration of exercise. Recommended frequency is 5 to 7 days per week.

19–A. Muscle strength peaks in the mid-twenties for both genders and remains fairly stable through the mid-forties. Muscle strength declines by approximately 15% per decade in the sixth and seventh decades and by approximately 30% per decade thereafter. However, older men and women demonstrate similar or even greater strength gains when compared with younger individuals in response to resistance training. These strength gains are related to improved neurologic function and, to a lesser extent, increased muscle mass.

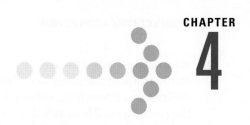

Pathophysiology/Risk Factors

MARK J. KASPER AND SUSAN M. PUHL

I. Cardiopulmonary Disorders

A. PULMONARY DISEASE

1. **Chronic Obstructive Pulmonary Disease (COPD)**

   COPD is actually a group of pulmonary disorders characterized by expiratory airflow obstruction, dyspnea (shortness of breath), and some capability for reversal or resolution of the condition. For example, an acute asthma attack can resolve spontaneously or as a result of medication (e.g., bronchodilator). COPD includes **bronchitis, emphysema, and asthma.**

   a. **Bronchitis**
      1) **Inflammation and edema of the trachea and bronchial tubes** are caused by an **irritant** (e.g., cigarette smoke, industrial pollution).
      2) The resultant **mucosal hypertrophy** with increased mucus secretion narrows and partially obstructs the airway.
      3) Impaired gas exchange leads to **arterial hypoxemia** (deficient blood oxygenation).
      4) **Arterial hypoxemia causes vasoconstriction** of smooth muscle in the pulmonary arterioles and venules, compounding the obstruction.
      5) Continued vasoconstriction may **lead to complications, such as pulmonary hypertension, right ventricular hypertrophy, and right heart failure** (cor pulmonale).
      6) **Symptoms** of bronchitis include **chronic cough, sputum production, and dyspnea.**

   b. **Emphysema**
      1) Alveolar wall integrity is damaged by an irritant (e.g., cigarette smoke, pollution) and results in **loss of alveolar surface area, impaired gas exchange, and hypoventilation.**
      2) This process results in **wasted ventilation,** or ventilation of areas within the lungs where no perfusion occurs (also referred to as dead space). Alveolar destruction is not uniform, and some areas are better ventilated than others.
      3) Hypoventilation of the alveoli leads to **hypoxia and hypercapnia** (excess carbon dioxide in the blood), with increased minute ventilation.
      4) An abnormally high minute ventilation is required to maintain adequate perfusion. These patients are often called **pink puffers** (secondary to a pink rather than to a blue or cyanotic skin color). Destruction of alveoli also destroys small blood vessels of the pulmonary system, leading to **increased pulmonary resistance, elevated pulmonary arterial pressure, and eventually, right heart failure.**
      5) **Dyspnea** is the major **symptom** associated with emphysema.

   c. **Asthma**
      1) Asthma is a reversible condition of **increased airway reactivity** or sensitivity to an initiating factor or trigger (e.g., dust, pollen, hyperventilation), which results in narrowing of the bronchial airways.
      2) The trigger causes increased calcium influx into mast cells, resulting in **release of chemical mediators** (e.g., histamine) that trigger **bronchoconstriction and an inflammatory response** (tissue swelling). Bronchoconstriction also may result from the chemical mediators directly stimulating the vagus nerve.
      3) Clinical manifestations of asthma include **dyspnea** and, possibly, **hypoxia and hypercapnia.**
      4) An **asthma attack can be self-limiting or may necessitate drug therapy** to prevent respiratory failure.

2. **Restrictive Lung Disease**

Restrictive lung disease involves **disorders that restrict or reduce lung volume by affecting the parenchyma**. These include conditions that may affect the **rib cage, spine** (scoliosis, ankylosing spondylitis), **respiratory muscles and nerves** (muscular dystrophy, spinal cord injury), the **pleura, and alveolar septum** (mesothelioma, interstitial fibrosis). Morbid obesity can also affect the thorax and respiratory muscles.

a. These disorders **compromise both resting and exercise lung volumes**.

b. **Chronic restriction** can lead to dyspnea, hypoxia, hypercapnia, and respiratory failure.

3. **Pulmonary Vascular Disease**

a. **Pulmonary Embolism**

1) A pulmonary embolism is a **blood clot** that typically lodges in a major branch of the pulmonary artery. Clots are **common in patients with congestive heart failure, atrial fibrillation, phlebitis** (inflammation of a vein), **and varicose veins and are a complication of surgery**.

2) **A large pulmonary embolism can be fatal**; a smaller clot may grow and increase pulmonary artery pressure, leading to right heart failure.

b. **Pulmonary Edema**

Pulmonary edema involves **excessive fluid retention in the lungs**, which can be caused by any factor that results in left heart failure, causing pooling of blood in the lungs which forces fluid into the alveolar spaces.

c. **Pulmonary Hypertension**

1) Increased pressure within the pulmonary circulation, usually greater than 30 mm Hg systolic and 12 mm Hg diastolic.

2) Causes

a) Conditions of the left atrium (e.g., mitral valve stenosis, left ventricular failure)

b) Ventricular or atrial septal defects (e.g., patent ductus arteriosus)

c) Any factor that increases pulmonary vascular resistance (right heart failure; e.g., COPD, pulmonary embolism).

B. CORONARY ARTERY DISEASE (CAD)

The coronary arteries undergo anatomic changes caused by genetic predisposition (through genome expression), the aging process, and multiple lifestyle risk factors.

Figure 4-1 depicts the normal coronary arterial wall.

1. **Arteriosclerosis and Atherosclerosis**

a. **Arteriosclerosis** is a loss of elasticity (or hardening) of the arteries that begins at birth and progresses throughout life.

b. **Atherosclerosis** is a form of arteriosclerosis characterized by accumulation of obstructive lesions within the intima of the arterial wall. (**Risk factors** are identified and discussed in section II.)

1) **Results of Arterial Injury (Inflammation)** *(Figure 4-2)*

a) **Endothelial cells lose selective permeability**, enabling cells and molecules to pass into the subendothelial space.

b) **Endothelial cells lose antithrombotic properties**, resulting in **increased risk of clot formation and thrombus**.

c) **Reduced secretion of vasodilating substances** (e.g., endothelium-derived relaxing factor nitric oxide) leads to abnormal vasoreactivity

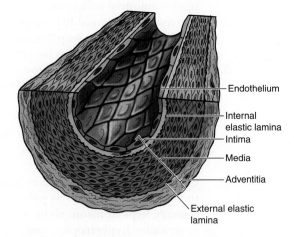

Endothelium

Internal elastic lamina

Intima

Media

Adventitia

External elastic lamina

FIGURE 4-1. The normal coronary arterial wall. The **lumen** is the inside cavity or channel where blood flows. The **endothelium** is a single layer of cells that form a tight barrier between the blood and the arterial wall. It resists thrombosis, promotes vasodilation, and inhibits smooth muscle cells from migration and proliferation into the intima. Damage to the endothelium increases susceptibility of the artery to atherosclerosis. The **intima** is the very thin, innermost layer of the arterial wall. Comprised of predominantly connective tissue with some smooth muscle cells, it is where atherosclerotic lesions are formed. The thickest, middle layer of the arterial wall, the **media** is comprised of predominantly smooth muscle cells. It is responsible for vasoconstriction or vasodilation of the artery, and it can contribute to the atherosclerotic process through migration and proliferation of smooth muscle cells to the intima. The **adventitia** is the outermost layer of the arterial wall. It provides the media and intima with oxygen and nutrients and is not believed to have a significant role in the development of atherosclerosis.

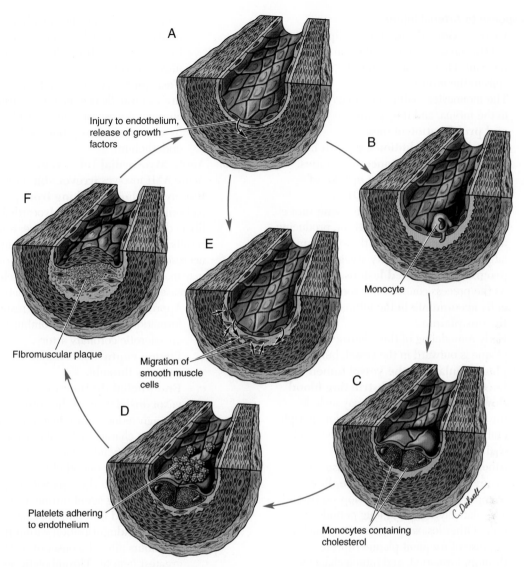

FIGURE 4-2. The atherosclerotic process–response to injury. A. Injury to endothelium with release of growth factors (small arrow). B. Monocytes attach to endothelium. C. Monocytes migrate to the intima, take up cholesterol, and form fatty streaks. D. Platelets adhere to endothelium and release growth factors. F. The result is a fibromuscular plaque. An alternative pathway is shown with arrows from A to E to F, with growth factor–mediated migration of smooth muscle cells from the media to the intima (E).

(increased vasoconstriction and/or decreased vasodilation).

d) **Endothelial cells secrete platelet-derived growth factor,** resulting in movement of smooth muscle cells into the intima.

e) **Endothelial cells attract other cells** toward the intima that are involved in the development of atherosclerosis.

f) The larger outcome of arterial (or endothelial) injury and insult is a resulting **endothelial dysfunction** that alters the homeostasis around the vessel wall. The end result can be ongoing, progressive atherosclerotic changes in the vessel and development of multiple lesions.

g) **Endothelial dysfunction can be reversed,** and many lifestyle behaviors relate specifically to either dysfunction or improved function (e.g., exercise, dietary fat content, appropriate management of stress-related events, maintaining optimal blood pressure, blood lipids and blood glucose).

2. **Response to Arterial Injury**
   a. Excess, **oxidized low-density lipoprotein (LDL) particles accumulate** in the arterial wall. They attract monocytes and other cells to the intima.
   b. The monocytes mature into macrophages in the intima, and they **promote mitosis and proliferation** of these cells.
   c. The **release of additional growth factors and vasoactive substances continues.**
   d. **Monocytes promote the uptake of more lipids,** particularly LDL.
   e. These **cells and connective tissue move from the media to the intima,** producing fatty streaks or lesions. As they ingest more fatty substances, the **fatty streaks progress to fat-filled lesions.**
   f. As the process continues, **smooth muscle cells accumulate** in the intima and form a **fibrous plaque.**
   g. Early remodeling of the atherosclerotic plaque is outward in the vessel, but as the **plaque enlarges, the vessel lumen becomes occluded, obstructing blood flow.** Other complications may include thrombus formation with occlusion, peripheral emboli, and weakening of the vessel wall.
   h. Atherosclerosis **does not necessarily occur or progress in a stable, linear manner.** Some lesions develop slowly and are relatively stable for long periods of time. Other lesions progress very quickly because of frequent plaque rupture, thrombi formation, and intima changes.
   i. **Regression of fatty, soft lesions is possible** with aggressive, multifactorial risk reduction. Modest results have been observed.

3. **Myocardial Ischemia**
   a. Insufficient blood flow to the myocardium occurs when **myocardial oxygen demand exceeds the oxygen supply.**
   b. Ischemia is **an outcome of significant coronary atherosclerosis** and can be silent (asymptomatic) or symptomatic (see *Angina Pectoris* below).

4. **Angina Pectoris**
   Angina pectoris is **discomfort generally associated with myocardial ischemia.** It is most commonly located in the areas of the chest, neck, cheeks/jaw, shoulder, and upper back or arms, and it is most often described as a constricting, squeezing, burning, or heavy feeling.
   a. **Classic (typical) angina** is initiated by factors such as exercise or stress, excitement, cold or hot weather, or food intake (especially large meals or heavy, high-fat meals). It is relieved by rest or nitroglycerin.
   b. **Vasospastic (variant or Prinzmetal's) angina** usually occurs at rest; results from coronary vasospasm, and is likely initiated by vasoconstrictors produced by the injured endothelium.

5. **Acute Myocardial Infarction (AMI)**
   Acute AMI involves **irreversible necrosis of the myocardium resulting from prolonged ischemia (>60 minutes).** Myocardial muscle fibers die within the ischemic zone; remodeling results in fibrous tissue residing among the necrosed myocardial tissue. The area of necrosis may increase secondary to residual ischemia or decrease because of collateral circulation.
   a. Approximately 90% of AMIs result from formation of an acute thrombus in an atherosclerotic coronary artery.
   b. **Plaque rupture is a major cause** of coronary thrombi.
   c. **Endothelial dysfunction contributes to vasoconstriction** of the coronary artery through reduced vasodilator substances as well as a characteristic, abnormal vasoreactivity inherent in the dysfunctioning endothelium.
   d. **Thrombolytic therapy** with a specific clot-dissolving agent during acute MI may restore blood flow and limit myocardial necrosis. Administration within the first 1 to 2 hours after the onset of AMI yields the greatest benefit. Thrombolytic agents used include streptokinase and recombinant tissue plasminogen activator (t-PA).
   e. Possible Complications
      1) **Extension of the zone of ischemia to the surrounding tissue, widening the necrosis.**
      2) **Ventricular Aneurysm**
         Necrotic muscle fibers of the heart degenerate and remodel the ventricular wall; as a result, the myocardial wall may become thinned. During systole, these nonfunctional muscle fibers do not contract but, rather, bulge outward (aneurysm), increasing the risk of thrombus, ventricular arrhythmias, and heart failure.
      3) **Rupture**
         a) Involves a mechanism similar to ventricular aneurysm, but in this case, the ventricular wall ruptures.

b) Rupture of the ventricular free wall is often fatal and may be associated with cardiac tamponade and/or a large area of infarction in the ventricular free wall.

c) Rupture of the ventricular septal wall is less often fatal and may be associated with congestive heart failure.

4) **Papillary Necrosis**
This necrosis of the papillary muscle affects valvular function and results in heart failure or pulmonary edema.

5) **Left Ventricular Dysfunction**
Left ventricular dysfunction may be caused by weakening of the left ventricle because of necrotic myocardium and is often associated with chronic congestive heart failure.

C. SIGNS AND SYMPTOMS OF CARDIOPULMONARY DISEASE

Major signs and symptoms suggestive of cardiovascular and pulmonary disease are listed in *Table 4-1.*

II. Risk Factors for CAD

A. NONMODIFIABLE PRIMARY RISK FACTORS

1. **Advancing Age**
   a. Risk increases steeply with advancing age in men and women because of accumulation of atherosclerosis.
   b. Approximately 50% of AMIs occur in persons older than 65 years of age, 45% in those 45 to 65 years of age, and 5% in those under 45 years of age.

2. **Male Sex**
   a. Although the percentage of deaths from heart disease is similar between men and women ($\approx$50%), men at any given age are at greater risk than women for CAD.
   b. Risk in women lags 10 to 15 years behind that of men, which is explained in part by the earlier onset of risk factors in men (e.g., lower high-density lipoprotein [HDL] cholesterol, hypertension).

3. **Family History**
   a. Children and siblings of a person with CAD are more likely to develop CAD themselves.
   b. A positive family history carries excess risk even when accounting for modifiable risk factors.
   c. Risk increases with the number of relatives affected and at younger ages of onset.

B. MODIFIABLE PRIMARY RISK FACTORS

1. **Smoking Tobacco**
   a. Smokers are at a roughly 2.5-fold greater risk for CAD than nonsmokers are, although individual risk varies with the extent of exposure (lifetime dosage).
   b. The risk of heart disease decreases 50% within 1 year of smoking cessation and approaches that of a lifetime nonsmoker within 15 years.
   c. Smoking has both acute (e.g., increased myocardial oxygen demand) and chronic effects (e.g., endothelial damage) on the myocardium and coronary vessels.
   d. Smoking negatively influences other CAD risk factors (e.g., lowers HDL).

2. **Dyslipidemia**
   a. A positive correlation exists between total cholesterol (TC) and LDL levels, fat, saturated fat, and cholesterol in the diet and CAD mortality and morbidity.
   b. Triglycerides, TC, and LDL contribute to the atherosclerotic process, whereas HDL is cardioprotective. The National Cholesterol Education Program Adult Treatment Panel III (ATPIII) provides recommendations for the detection, evaluation, and treatment of high blood cholesterol in adults. The aggressiveness of lipid management is determined by the absolute risk of developing CAD (e.g., AMI, CAD death) over the next 10 years. The primary target for management is LDL, especially in those with established CAD.

3. **Hypertension**
   a. Blood pressure classifications of the 2003 *Seventh Report of the Joint Committee on Prevention, Detection, Evaluation, and Treatment of High Blood Pressure* (JNC 7) are provided in Chapter 2, *Table 2-3.* Recommendations on treatment are also available from this document.
   b. **As blood pressure increases, so does the risk of cardiovascular disease.** This holds true across all blood pressure ranges, including individuals who are classified as normal or prehypertensive.
   c. Hypertension has both **acute** (e.g., increased myocardial oxygen demand) **and chronic effects** (e.g., endothelial and renal dysfunction) on the myocardium.
   d. **Treatment of hypertension does not remove all of the cardiovascular risk** associated with elevated blood pressure.

TABLE 4-1. Major Symptoms or Signs Suggestive of Cardiopulmonary or Metabolic Disease

Symptom: Pain or discomfort in the chest or surrounding areas that appears to be ischemic in nature.
Clarification/Significance: One of the cardinal manifestations of cardiac disease, particularly coronary artery disease. Key features favoring an ischemic origin include:

- Character—constricting, squeezing, burning, "heaviness" or "heavy feeling."
- Location—substernal; across midthorax, anteriorly; in both arms, shoulders; in neck, cheeks, teeth; in forearms, fingers; in interscapular region.
- Provoking factors—exercise, excitement, other forms of stress, cold weather, occurrence after meals.

Key features **against** an ischemic origin include:

- Character—dull ache; "knife-like," sharp, stabbing; "jabs" aggravated by respiration.
- Location—in left submammary area, in left hemithorax.
- Provoking factors—after completion of exercise, provoked by a specific body motion.

Symptom: Unaccustomed shortness of breath, or shortness of breath with mild exertion.
Clarification/Significance: Dyspnea (defined as an abnormally uncomfortable awareness of breathing) is one of the principal symptoms of cardiac and pulmonary disease. It commonly occurs during strenuous exertion in healthy, well-trained persons and during moderate exertion in healthy, untrained persons. It should be regarded as abnormal, however, when it occurs at a level of exertion that is not expected to evoke this symptom in a given individual. Abnormal exertional dyspnea suggests the presence of cardiopulmonary disorders, particularly left ventricular dysfunction or chronic obstructive pulmonary disease.

Symptom: Dizziness or syncope.
Clarification/Significance: Syncope (loss of consciousness) is most commonly caused by a reduced perfusion of the brain. Dizziness and, particularly, syncope *during* exercise may result from cardiac disorders that prevent the normal rise (or an actual fall) in cardiac output. Such cardiac disorders are potentially life-threatening and include severe coronary artery disease, hypertrophic cardiomyopathy, aortic stenosis, and malignant ventricular arrhythmias. Although dizziness or syncope shortly *after* cessation of exercise should not be ignored, these symptoms may occur even in healthy persons as a result of a reduction in venous return to the heart.

Symptom: Orthopnea and paroxysmal nocturnal dyspnea.
Clarification/Significance: Orthopnea refers to dyspnea occurring at rest in the recumbent position that is relieved promptly by sitting upright or standing. Paroxysmal nocturnal dyspnea refers to dyspnea that usually begins 2 to 5 hours after the onset of sleep and that may be relieved by sitting on the side of the bed or by getting out of bed. Both are symptoms of left ventricular failure. Although nocturnal dyspnea may occur in persons with chronic obstructive pulmonary disease, it differs in that it is usually relieved after the reduction or alleviation of secretions rather than specifically by sitting up.

Sign: Ankle edema.
Clarification/Significance: Bilateral ankle edema that is most evident at night is a characteristic sign of heart failure or bilateral chronic venous insufficiency. Unilateral edema of a limb often results from venous thrombosis or lymphatic blockage in the limb. Generalized edema (anasarca) occurs in persons with nephrotic syndrome, severe heart failure, or hepatic cirrhosis. Edema around the eyes and of the face is characteristic of several conditions, including nephrotic syndrome, acute glomerulonephritis, angioneurotic edema, hypoproteinemia, and myxedema.

Symptom/Sign: Palpitations or tachycardia.
Clarification/Significance: Palpitations (an unpleasant awareness of the forceful or rapid beating of the heart) may be induced by various disorders of cardiac rhythm. These include tachycardia, bradycardia of sudden onset, ectopic beats, compensatory pauses, and accentuated stroke volume caused by valvular regurgitation. Palpitations also often result from anxiety states and high cardiac output (or hyperkinetic) states (e.g., anemia, fever, thyrotoxicosis, arteriovenous fistula, idiopathic hyperkinetic heart syndrome).

Symptom: Claudication.
Clarification/Significance: Intermittent claudication refers to the pain that occurs in a muscle with an inadequate blood supply (usually as a result of atherosclerosis) that is stressed by exercise. The pain does not occur with standing or sitting, is reproducible from day to day, is more severe when walking upstairs or up a hill, and is often described as a cramp that disappears within 1 or 2 minutes after stopping exercise. Coronary artery disease is more prevalent in persons with intermittent claudication. Persons with diabetes are at increased risk for this condition.

Sign: Known heart murmur.
Clarification/Significance: Although some cases may be innocent, heart murmurs may indicate valvular or other cardiovascular disease. From the standpoint of exercise safety, it is especially important to exclude hypertrophic cardiomyopathy and aortic stenosis as underlying causes, because these are among the more common causes of exertion-related sudden cardiac death.

These symptoms and signs must be interpreted in the clinical context in which they appear, because not all of them are specific for cardiopulmonary or metabolic disease. (Data from American College of Sports Medicine: *Guidelines for Exercise Testing and Prescription*, 6th ed. Philadelphia, Lippincott Williams & Wilkins, 2000; Braunwald E, Isselbacher KJ, Petersdorf RG, et al. (eds): *Harrison's Principles of Internal Medicine*. New York, McGraw-Hill, 1988; and Braunwald E: The history. In *Heart Disease: A Textbook of Cardiovascular Medicine*. Philadelphia, WB Saunders, 1988.)

4. **Sedentary Lifestyle**
   a. A sedentary lifestyle carries a risk for CAD similar to that from hypertension, dyslipidemia, and cigarette smoking.
   b. **A sedentary lifestyle can influence other risk factors** (e.g., increased blood pressure, decreased HDL cholesterol, decreased sensitivity to insulin resulting in elevated blood glucose levels, increased overweight/obesity).
   c. **Persons who are physically inactive after an AMI have significantly higher mortality rates** compared with those of active individuals.

5. **Overweight/Obesity**
   a. Overweight/obesity has a strong positive

relationship with other risk factors for CAD (e.g., hypertension, dyslipidemia, type 2 diabetes mellitus [DM]).

   b. The risk for CAD is **greater in persons with central** (android or upper body) **obesity** than in those with peripheral (gynoid or lower body) obesity.
      1) **Waist-to-hip ratio (WHR) provides an index of central obesity.** Health risk increases with WHR, and standards for risk vary with age and gender.
      2) A waist circumference greater than 100 cm (men) or >88 cm (women) is an indicator of risk.
   c. Classification of disease risk can also be based on body mass index (BMI).
      1) Obesity is also defined as a BMI of greater than 30 kg/m^2.
      2) Overweight is defined as a BMI of between 25 and 29.9 kg/m^2.

6. Diabetes Mellitus
   a. Persons with DM are two- to fourfold more likely to develop CAD than are those without diabetes. The risk of AMI is 50% greater in diabetic men and 150% greater in diabetic women.
   b. Aggressive behavior modification and pharmacological therapy to reduce hyperglycemia can **lower the risk of microvascular complications** (e.g., retinopathy, nephropathy, automatic neuropathy), and recent studies suggest a **lower incidence of cardiovascular diseases** (e.g., nonfatal MI and stroke)
   c. Commonly, DM is associated with central obesity, elevated triglyceride and LDL levels, and hypertension (known as syndrome X the metabolic syndrome.
   d. The ATPIII lists DM as "CAD equivalent"; that is, persons with DM are treated as if they have clinically diagnosed CAD.

C. EMERGING RISK FACTORS
Emerging risk factors are those associated with an increased risk of CAD but with a causal link that has not been proved with certainty. Those receiving the most attention include:
   1. Homocysteine.
   2. Lipoprotein(a).
   3. Fibrinogen.
   4. t-PA.
   5. C-reactive protein.
   6. Infectious agents.
   7. Impaired fasting glucose.
   8. Subclinical atherosclerosis.

D. METABOLIC SYNDROME
   1. Metabolic syndrome is considered to be **"CAD equivalent"** by the American Heart Association (AHA) and Framingham Risk Stratification Model. Therefore, a person with metabolic syndrome is considered to have CAD for both risk assessment and therapeutic guidelines.
      a. **Metabolic syndrome is defined as having three or more of the following:**
         1) Waist circumference greater than 40 inches (102 cm) for men and greater than 35 inches (88 cm) for women.
         2) Serum triglyceride levels greater than 150 mg/dL (1.69 mmol/L).
         3) HDL cholesterol levels less than 40 mg/dL (1.04 mmol/L) in men or less than 50 mg/dL (1.29 mmol/L) in women.
         4) Blood pressure greater than 130/80 mm Hg.
         5) Blood sugar (serum glucose) levels greater than 110 mg/dL (6.1 mmol/L).
      b. In most sets of established guidelines (AHA, JNC 7, ATPIII), people with metabolic syndrome are managed therapeutically as if they had CAD.
      c. **Metabolic syndrome is preventable and reversible** through diet and exercise.

III. Diagnosis of CAD

A. ELECTROCARDIOGRAPHY (ECG)
   1. Is a noninvasive, diagnostic test that records cardiac electrical currents by placing electrodes on the surface of the body (see Chapter 12 for an extensive discussion of ECG).
   2. Can be administered at rest or during exercise
   3. Can be administered with a variety of pharmacological agents that impose physiologic stress on the myocardium.
   4. Used to assess rhythm and conduction disturbances, chamber enlargement, ischemia, infarction, and ventricular function.
   5. Various changes and combinations of ST-segment abnormalities, presence of significant Q waves, and absence of R waves point to acute, recent, or old MI.
      a. ST-segment depression suggests subendocardial ischemia.
      b. ST-segment elevation suggests acute ischemia.
   6. Certain cardiac conditions, illnesses, and medications may make interpretation of resting or exercise ECG difficult. More sensitive and specific tests (e.g., radionuclide imaging, echocardiography, coronary angiography) may

be needed to confirm or rule out ischemia. (See Chapter 6, section IIIF, for definitions of sensitivity and specificity in exercise testing.)

B. RADIONUCLIDE IMAGING

1. Is the use of imaging agents to visualize anatomic and/or physiologic function of the myocardium.
2. Is more sensitive and specific test than exercise testing
3. Is the standard diagnostic test for CAD.
   a. **Perfusion Imaging**
      This test **assesses the extent and location** of both transient (ischemic) and fixed (necrotic) myocardial perfusion defects.
      1) A radioisotope such as thallium-201, technetium-99m, or sestamibi (Cardiolite) is injected intravenously. In a **pharmacologic stress test**, the radioisotope is used in combination with dipyridamole, dobutamine, or adenosine to **impose physiologic stress on the myocardium.** This is often used in place of or in addition to exercise as a stressor.
      2) Images are taken **at rest and under the influence of the stressor** (pharmacologic or exercise) using planar, single-photon emission computed tomography (SPECT) or positron-emission tomography (PET) scans.
         a) In a **normal heart**, full perfusion is revealed in both scans.
         b) In an **ischemic heart**, unequal perfusion (a defect or cold spot) is identified but is reversible.
         c) In a **necrotic heart**, unequal perfusion is shown in areas where scarring has occurred that has no reversibility; thus, infarcted (scar) tissue is identified.
   b. The **sensitivity and specificity** for each type of scan are:
      1) Planar: sensitivity, 83%; specificity, 88%.
      2) SPECT: sensitivity, 89%; specificity, 76%.
      3) PET: sensitivity, 78%–100%; specificity, 87%–97%.
2. **Radionuclide Ventriculography**
   a. Is commonly called a multiple-gated acquisition scan (MUGA).
   b. Is used to **assess heart wall motion abnormalities, ejection fraction, systolic and diastolic function, and cardiac output.**

1) In MUGA, a bolus (first-pass technique) of radioisotope is ejected in a central vein. In MUGA with pharmacologic testing (commonly done to assess complications of AMI), dipyridamole, dobutamine, or adenosine is administered to create myocardial stress for those who are unable to exercise or in whom exercise might be overly demanding.
2) The real-time exercise scans are recorded and compared to resting scans.

C. ECHOCARDIOGRAPHY

1. This test **assesses heart wall motion abnormalities, valvular disease, ejection fraction, systolic and diastolic function, and cardiac output** by use of sound waves.
2. Resting or exercise images are used. Radioactive isotopes and pharmacological agents may also be used.

D. CORONARY ANGIOGRAPHY

1. A **catheter** is inserted into a chamber of the heart or into the coronary artery system through a large vein of the groin or arm. A **radiopaque dye** with a vasodilator effect is injected and then depicted radiographically so that images of the chamber or the artery can be viewed
2. Coronary angiography is most efficacious in patients with a high pretest likelihood of CAD.
3. Coronary angiography is often used in combination with ventriculography to assess heart wall motion abnormalities, cardiac ejection fraction, systolic and diastolic function, and cardiac output.

E. ELECTRON-BEAM COMPUTED TOMOGRAPHY (EBCT)

1. Atherosclerotic plaque in the coronary arteries accumulates **calcium.**
2. The noninvasive EBCT is a means to **quantify coronary calcium** and, thus, calcified coronary plaque.
3. Additional research is warranted to determine the sensitivity, specificity, and predictive value of EBCT before recommendation for widespread use, but in specific populations, it can be a useful screening tool for CAD.

IV. Treatment of CAD

A. RISK FACTOR MODIFICATION

Aggressive control of modifiable risk factors **may slow, halt, or even reverse the progression of atherosclerosis** through a reduction of ischemia, angina, recurrent cardiac events, and revascularization.

B. **PHARMACOLOGIC THERAPY**

1. **Platelet Inhibitors**

    Platelet-inhibiting agents such as aspirin, warfarin (Coumadin), or clopidogrel (Plavix) significantly **reduce cardiovascular events** (mortality and morbidity), acute thrombotic events following angioplasty, and thrombotic events affecting patency of saphenous and other vein grafts.

2. **Anti-Ischemic Agents**

    a. **β-Adrenergic Blockers**

    1) **Reduce ischemia by lowering myocardial oxygen demand** for any given workload.

    2) **Lower blood pressure.**

    3) **Control ventricular arrhythmias.**

    4) Reduce the first-year mortality rate in patients after MI by 20% to 35%.

    b. **Calcium-Channel Blockers**

    1) Reduce ischemia at any given workload by **altering the major determinants of myocardial oxygen supply and demand.** Some calcium-channel blockers reduce resting and exercise heart rate. All calcium-channel blockers reduce resting and exercise blood pressure.

    2) Have not been shown to reduce post-MI mortality.

    c. **Nitrates**

    1) Reduce ischemia by **reducing myocardial oxygen demand** with a small, concomitant increase in oxygen supply.

    2) Are used in both short- and long-acting forms to treat typical and variant angina.

    3) Have not been shown to reduce mortality after MI.

3. **Other Agents**

    a. **Angiotensin-Converting Enzyme Inhibitors**

    1) Reduce myocardial oxygen demand by **reducing systemic vascular resistance** and, thus, may increase exercise tolerance in those with left ventricular dysfunction.

    2) **Reduce resting and exercise blood pressure through vasodilation** of the systemic vasculature.

    b. **Digitalis**

    1) **Enhances contractility** (positive inotropic) of the myocardium, resulting in increased stroke volume.

    2) **Blunts sinoatrial- and atrioventricular-node conduction,** which results in a lower ventricular response (chronotropic effect) in those with atrial fibrillation or tachycardia.

    3) Are used in the management of congestive heart failure.

    c. **Diuretics**

    1) Reduce blood pressure by **increasing the renal excretion of sodium, potassium, and other ions,** which results in a loss of water as urine.

    2) Are used when a mild reduction in blood pressure is warranted.

    3) Exert a slight effect on resting and exercise blood pressure but no effect on resting or exercise heart rate.

    4) May increase exercise tolerance in those with congestive heart failure.

4. **Lipid-Lowering Therapy**

    a. The goal is to reduce the availability of lipids to the injured endothelium.

    b. Lowering LDL and TC is effective in decreasing progression and increasing regression of atherosclerosis.

    c. Various classifications of lipid-lowering drugs are based on their different mechanisms of action.

    1) **Bile acid sequestrants** such as cholestyramine (Questran), colestipol (Colestid), and colesevelam (Welchol) lower LDL but tend to elevate triglycerides. These agents **bind bile acids and reduce recirculation through the liver.**

    2) **Niacin** (Nicobid) lowers LDL by **inhibiting lipoprotein secretion from the liver.** It has no influence on triglycerides but increases HDL.

    3) The **statin** drugs such as lovastatin (Mevacor), pravastatin (Pravachol), simvastatin (Zocor), atorvastatin (Lipitor), and rosuvastatin (Crestor) are also effective for lowering LDL and TC. They are less effective for decreasing triglycerides and elevating HDL, but the newer statins are relatively more effective at raising HDL. These compounds are also called 3-hydroxy-3-mthylgultaryl–coenzyme A reductase inhibitors and work by **affecting a primary metabolic pathway in the production of cholesterol as well as by increasing the number of LDL receptors** in the liver and, perhaps, directly reducing circulating LDL particles.

4) **Fibric acid** drugs such as **gemfibrozil** (Lopid) and **clofibrate** (Atromid) are effective for lowering elevated triglyceride levels, with a moderate reduction in LDL and elevation of HDL. They work by **promoting lipolysis of very-low-density lipoprotein (VLDL)** triglycerides.

C. PERCUTANEOUS TRANSLUMINAL CORONARY ANGIOPLASTY (PTCA)

1. A catheter with a deflated balloon is inserted into the narrowed portion of the coronary artery. The balloon is inflated, and **plaque is "flattened" inside the walls of the artery,** increasing the inner diameter of the artery. The balloon is then deflated, and the catheter is removed. Today, most of these procedures also involve the placement of a coronary artery stent (see below).
2. In patients with acute MI, PTCA can be used to interrupt an active infarction.
3. Typically, PTCA was reserved for younger patients, those with single-vessel disease, and those with stenosis distal to the occluded artery. Today, it is commonly used in higher-risk individuals.
4. Restenosis with PTCA alone occurs within 6 months in approximately 30% to 50% of patients.
5. Used alone, PTCA carries a greater risk of restenosis than either PTCA/stent or coronary artery bypass graft surgery (CABGS).

D. CORONARY ARTERY STENT

1. A coronary artery stent is a **mesh tube that acts as a scaffold to hold open the walls of the artery after PTCA,** improving blood flow and relieving the symptoms of CAD. The stent is mounted on a balloon catheter that is inserted into the artery, inflated/expanded at the blockage site, and permanently implanted in the artery. **Stents are typically used in conjunction with PTCA** in interventional therapy for CAD or MI.
2. Restenosis occurs within 6 months in as many as 10% to 15% of patients.
3. The lower rate of restenosis of PTCA/stent has made the use of PTCA alone rare.
4. Newer drug-eluting stents coated with time-release immunosuppressant (Sirolimus) or chemotherapeutic (Paclitaxel) agent have very low rates of restenosis (perhaps as low as 3%–4%).

E. ATHERECTOMY

1. Atherectomy is a procedure similar to PTCA.
2. A rotational atherectomy uses a high-speed, rotating shaver to grind the plaque.
3. A transluminal extraction atherectomy cuts and vacuums away the plaque.
4. Atherectomy may be used in conjunction with PTCA/stent.
5. Long-term outcomes are similar to those with PTCA.

F. LASER ANGIOPLASTY

1. Laser angioplasty is a procedure similar to PTCA.
2. The end of catheter emits pulses of photons that vaporizes plaque.
3. Laser angioplasty is useful when the PTCA catheter cannot be passed through an artery or if calcification is present.
4. Laser angioplasty may be used in conjunction with PTCA/stent.
5. Long-term outcomes are similar to those with PTCA.

G. CORONARY ARTERY BYPASS GRAFT SURGERY

1. In CABGS, the left mammary artery (LIMA), saphenous vein (SVG), or other large vein is removed and attached to the base of the aorta and at other points below the stenosis of a coronary artery caused by plaque.
2. This surgery is indicated for:
   a. Patients who are unresponsive to pharmacological treatment,
   b. Patients who have failed PTCA/stents
   c. Other higher-risk patients with CAD (e.g., patients with left main or multiple-vessel disease or left ventricular dysfunction).
3. LIMA grafts are superior to SVG grafts in terms of patency (90% for arterial grafts versus <50% for venous grafts at 10 years).

V. Risk Stratification

A. DEFINITION
Risk stratification consists of placing an individual in a risk group for untoward events based on sets of known risk factors.

B. PURPOSE
The purpose of risk stratification is to provide:
1. **Guidance on the need for a medical examination and exercise test** before participation in a moderate-to-vigorous exercise program.
2. **Guidelines for monitoring and supervision** during exercise testing and training.

3. Recommendations for occupational, recreational, or daily activity participation and any necessary restrictions.
4. **Therapeutic guidelines** for CAD or lipid management.

C. GOAL

1. **To increase the safety of exercise training** in adult fitness and exercise-based cardiac rehabilitation programs.
2. **To increase the efficacy of secondary prevention** in exercise-based cardiac rehabilitation programs.

D. CRITERIA

1. The criteria for an **initial** risk stratification are published by the ACSM and are discussed in Chapter 6.
2. Cardiac patients may be further stratified for risk of untoward events during exercise and for progression of disease using criteria published by the American Association of Cardiovascular and Pulmonary Rehabilitation (AACVPR) (*Table 4-2*).
3. The AACVPR stratification can be used in conjunction with *Table 4-3* to provide recommendations for ECG monitoring and supervision during exercise.

TABLE 4-2. American Association of Cardiovascular and Pulmonary Rehabilitation Risk Stratification Criteria for Cardiac Patients

---

Characteristics of patients at lowest risk for exercise participation (all characteristics listed must be present for patient to remain at lowest risk)
- Absence of complex ventricular dysrhythmias during exercise testing and recovery.
- Absence of angina or other significant symptoms (e.g., unusual shortness of breath, light-headedness or dizziness during exercise testing and recovery).
- Presence of normal hemodynamics during exercise testing and recovery (appropriate increases and decreased in heart rate and systolic blood pressure with increasing workloads and recovery).
- Functional capacity of 7.0 METs or greater.

Nonexercise testing findings
- Rest ejection fraction of 50% or greater.
- Uncomplicated myocardial infarction or revascularization procedure.
- Absence of complicated ventricular dysrhythmias at rest.
- Absence of congestive heart failure.
- Absence of signs or symptoms of postevent/postprocedure ischemia.
- Absence of clinical depression.

Characteristics of patients at moderate risk for exercise participation (any one or a combination of these places a patient at moderate risk)
- Presence of angina or other significant symptoms (e.g., unusual shortness of breath, light-headedness or dizziness at low levels of exertion [<5.0 METs] during recovery).
- Mild to moderate level of silent ischemia during exercise testing or recovery (ST-segment depression < 2.0 mm from baseline).
- Functional capacity less than 5.0 METs.

Nonexercise testing findings
- Rest ejection fraction between 40% and 49%.

Characteristics of patients at high risk for exercise participation (any one or a combination of these places a patient at high risk)
- Presence of complex ventricular dysrhythmias during exercise testing or recovery.
- Presence of angina or other significant symptoms (e.g., unusual shortness of breath, light-headedness or dizziness during exercise testing and recovery).
- High level of silent ischemia (ST-segment depression of 2.0 mm or greater from baseline) during exercise testing or recovery.
- Presence of abnormal hemodynamics with exercise testing (chronotropic incompetence or flat or decreasing systolic blood pressure with increasing workloads) or recovery (severe postexercise hypotension).

Nonexercise testing findings
- Resting ejection fraction less than 40%.
- History of cardiac arrest or sudden death.
- Complex dysrhythmias at rest.
- Complicated myocardial infarction or revascularization procedure.
- Presence of congestive heart failure.
- Presence of signs or symptoms of postevent/postprocedure ischemia.
- Presence of clinical depression.

MET, metabolic equivalent.

(From American Association of Cardiovascular and Pulmonary Rehabilitation: *Guidelines for Cardiac Rehabilitation ad Secondary Prevention*, 4th ed. Human Kinetics Publishers, 2004.)

TABLE 4-3. Recommendations for Intensity of Supervision and Monitoring Related to Risk of Exercise Participation

Patients at lowest risk for exercise participation
- Direct staff supervision of exercise should occur for a minimum of 6 to 18 sessions or 30 days postevent or postprocedure, beginning with continuous ECG monitoring and decreasing to intermittent ECG monitoring as appropriate (e.g., 6–12 sessions)
- For a patient to remain at lowest risk, his or her ECG and hemodynamic findings should remain normal, there should be no development of abnormal signs and symptoms either within or away from the exercise program, and progression of the exercise regimen should be appropriate.

Patients at moderate risk for exercise participation
- Direct staff supervision of exercise should occur for a minimum of 12 to 24 sessions or 60 days postevent or postprocedure, beginning with continuous ECG monitoring and decreasing to intermittent ECG monitoring as appropriate (e.g., 12–18 sessions).
- For a patient to move to the lowest risk, his or her ECG and hemodynamic findings should be normal, there should be no development of abnormal signs and symptoms either within or away from the exercise program, and progression of the exercise regimen should be appropriate.
- Abnormal ECG or hemodynamic findings during exercise, development of abnormal signs and symptoms either within or away from the exercise program, or need to decrease exercise levels severely may result in the patient remaining in the moderate-risk category or even moving to the high-risk category.

Patients at moderate risk for exercise participation
- Direct staff supervision of exercise should occur for a minimum of 18 to 36 sessions or 90 days postevent or postprocedure, beginning with continuous ECG monitoring and decreasing to intermittent ECG monitoring as appropriate (e.g., 18, 24, or 30 sessions).
- For a patient to move to moderate risk, his or her ECG and hemodynamic findings should be normal, there should be no development of abnormal signs and symptoms either within or away from the exercise program, and progression of the exercise regimen should be appropriate.
- Abnormal ECG or hemodynamic findings during exercise, development of abnormal signs and symptoms either within or away from the exercise program, or need to decrease exercise levels severely may result in the patient discontinuing the exercise program until appropriate evaluation and intervention, where necessary, can take place.

(see p. 49 AACVPR Guidelines 3rd ed., table 4.4.)

4. The AHA (*Table 4-4*) also provides recommendations for patient monitoring, supervision, and activity restriction.

VI. Effects of Exercise on Cardiopulmonary and Other Disorders

A. PULMONARY DISEASE
1. Exercise can **improve musculoskeletal and psychosocial factors** that typically limit exercise in persons with pulmonary disease.
2. Because pulmonary disease is commonly associated with CAD and CAD risk factors, exercise training can reduce the risk of CAD in persons with pulmonary disease.

B. CORONARY ARTERY DISEASE
Exercise helps to reduce mortality in persons with CAD. The **mechanisms responsible for a reduction in CAD deaths** include:
1. **Effects of exercise on other risk factors.**
2. **Reduction in myocardial oxygen demand** at rest and at submaximal workloads, resulting in an increased ischemic and angina threshold.
3. **Reduction in platelet aggregation.**
4. **Improved endothelial-mediated vasomotor tone.**

C. OBESITY
1. An **increase in caloric expenditure** through exercise (combined with a reduction in caloric intake) results in a caloric deficit. Over time, a caloric deficit results in a reduction of overall body fat and a likely reduction of central fat deposits.
2. **Decreased body fat**, especially reduced central obesity, **can reduce risk factors for CAD**, including dyslipidemia, type 2 DM, and hypertension.
3. Exercising to induce a caloric deficit **can preserve lean body mass.** Dieting alone to produce a caloric deficit usually results in a **loss of lean body mass.** A combination of exercise and diet is best for initial and long-term weight loss and maintenance of target weight.
4. The ACSM's *Appropriate Intervention Strategies for Weight Loss and Prevention of Weight Regain for Adults* recommends strategies to be incorporated into weight-loss interventions.

D. DYSLIPIDEMIA
1. **Exercise has the beneficial effect of lowering triglycerides and raising HDL.**
   a. Exercise **increases the activity of lipoprotein lipase,** which frees VLDL triglycerides. Triglyceride levels are then decreased when they are used in metabolism by skeletal muscles during exercise. In addition, VLDL remnants serve as precursors to HDL, which is cardioprotective.
   b. Exercise **moderates the postprandial lipemia** that ensues after a high-fat or moderately high-fat meal.
   c. To induce these beneficial changes, the **volume (duration and frequency) of**

TABLE 4-4. American Heart Association Risk Stratification Criteria

Class A: Apparently healthy
- Individuals younger than 40 years with no symptoms or known presence of heart disease or major coronary risk factors, and individuals of any age without known heart disease or major risk factors and who have a normal exercise test.
- Activity guidelines: No restrictions other than basic guidelines.
- ECG and blood pressure monitoring: Not required.
- Supervision required: None.

Class B: Documented, stable cardiovascular disease with low risk for vigorous exercise but slightly greater risk than that for apparently healthy individuals
- Moderate activity is not believed to be associated with increased risk in this group.
- Includes individuals with (1) CAD (MI, CABGS, PTCA, angina pectoris, abnormal exercise test, abnormal coronary angiograms) whose condition is stable and who have the clinical characteristics outlined below, (2) valvular heart disease, (3) congenital heart disease, (4) cardiomyopathy, and (5) exercise test abnormalities that do not meet the criteria outlined in class C below.
- Clinical characteristics: (1) NYHA class 1 or 2, (2) exercise capacity greater than 6 METs, (3) no evidence of heart failure, (4) free of ischemia or angina at rest or on the exercise test at 6 METs or less, (5) appropriate rise in systolic blood pressure during exercise, (6) no sequential ectopic ventricular contractions, and (7) ability to satisfactorily self-monitor intensity of activity.
- Activity guidelines: Activity should be individualized. with exercise prescription by qualified personnel trained in basic CPR or with electronic monitoring at home.
- ECG and blood pressure monitoring: Only during the early prescription phase of training, usually 6 to 12 sessions.
- Supervision required: Medical supervision during prescription sessions and nonmedical supervision for other exercise sessions until the individual understands how to monitor his or her activity.

Class C: Those at moderate to high risk for cardiac complications during exercise and/or unable to self-regulate activity or to understand recommended activity level
- Includes individuals with (1) CAD having the clinical characteristics outlined below, (2) cardiomyopathy, (3) valvular heart disease, (4) exercise test abnormalities not directly related to ischemia, (5) previous episode of ventricular fibrillation or cardiac arrest that did not occur in the presence of an acute ischemic event or cardiac procedure, (6) complex ventricular arrhythmias that are uncontrolled at mild to moderate work intensities with medication, (7) three-vessel disease or left main disease, and (8) low ejection fraction (<30%).
- Clinical characteristics: (1) Two or more MIs, (2) NYHA class 3 or greater, (3) exercise capacity less than 6 METs, (4) ischemic horizontal or downsloping ST depression of 4 mm or more or angina during exercise, (5) fall in systolic blood pressure with exercise, (6) a medical problem the physician believes may be life-threatening, (7) previous episode of primary cardiac arrest, and (8) ventricular tachycardia at a workload less than 6 METs.
- Activity guidelines: Activity should be individualized with exercise prescription by qualified personnel.
- ECG and blood pressure monitoring: Continuous during exercise sessions until safety is established, usually 6 to 12 sessions (or more).
- Supervision required: Medical supervision during all exercise sessions until safety is established.

Class D: Unstable disease with activity restriction
- Includes individuals with (1) unstable ischemia, (2) uncompensated heart failure, (3) uncontrolled arrhythmias, (4) severe and symptomatic aortic stenosis, and (5) other conditions that could be aggravated by exercise.
- Activity guidelines: No activity is recommended for conditioning purposes. Attention should be directed to treating and restoring subjects to class C or higher. Daily activities must be prescribed based on individual assessment by a subject's personal physician.

CABGS, coronary artery bypass graft surgery; CAD, coronary artery disease; CPR, cardiopulmonary resuscitation; ECG, electrocardiography; MET, metabolic equivalent; MI, myocardial infarction; NYHA, New York Heart Association; PTCA, Percutaneous transluminal coronary angioplasty.

(Modified from Fletcher GA, Balady G, Froelicher VF, et al.: Exercise standards: A statement for health care professionals from the American Heart Association. *Circulation* 91:580–615, 1995.)

aerobic activity is more important than the intensity of activity.

2. **Exercise can indirectly lower TC and LDL.** Lowering TC and LDL is related more to caloric restriction; dietary fat, saturated fat, and cholesterol reduction; and body fat reduction than to exercise training alone. However, because exercise training can result in body fat reduction, it can have an indirect effect on TC and LDL levels.

E. DIABETES MELLITUS
1. Exercise can **improve insulin sensitivity and glucose metabolism in** people with type 1 DM.
2. In people with type 2 DM, exercise can **enhance fat loss,** resulting in improved insulin sensitivity and glucose metabolism.

3. Exercise can **favorably alter other risk factors** typically associated with DM, including dyslipidemia and hypertension, and thus decrease the overall risk of CAD.
4. Aggressive pharmacologic therapy and behavior modification, including exercise training to reduce hyperglycemia, can lower the risk of microvascular complications (e.g., retinopathy, nephropathy, automatic neuropathy), and recent studies suggest a lower incidence of cardiovascular diseases (e.g., nonfatal MI and stroke).

F. HYPERTENSION
1. By **reducing circulating catecholamines, plasma renin, and heart rate and by increasing vasodilator substances,** exercise can reduce cardiac output and total peripheral

resistance and, thus, reduce blood pressure. An average reduction of approximately 10 mm Hg in both systolic and diastolic blood pressure has been observed in patients with mild to moderate hypertension as a result of aerobic exercise training.

2. Exercise can **reduce intra-abdominal visceral fat and hyperinsulinemia,** decreasing the total peripheral resistance.

3. Exercise training at a **lower intensity level** (40%–70% maximal aerobic capacity) appears to lower blood pressure as much as, if not more than, exercise at higher intensity.

G. PERIPHERAL ARTERY DISEASE

1. Exercise training can **improve oxygen extraction from skeletal muscle.** Increased oxygen extraction improves the relationship between oxygen supply and oxygen demand. When oxygen supply equals or exceeds oxygen demand, claudication is less likely to occur.

2. Exercise may **improve the mechanical efficiency** of walking, which (together with changes in the oxygen supply:demand ratio) improves the ability to walk longer or at higher intensities.

3. Maintenance of exercise training reduces the ill effects of deconditioning and risk factors associated with peripheral artery disease (e.g., hypertension, insulin resistance).

H. OSTEOPOROSIS

1. Exercise reduces the deleterious effects of deconditioning and the risk factors for osteoporosis associated with physical inactivity.

2. Exercise may help to **delay or halt the age-related decline in bone mass.**

3. **Resistance training may be more beneficial** than aerobic training.

4. **Weight-bearing exercise may be more effective** than nonweight-bearing exercise at increasing bone mass.

5. Adaptations in bone are **site-specific to the limbs exercised.**

6. Exercise training may also reduce the risk of falls by increasing muscle strength, posture, and balance.

VII. Environmental Risk Factors and Exercise

A. HEAT

1. High ambient temperature and high relative humidity increase the risk of **heat-related disorders** (e.g., heat cramps, heat syncope, dehydration, heat exhaustion, heat stroke). Persons with hypertension or diabetes, obese individuals, unfit persons, pregnant women,

children, the elderly, and individuals using certain medications or alcohol may have particular difficulty adapting to high ambient temperature and high humidity and, thus, are at increased risk for heat-related disorders.

2. High ambient temperature and high humidity may produce **increased heart rate response** at submaximal workloads and **decreased oxygen consumption** at maximal workloads.

3. The **wet bulb globe temperature** is an index of environmental heat stress derived from measures of ambient temperature, relative humidity, and radiant heat. It provides guidance for exercise prescription to minimize the risk of developing heat-related illnesses.

4. General **guidelines for safe exercising** in high ambient temperatures and humidity are listed in *Table 4-5*.

B. COLD

1. Cold exposure results in vasoconstriction with resulting blood pressure elevation. The elevation in blood pressure increases the oxygen demand on the heart. This lowers the angina threshold in patients who are prone to angina and **may provoke resting angina** (variant or Prinzmetal's).

2. Breathing large volumes of cold, dry air may provoke **exercise-induced asthma,** general dehydration, and dryness or burning of the mouth and throat.

3. **Use the wind-chill equivalent,** not the actual temperature, when gauging the risk of hypothermia and frostbite.

C. ALTITUDE

1. The primary consideration in exercise prescription at high altitude is to **lower the exercise intensity** (absolute workload) for the following reasons:

   a. Acute exposure to high altitude causes an increase in pulmonary ventilation, heart rate, and cardiac output at submaximal workloads.

TABLE 4-5. General Guidelines for Safe Exercise in High Temperatures and Humidity

Decrease the intensity and, possibly, the duration of the exercise session; if necessary, schedule intermittent rest periods.
Exercise in cool areas (e.g., an air-conditioned room) or during a cooler time of day (e.g., early morning, evening).
Be familiar with and alert for the signs and symptoms of heat-related disorders, and know the appropriate first-aid procedures.
Wear minimal, loose-fitting, light-colored clothing.
Ensure adequate hydration before, during, and after exercise.
Reduce the risk of developing heat-related illness through gradual acclimation to exercise in hot environments (~2 weeks)

b. After acclimatization to high altitude, persons generally experience a continued **increase in pulmonary ventilation and heart rate response** at submaximal workloads but a reduced cardiac output, stroke volume, and heart rate at maximal exercise.

c. Even after exposure and training, a reduction occurs in maximal oxygen consumption of approximately 10% per 1,000 m of altitude above 1,500 m. These changes **may lower the angina threshold.**

2. Individuals with pulmonary hypertension, congestive heart failure, unstable angina, recent MI, or severe anemia may be at greater risk for traveling or exercising at high altitudes.

D. CARBON MONOXIDE

1. Prolonged exposure to carbon monoxide can **reduce maximal oxygen consumption.**
2. Individuals with CAD have a **lower angina threshold and are prone to arrhythmias** induced by carbon monoxide exposure.
3. Guidelines for exercise prescription include avoiding carbon monoxide exposure or decreasing the intensity and duration of exercise during periods or in areas of high ambient carbon monoxide levels (e.g., heavy motor vehicle traffic).

VIII.   Influence of Drugs on Exercise

Classes of drugs and their effects on resting and exercise ECG, heart rate, blood pressure, symptomatology, and exercise capacity are listed in Chapter 8, *table 8-8.*

Review Test

DIRECTIONS: Carefully read all questions, and select the BEST single answer.

1. Angina that occurs at rest is termed
   A) Silent.
   B) Stable.
   C) Variant.
   D) Typical.

2. A group of pulmonary disorders characterized by expiratory airflow obstruction, dyspnea (shortness of breath), and some degree of airway reversal is known as
   A) Bronchitis.
   B) Asthma.
   C) Emphysema.
   D) COPD.

3. The primary effects of chronic exercise training on lipid values are
   A) Decreased triglycerides and increased HDL.
   B) Decreased TC and LDL.
   C) Decreased HDL and increased LDL.
   D) Decreased TC and increased HDL.

4. Which of the following would be the best recommendation for exercise training in a hot and humid, outdoor environment?
   A) Wait for approximately 2 weeks to become acclimated to the heat before exercising.
   B) Use a mode of activity that would increase heat loss by convection (e.g., bicycling, running).
   C) Reduce the exercise intensity.
   D) Increase evaporative cooling by wiping away sweat that forms on the body.

5. Which of the following best explains the pathophysiology of CAD?
   A) Injury to the arterial wall begins in the media.
   B) Platelets and thrombi form in the adventitia.
   C) The endothelium takes up lipids, especially LDL.
   D) Atherosclerotic lesions form in the intima.

6. A cardiac patient is taking a β-blocker medication. During an exercise test, you would expect
   A) A radioisotope (e.g., Cardiolite) to be administered, because β-blockers depress the ST segment on the resting ECG.
   B) An increase in the angina threshold compared to a test without the medication.

C) No change in heart rate or blood pressure compared to a test without the medication.
   D) A slight decrease or no effect on blood pressure compared to a test without the medication.

7. The aging-related loss of elasticity (or "hardening") of the arteries is known as
   A) Atherosclerosis.
   B) Arteriosclerosis.
   C) Atheroma.
   D) Adventitia.

8. The deficiency of blood flow to the myocardium that results when oxygen demand exceeds oxygen supply is known as
   A) Infarction.
   B) Angina.
   C) Ischemia.
   D) Thrombosis.

9. What procedure uses a clot-dissolving agent during acute MI to restore blood flow and limit myocardial necrosis?
   A) PTCA.
   B) Thrombolytic therapy.
   C) Radionuclide imaging.
   D) CABGS.

10. All of the following are suggestive of cardiovascular and pulmonary disease EXCEPT
    A) Palpitations that occur at rest.
    B) Dyspnea during strenuous exertion.
    C) Syncope during moderate-intensity exercise training.
    D) Substernal burning during exertion that dissipates with rest.

11. Modifiable primary risk factors for CAD include
    A) Hypertension, dyslipidemia, advancing age, and tobacco smoking.
    B) Homocysteine, lipoprotein(a), C-reactive protein, and t-PA.
    C) Obesity, DM, tobacco smoking, and sedentary lifestyle.
    D) Tobacco smoking, dyslipidemia, hypertension, and homocysteine.

12. What is the current state of knowledge on progression or regression of atherosclerosis in human coronary arteries?
    A) Regression of atherosclerosis has been observed in clinical studies.
    B) Regression of atherosclerosis has yet to be observed in clinical studies.

C)   Progression of atherosclerosis begins at puberty.

D)   The rate of progression or regression between those who undergo usual medical care is no different from that in those who aggressively control risk factors.

13. What is the correct term and definition to describe a potential complication that may occur after an acute MI?
A)   Expansion—another MI.
B)   Aneurysm—bulging of the ventricular wall.
C)   Extension—left ventricular dilation.
D)   Rupture—coronary artery breaks open.

14. The goal of risk stratification is to
A)   Determine the prognosis.
B)   Assess the disease severity.
C)   Confirm the diagnosis.
D)   Increase the safety of exercise participation.

15. A classic sign of subendocardial ischemia is
A)   Angina.
B)   ST-segment depression.
C)   ST-segment elevation.
D)   A pathologic Q wave.

16. Which of the following is the one true statement concerning the surgical treatment of CAD?
A)   A coronary artery stent carries a lower rate of restenosis than does PTCA.
B)   Atherectomy is a prerequisite requirement for PTCA.
C)   Venous grafts are significantly superior to arterial grafts in terms of patency.
D)   Long term outcome of laser angioplasty is unknown and, thus, are rarely used.

17. A possible mechanism by which chronic exercise training may reduce resting blood pressure in hypertensive individuals is through
A)   An increase in plasma renin.
B)   A higher cardiac output.
C)   A reduced heart rate.
D)   A lower stroke volume.

18. An embolism
A)   Can increase pulmonary vascular resistance.
B)   Is excessive fluid retention.
C)   Can be triggered by a chemical mediator (e.g., histamine).
D)   Is an outward bulging of the ventricular wall.

19. A sedentary lifestyle
A)   Has a risk similar to that of hypertension, high cholesterol, and cigarette smoking.

B)   Increases HDL cholesterol.
C)   Increases the sensitivity to insulin.
D)   Has little influence on post-MI mortality rates.

20. Body fat appears to be most dangerous when
A)   Weight for height exceeds 20% above recommended.
B)   It exceeds 25% for males and 30% for females.
C)   Central (android) obesity is present.
D)   The BMI exceeds 25 kg/m^2.

21. All of the following are considered possible causes of restrictive lung disease EXCEPT
A)   Scoliosis.
B)   Obesity.
C)   Muscular dystrophy.
D)   Cigarette smoke.

22. Which statement below best describes the condition of asthma?
A)   Narrowing of the bronchial airways.
B)   Alveolar destruction.
C)   Ventilatory dead space.
D)   Respiratory muscular atrophy.

23. Metabolic syndrome (also referred to a syndrome X or the deadly quartet) is comprised of
A)   Elevated TC, obesity, diabetes, and physical inactivity.
B)   Central obesity, elevated LDL cholesterol, diabetes, and physical inactivity.
C)   Low HDL cholesterol, cigarette smoking, hypertension, and physical inactivity.
D)   Central obesity, elevated triglycerides and low HDL cholesterol, hypertension, and insulin resistance.

24. All of the following risk factors for CAD can be modified by a regular and appropriate exercise training program EXCEPT
A)   Advancing age.
B)   DM.
C)   Hypertension.
D)   HDL cholesterol.

25. Emerging risk factors for CAD include
A)   Advancing age, family history, and male sex.
B)   Impaired fasting glucose, obesity, and hypertension.
C)   Lipoprotein(a), advancing age, and male sex.
D)   Homocysteine, lipoprotein(a), and fibrinogen.

ANSWERS AND EXPLANATIONS

1-C. Variant (or Prinzmetal's) angina is a form of unstable angina that occurs at rest because of coronary vasospasm. Typical (or classic) angina is usually provoked by physical activity and is relieved by rest or nitroglycerin. Stable angina is a form of typical angina that is predictable in onset, severity, and means of relief. Silent angina is not a medical term used to describe chest pain.

2-D. Bronchitis, asthma, and emphysema are all forms of COPD.

3-A. Chronic exercise training has its greatest benefit on lowering triglycerides and increasing HDL. Changes in TC or LDL cholesterol are influenced more by dietary habits and body weight than by exercise training.

4-C. Compared to a cool and dry environment, exercise in a hot and humid environment involves a higher metabolic cost at submaximal workloads. Thus, one should alter the exercise prescription by lowering the intensity of work. Evaporation of sweat cools the skin; therefore, wiping away sweat would decrease evaporative cooling and heat loss. Heat loss by convection, such as that which occurs when a breeze is created by running, can be beneficial, but not unless the workload of activity is reduced. One must exercise in the heat and humidity to become acclimated to the environment; it will not occur by being sedentary.

5-D. Atherosclerotic lesions are formed in the intima. Injury to the arterial wall does not begin in the media but, rather, in the endothelial layer, with subsequent platelet and clot formation. Monocytes adhere to the endothelium, move to the intima, and take up cholesterol. The adventitia is the outermost layer of the arterial wall and is not involved in the development of atherosclerosis.

6-B. β-Blockers increase the angina threshold by reducing myocardial oxygen demand at rest and during exercise. This occurs through a reduction in chronotropic (heart rate) and inotropic (strength of contraction) responses. Blood pressure is also reduced at rest and during exercise by a reduction in cardiac output (reduced chronotropic and inotropic response) and a reduction in total peripheral resistance. β-Blockers do not produce ST-segment changes on the resting ECG.

7-B. Arteriosclerosis is often associated with the aging process and its characteristic "hardening" of the arteries, which is actually a loss of arterial elasticity. Atherosclerosis is a form of arteriosclerosis characterized by an accumulation of obstructive lesions within the arterial wall. The adventitia (the outermost layer of the arterial wall) provides the media and intima with oxygen and other nutrients.

8-C. An outcome of significant coronary atherosclerosis, ischemia occurs when the oxygen supply does not meet oxygen demand, resulting from decreased blood flow to the myocardium. This process often leads to angina (symptoms) or infarction caused by a thrombosis.

9-B. Administration of streptokinase or t-PA within the first 1 to 2 hours after MI may dissolve the clot causing the injury. This type of therapy, called thrombolytic therapy, is designed to restore blood flow and limit myocardial necrosis.

10-B. Dyspnea (shortness of breath) commonly occurs during strenuous exertion in healthy, well-trained persons and during moderate exertion in healthy, untrained persons. It should be regarded as abnormal, however, when it occurs at a level of exertion that is not expected to evoke this symptom in a given individual. Underlying cardiac arrhythmias may cause palpitations, even at rest. Syncope is loss of consciousness and is abnormal at rest or during any level of exertion. The location (substernal), character (burning), and provoking factor (exertion that dissipates with rest) of substernal burning are features of classic ischemia.

11-C. The primary modifiable risk factors for CAD are smoking tobacco, dyslipidemia, hypertension, sedentary lifestyle, obesity, and DM. The primary nonmodifiable risk factors for CAD are advance age, male gender, and family history. Emerging risk factors for CAD are numerous and include, for example, homocysteine, fibrinogen, t-PA, lipoprotein(a), and C-reactive protein.

12-A. Clinical studies of cardiac patients have shown that long-term, aggressive control of CAD risk factors can reduce or even halt the rate of progression and may actually result in regression of atherosclerotic plaque. Individuals who aggressively attack, reduce, and control risk factors are more likely to see favorable results compared to individuals who undergo usual medical care. The process of atherosclerosis begins at birth.

13-B. A ventricular aneurysm is a bulging of the ventricular wall. Expansion is dilation of the left ventricle; extension is another MI. Rupture is an aneurysm that breaks open in the ventricular wall, not the coronary artery.

14-D. The goal of risk stratification is to increase the safety of exercise training in adult fitness and exercise-based cardiac rehabilitation programs. Initial risk stratification tables are available from the ACSM. Cardiac patients may be further stratified using tables available from the AHA and the AACVPR. Although risk stratification is based on the likelihood of experiencing an untoward cardiac event, it does not attempt to diagnose disease, predict prognosis, or determine severity of disease. Different nomograms and tables are available for such information.

15-B. A classic sign of ischemia is ST-segment alteration. The ST-segment depression suggests subendocardial ischemia, whereas the ST-segment elevation indicates transmural ischemia. Pathologic Q waves point to transmural MI. Angina is a classic symptom, not a sign, of ischemia.

16-A. Restenosis occurs within 6 months in approximately 30% to 50% of patients with PTCA, whereas a stent has a failure rate of approximately 25% and the drug-eluting stent in the low single digits. Atherectomy can be used along with PTCA and is useful when the PTCA catheter cannot pass through the artery, but atherectomy is not a prerequisite for PTCA. Internal mammary artery grafts are preferred over saphenous venous grafts because of superior patency (90% versus less than 50% at 10 years). Approximately 25% to 50% of patients will experience restenosis within 6 months of laser angioplasty.

17-C. Blood pressure is the product of cardiac output and total peripheral resistance. A benefit of exercise training is a reduction in cardiac output and total peripheral resistance at any given workload, including rest. A lower cardiac output is probably caused by a reduction in heart rate as a result of an increased stroke volume and arteriovenous oxygen difference. Plasma renin is a catalyst for vasoconstriction. It is reduced, not increased, with exercise training.

18-A. An embolism is a blood clot. Blood clots in the lungs are often fatal, but do increase pulmonary

vasculature resistance. Excessive fluid retention is called "edema". Histamine more often is implicated in increased bronchial constriction in conditions such as exercise-induced bronchoconstriction (EIB). Outward bulging of the ventricular wall is called an "aneurysm".

19-A. The risk ratios of hypertension (2.1), high cholesterol (2.4), cigarette smoking (2.5) and physical inactivity (1.9) are similar. A sedentary lifestyle is associated with low HDL cholesterol and sensitivity to insulin (higher plasma glucose values). Studies have shown that in patients after MI, a regular exercise training program can significantly reduce mortality rates as compared to individuals who are less active after MI.

20-C. The distribution of body fat, rather than the overall quantity of fat, appears to be the most important predictor of the health risks associated with obesity. Individuals with abdominal fat (central or android obesity) are especially at increased risk for a variety of cardiovascular conditions compared to individuals with similar body fat levels but with more of their fat on the extremities. A WHR or waist-to-hip ratio can be used to assess risk of central obesity. Weight-for-height tables, body composition assessment, and BMI provide indices of total excess weight or total fat weight but do not provide the distribution of body fat.

21-D. Restrictive lung disease can be caused by a variety of factors that compromise the ability of the lungs and rib cage to expand outward and upward, including, for example, scoliosis, muscular dystrophy, and obesity. Cigarette smoke is a risk factor for obstructive lung disease, which is a condition characterized by inflammation of the airways or impaired gas exchange.

22-A. Asthma is a narrowing or vasoconstriction of the bronchial airways initiated by some trigger (e.g., dust, cigarette smoke). Destruction of the alveoli and impaired ventilation (dead space) is the pathophysiology of emphysema. When the muscles of respiration are compromised (e.g., muscular dystrophy), restrictive lung disease can occur.

23-D. The metabolic syndrome is a cluster of lipid and nonlipid risk factors of metabolic origin. Excess body fat, particularly abdominal obesity, raised blood pressure, insulin resistance (with or without glucose intolerance), and dyslipidemia (elevated triglycerides and low HDL cholesterol) comprise this deadly quartet. The metabolic syndrome increases the risk for heart disease exponentially.

24-A.   A modifiable risk factor is one that can be influenced by either surgical, pharmacologic, or behavioral intervention. A regular and appropriate exercise program can reduce the risk of developing (or be used as an adjunct treatment for) DM, hypertension, and unfavorable HDL levels.

25-D.   Primary risk factors are those that have shown a consistent causal link over time and that have been proved with much certainty (e.g., advancing age, obesity, hypertension). Emerging risk factors are those that been shown to be related to an increased risk; however, their link has not been causal or consistent in nature. Although such factors (e.g., homocysteine, lipoprotein[a], fibrinogen) show promise as independent causes of CAD, additional studies are warranted to assess their complete significance to CAD.

Human Behavior and Psychology

CHAPTER 5

ANDREA L. DUNN AND BESS H. MARCUS

I. Psychological Theories: The Foundation for Behavioral Change

A. WHAT IS A THEORY?

1. A **theory** is a set of assumptions that account for the relationships between certain variables and the behavior of interest.
2. **Explanatory theories** have been developed to explain certain behaviors.
3. **Other theories** have been developed to **guide interventions**, such as trying to create some change in behavior (e.g., increasing physical activity).

B. HOW ARE PSYCHOLOGICAL THEORIES USED IN THE HEALTH AND FITNESS SETTING?

1. Psychological theories provide the foundation for effective use of the strategies and techniques of **counseling and motivational skill-building for exercise adoption and maintenance**.
2. Psychological theories provide **a conceptual framework** for assessments, development of programs or interventions, application of cognitive-behavioral principles, and evaluation of program effectiveness.
   a. Assessments
      1) Assessments are performed **to establish baseline measures** of behavioral or psychological constructs and **to assess change**.
      2) Assessments help us **to understand in what areas assistance might be required** (e.g., building confidence).
      3) Assessments **naturally lead to focusing on intervention strategies** (e.g., setting and achieving realistic fitness goals to build confidence).
   b. Development of Programs or Interventions Interventions or programs can be designed to:
      1) Build the skills of participants.
      2) Correct misunderstandings.
      3) Clarify relationships.
      4) Negotiate and solve problems.
      5) Establish a supportive relationship.
      6) Provide a target for follow-up.
   c. Application of Cognitive-Behavioral Principles
      1) Cognitive-behavioral principles are the **methods used within programs** to improve motivational skills as suggested by the assessment.
      2) **Example:** Setting **several small, short-term goals** to attain a long-term goal is likely to increase self-efficacy (self-confidence; discussed in greater detail later) as the person successfully reaches each short-term goal on the way to attaining the long-term goal.
   d. **Evaluation of Program Effectiveness**
      1) The same cognitive-behavioral principles can be used to determine improvement.
      2) **Example:** If baseline self-efficacy for exercise is low, then appropriate application of behavioral tools should increase self-efficacy.

C. WHAT ARE THE LIMITATIONS OF PSYCHOLOGICAL THEORIES?

1. Most psychological theories have been developed to explain the behaviors of individuals or small groups. They **cannot always explain the behavior of larger groups** (e.g., communities).
2. Psychological theories **may leave out important elements that may influence behavior** (e.g., sociocultural elements).

II. Theories Used to Encourage Exercise Adoption and Maintenance and to Improve Adherence

In 1996, the Surgeon General's Report on Physical Activity and Health cited studies of various psychological theories of behavioral change.

A. LEARNING THEORIES

1. Propose that an overall **complex behavior arises from many small, simple behaviors**.
2. Propose that it is possible to **shape** the desired behavior by **reinforcing "partial behaviors"** and **modifying cues** in the environment.
   a. Reinforcing "Partial" Behaviors
      1) **Reinforcement is the positive or negative consequence for performing or not performing a behavior.**
      2) **Reinforcement can be simple,** such as saying "Good job!" to participants who have performed an exercise correctly or achieved an exercise goal.
      3) **Reinforcement can be complex,** such as earning points to earn incentives (e.g., T-shirts for exercising 3 days or more a week for a period of 1 month).
      4) **Positive consequences are rewards that motivate behavior.**
         a) **Intrinsic rewards** are the benefits gained because of the rewarding nature of the activity. For example, an intrinsic reward would be feeling good about being able to perform an activity or skill, such as finally being able to run 1 mile or to increase the speed of walking 1 mile.
         b) **Extrinsic or external rewards** are the positive outcomes received from others. This can include encouragement and praise or material reinforcements (e.g., T-shirts, money).
   b. Modifying Cues in the Environment
      External or internal stimuli (cues) can signal behaviors. For example, many traditional, gym-based programs have participants keep their gym clothes packed (cues) to remind them that they are ready to go to the gym.
      1) Behaviors can be **habitual,** such as coming home from work, turning on the television, and sitting down for the remainder of the evening.
      2) Behaviors can be **cued from the engineered environment.** For example, the easy availability of elevators compared with stairways discourages stair-climbing.
      3) **Internal cues** (e.g., fatigue, boredom) can make one feel "too tired" to exercise.
   c. Limitations of Reinforcing Behaviors and Modifying Cues
      1) The techniques of modifying cues and providing reinforcement seem to be **more effective for helping people adopt a behavior than for maintaining a behavior.**
      2) For people who are not ready to start an exercise program or who need help maintaining an exercise program, **additional tools or strategies for change are required.**

B. THE HEALTH BELIEF MODEL

1. The Health Belief Model assumes that people will engage in a behavior (i.e., exercise) when:
   a. There is a perceived threat of disease.
   b. There is the belief of susceptibility to disease.
   c. The threat is severe.
2. Taking action depends on whether the **benefits outweigh the barriers.**
3. This model also incorporates **cues to action** as being critical to adopting and maintaining behavior.
4. This model also incorporates the concept of **self-efficacy** (self-confidence).

C. THE TRANSTHEORETICAL MODEL OF CHANGE (STAGES OF CHANGE OR MOTIVATIONAL READINESS)

This model incorporates constructs from other theories, including intention to change and processes (or strategies) of change.

1. The basic concepts of this model are:
   a. **People progress through five stages of change at varying rates.**
   b. In the process of changing, **people move back and forth along the stage continuum.**
   c. People use different cognitive and behavioral processes or strategies.
2. **Stages of change or motivational readiness** describe five categories of readiness to change or maintain behavior. As applied to physical activity or exercise, they are:
   a. **Stage 1: Precontemplation**
      No physical activity or exercise is occurring, and the person has **no intention to start** within the next 6 months.
   b. **Stage 2: Contemplation**
      No physical activity or exercise is occurring, but the person has an **intention to start** within the next 6 months.
   c. **Stage 3: Preparation**
      Participation in some physical activity or exercise is occurring, but not at levels

that meet the Centers for Disease Control and Prevention/ACSM (CDC/ACSM) 1995 recommendations or current ACSM exercise prescription guidelines.

    d. **Stage 4: Action**
    The person is engaged in **physical activity or exercise that meets CDC/ACSM recommendations** for physical activity or ACSM guidelines, but the person has not maintained this program for 6 months or longer.

    e. **Stage 5: Maintenance**
    Exercise or activity has been occurring **for 6 months or longer.**

3. Other key components of the Transtheoretical Model are the **processes of behavioral change**.

    a. **Processes** are various behavioral or cognitive **skills or strategies** that are applied during the different stages of change.

    b. The model has numerous applications, depending on the **stage of readiness.**

    c. In general, **cognitive processes** are the most efficient strategies **for early stages**, and **behavioral processes** are the most efficient strategies **for later stages**.

        1) The **five cognitive processes** include:
            a) **Consciousness raising** (increasing knowledge).
            b) **Dramatic relief** (warning of risks).
            c) **Environmental reevaluation** (caring about consequences to oneself and to others).
            d) **Self-reevaluation** (comprehending benefits)
            e) **Social liberation** (increasing healthy opportunities)

        2) The **five behavioral processes** include:
            a) **Counterconditioning** (substituting alternatives).
            b) **Helping relationships** (enlisting social support).
            c) **Reinforcement management** (rewarding yourself).
            d) **Self-liberation** (committing yourself).
            e) **Stimulus control** (reminding yourself).

D. THE RELAPSE PREVENTION MODEL

1. The Relapse Prevention Model incorporates the **identification of high-risk situations** and the **development of plans** for coping with high-risk situations.

2. An important element of this model is to learn how to **restructure thinking to distinguish between a lapse and a relapse and to develop flexibility** in the approach for attaining exercise and physical activity goals.

E. THE THEORY OF REASONED ACTION (AND ITS LATER EXTENSION, THE THEORY OF PLANNED BEHAVIOR)

1. The Theory of Reasoned Action postulates that **intention** is the most important determinant of behavior.

2. In turn, attitudes and subjective norms influence intention (*Figure 5-1*).

    a. **Attitudes** are determined by positive and negative beliefs about the **outcome** or the **process of performing** the behavior.

    b. **Subjective norms** are influenced by perceptions about what others think or believe (**normative beliefs**).

    c. The **Theory of Planned Behavior** extends the Theory of Reasoned Action by incorporating **perceived behavioral control**, which is determined by **perceived power** and **control beliefs**.

F. SOCIAL COGNITIVE THEORY

1. The Social Cognitive Theory is one of the most widely used and comprehensive theories of behavioral change.

2. This dynamic model involves **three major interacting influences: behavior, personal, and environmental** (*Figure 5-2*).

3. The theory contains **several different concepts or constructs** that are implicated in the adoption and maintenance of healthy behavior

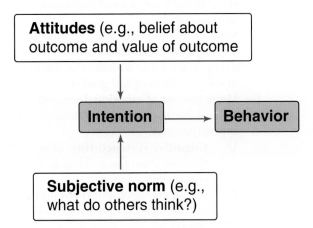

FIGURE 5-1. The Theory of Planned Behavior postulates that intentions influence behavior and that attitudes and subjective norms influence intentions. (Modified from Ajzen I, Fishbein M: *Understanding Attitudes and Predicting Social Behavior*. Upper Saddle River, NJ: Prentice Hall, 1980:8; adapted by permission of Prentice Hall.)

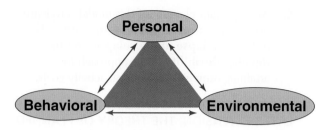

FIGURE 5-2. The Social Cognitive Theory takes into account reciprocal relationships between the personal, behavioral, and environmental factors.

and that are used for increasing and maintaining physical activity or exercise.

a. **Observational learning** says that people can learn by watching others **model** a behavior and by perceiving the rewards that another person receives for engaging in that behavior. This is sometimes called **vicarious reward**.

b. **Behavioral capability** means that the person has both the **knowledge** and the **skill** to perform the behavior.

c. **Outcome expectations and outcome expectancies** are the anticipated benefits from engaging in the behavior.
   1) **Outcome expectations** are what the person **anticipates the outcome will be** for performing the behavior.
   2) **Outcome expectancies** are the **values** of that outcome.

d. **Self-efficacy** is the confidence about performing a **specific behavior**. This construct has been **one of the strongest predictors for adopting a program of regular exercise** in many populations and in many settings.

e. **Self-control of performance** refers to self-regulatory skills when directed toward a specific goal. This includes the concepts of **self-monitoring** and **goal setting**.

f. **Management of emotional arousal** is the ability to deal with emotions appropriately by:
   1) **Cognitive restructuring**, as in thinking about the problem in a more constructive manner.
   2) **Stress management techniques**, as in controlling symptoms of emotional distress.
   3) **Learning methods of effective problem solving**.

g. **Reinforcement** is derived from **operant learning theories**, which state that

behavior is controlled by the consequences of the behavior and that the behavior will increase if **positive reinforcement is applied or a negative reinforcement is removed**. Social Cognitive Theory involves **three types of reinforcement**:
   1) **Direct reinforcement**, as described in operant conditioning.
   2) **Vicarious reinforcement**, as described in observational learning.
   3) **Self-reinforcement**, as one would apply in a self-control technique.

III. Applying Concepts from Theories to the Exercise Setting

A. ASSESSING PARTICIPANTS AND DEVELOPING STRATEGIES TO INCREASE EXERCISE ADHERENCE

Various assessments can be used to determine behavioral needs as well as strategies to encourage initiation, adherence, and return to participation if an individual has experienced a relapse.

1. **Assessing benefits and barriers** entails using a **decisional balance sheet**.
   a. All of the perceptions about exercise programs, both **negative** (lack of time) and **positive** (feeling more energetic), are written on a sheet of paper.
   b. Helping individuals see the **benefits of exercising** can increase the likelihood of participation in an exercise program.
   c. **Helping a client to problem-solve** by removing barriers to exercise, one by one, can help the client learn how to find time and enjoyment, and it can decrease the reasons for not being able to maintain a program of regular exercise.
   d. As a client finds more reasons to become active and reduces the number of reasons for inactivity, the **decisional balance tips in the positive direction** and improves adherence.

2. **Assessing self-efficacy (confidence)** means determining the degree to which individuals believe that they can perform the desired behavior.
   a. Self-efficacy can be assessed by the use of a **paper-and-pencil questionnaire**. Using a 1-to-5 or a 1-to-10 scale, individuals rank how confident they are that they could exercise when it is raining or snowing, when they feel they don't have the time, when they are tired, and so forth.

b. Four Ways to Increase Self-Efficacy
   1) **Performance Accomplishments**
      a) **Example:** Set a goal of walking 1 mile continuously within 1 month by gradually increasing the weekly walking distance.
      b) Assist by helping to set **realistic, specific short- and long-term goals**.
   2) **Vicarious Experience**
      Example: "This person is like me; if she can do it, then I probably can."
   3) **Verbal Persuasion**
      a) **Example:** Helping the person to see how he or she might be able to understand the feasibility of a goal and how to accomplish it.
      b) **Provide continuous reinforcement and feedback.**
   4) **Physiologic States**
      a) Get the person to recognize and monitor the number of positive feelings that come from exercise.
      b) Increase the use of **self-monitoring techniques**, such as keeping an exercise log and counting steps using a mechanical step-counter.

3. Techniques from learning theories, such as **shaping, reinforcement, and antecedent control**, have been used to increase adoption and maintenance of exercise.
   a. **Shaping** is setting a series of intermediate goals that lead to a long-term goal. Shaping is especially appropriate when:
      1) Applied to **increasing frequency, intensity, duration, or types** of activities.
      2) Initiating exercise programs in which the **long-term goals may be too difficult for a novice**.
   b. **Reinforcement** should be scheduled to occur both during and after exercise to offset any possible immediate negative consequences (e.g., feeling hot, sweaty, or out of breath). Reinforcement can take several forms:
      1) **Verbal encouragement**.
      2) **Material incentives** (based on **specific contingency contracts**).
      3) **"Natural" reinforcements** (e.g., stress relief, self-praise).

   c. **Antecedent control** uses techniques that prompt the initiation of behavior. Such prompts include:
      1) Telephone reminders.
      2) Packing a gym bag for the next day before going to bed.
      3) Scheduling time for exercise in a daily schedule.

4. **Cognitive restructuring techniques** involve changing thought processes about a particular situation. These are particularly important for **adoption and maintenance of activity** as well as for **relapse prevention**.
   a. **Relapse prevention strategies** include having the participant **identify high-risk situations** that may lead to a lapse. **Plans are developed before a lapse occurs**. Then, if the lapse occurs, the plan is in place and a relapse less likely.
   b. **Elimination of "All-or-None" Thinking**
      1) A momentary lapse in a regular exercise routine does not label a participant as a failure and, subsequently, lead to stopping the exercise routine altogether.
      2) This technique helps to label the lapse correctly as a slight disruption and to problem-solve the resumption of regular exercise.

B. UNDERSTANDING CONFIDENCE LEVEL, PERCEIVED BENEFITS, AND BARRIERS

1. This provides a focus for the exercise professional to **set realistic goals and gradually shape and increase** exercise behavior.
2. As the client progresses, it is important to continue **to set goals and to plan for possible lapses**.

C. USING THE STAGES OF CHANGE MODEL TO INCREASE ADHERENCE

See also the previous discussion of the Transtheoretical Model.

1. **Precontemplation**
   Discussing benefits, what can be learned from previous attempts, and the change process may assist during this stage. For example, many people decide to become a regular exerciser and then have difficulty in maintaining a regular program.
   a. Clients at this stage **may not be aware of the risks** associated with being sedentary, or they **may have become discouraged** by previous attempts to stay active and have feelings of failure. Multiple attempts may be required to succeed.

b. The exercise professional should not assume that the participant at the precontemplation stage is ready for an exercise program.

c. **Counseling should center on achievable goals** at which success is relatively certain (e.g., 2-minute walk during the workweek). This may not be the desired or long-term outcome, but by using a gradual process of shaping, the exercise behavior can become more frequent and of longer duration.

2. **Contemplation**
Contemplators believe the reasons for being inactive (e.g., "I am too tired," "Exercise takes too much time") outweigh the benefits of initiating exercise. Useful approaches at this stage include:

a. **Discuss the benefits of exercise, and help the client problem-solve** to eliminate barriers. These techniques should increase the client's confidence level and self-efficacy.

b. **Encourage setting specific short-term goals** (e.g., exercise for 10 minutes on one to seven specific days).

3. **Preparation**
Irregular exercise behavior is the hallmark of people at this stage.

a. Discussing **further reductions of barriers and continued building of self-efficacy** are important.

b. **Monitoring gains and rewarding the achievement of goals** are two methods for increasing confidence.

c. **Shaping by reinforcing small steps** toward action is also important. Gradually increasing the time for, intensity of, and adherence to exercise will assist in achieving recommended levels of exercise behavior.

4. **Action**
People in the action stage are at the **greatest risk of relapse**.

a. Instruction on **avoiding injury, exercise boredom, and burnout** is important to those who have recently begun an exercise program.

b. **Social support** (e.g., asking how it is going) and **praise** are the most important contributors to maintained activity.

c. **Planning for high-risk relapse situations** (e.g., vacations, sickness, bad weather, and increased demands on time) is important. The exercise professional can emphasize that a short lapse in activity can be a learning opportunity and is not failure. Planning can help to develop coping strategies and to eliminate the "all-or-none" thinking that sometimes is typical of people who miss several exercise sessions and think they need to give up.

5. **Maintenance**
After 6 months of regular activity, individuals are considered to be in the maintenance stage of exercise adoption.

a. At this stage, some coping strategies have been developed, but **risk for dropping out remains present**.

b. **Scheduling check-in appointments** can help the maintainer to stay motivated.

c. **Continued feedback** is important. If a maintainer is absent for several sessions, a **prompt such as a telephone call or letter noting the absence** can help to reestablish maintenance.

d. **Planning for high-risk situations** (e.g., alternate activities, plans to begin exercise after a lapse, finding someone to exercise with, lowering initial exercise goals after a lapse) is also important.

e. **Revisit the benefits** of physical activity.

f. Gradually shift the exercise program with the exercise professional to the maintenance environment.

g. **Reassess the goals** of physical activity.

h. **Avoid boredom** by including a variety of activities.

IV. Understanding Variables that Influence Activity Levels

A. DEMOGRAPHIC VARIABLES

1. Women tend to participate in less vigorous activity than men. Therefore, many women may respond better to programs that incorporate moderate-intensity activity.

2. Older age is associated with lower levels of physical activity, especially vigorous activity. Older individuals may respond better to programs that incorporate moderate-intensity activity.

B. COGNITIVE AND EXPERIENTIAL VARIABLES

1. **Past experiences** with physical activity can influence initiation of an exercise program.

2. An individual's **perception of his or her current health status** can affect current physical activity levels.

3. **Perceived enjoyment of physical activity** can affect adoption of and adherence to an exercise program.

4. **Access to exercise facilities** and convenience of exercise program can also affect adoption of and adherence to such a program.

C. ENVIRONMENTAL AND PROGRAM FACTORS

1. **Social support** from family, peers, and coworkers.
2. **Weather** that is either too hot or too cold.
3. **Increased flexibility/adaptability** of the exercise program (e.g., adding lifestyle components, home exercise, location, intensity, frequency).
4. **Reminders** in the environment to exercise.
5. **Neighborhood factors** (e.g., sidewalks, stray animals, crime, streetlights).

V. Effective Counseling Tips

A. USING A THREE-FUNCTION MODEL OF PARTICIPANT-CENTERED EDUCATION AND COUNSELING

1. During **information gathering**, any or all of the following areas should be assessed for participants:
   a. Current level of knowledge.
   b. Attitudinal beliefs, intentions, and readiness to change.
   c. Past experiences with exercise or physical activity skills.
   d. Behavioral skills.
   e. Available social support.
2. In **developing a helping relationship**, it is important to **understand the process** and to **establish support**.
   a. An effective process is **interactive**, assesses information central to the issues, **asks questions** of the participant, **instructs**, and takes into account a willingness to **negotiate**. Effective listening skills are essential in developing a helping relationship.
   b. **Exhibiting feelings of acceptance develops a supportive relationship.** If the exercise professional is judgmental, participants may not share information regarding their exercise behavior and lifestyle.
   c. Establishing a Supportive Relationship
      1) **Exhibit empathy** by restating expressed emotion (e.g., "This seems frustrating to you").
      2) **Legitimize concerns** (e.g., "I can understand why you might be concerned with travel out of town").
      3) **Respect abilities and positive efforts** (e.g., "You've worked hard to get this far").
      4) **Support by providing reinforcement and follow-up** (e.g., "I'll be available to help you get on track and stay on track").
      5) **Partner with the individual** by stating your willingness to work together (e.g., "You won't be alone; I will be there to help you").
      6) **Pay attention to nonverbal communication** (e.g., eye contact, body posture, vocal quality).
3. **Participant education and counseling** is a multifactorial process that may involve various situations and issues. To counsel effectively about readiness to change, it is necessary to understand that **waning motivation to exercise is universal**. Effective counseling can assist a person who is experiencing a **lapse** (short break) to prevent it from turning into a **relapse** (longer period of inactivity) or a collapse (no plans for returning to exercise).
   a. During each counseling session, the **five A's** should be used:
      1) **Address the agenda** (e.g., "I'd like to talk to you about... ").
      2) **Assess** (e.g., "What do you know about... ?" "How do you feel?" What are you considering... ?").
      3) **Advise** (e.g., "I'd advise...").
      4) **Assist** (e.g., "How would you like for me to help you?" "What problems do you foresee?")
      5) **Arrange follow-up** (e.g., "We will set up a time for you to let me know how you did...").
   b. Most sedentary people are not motivated to initiate exercise programs, and if exercise is initiated, they are likely to stop within 3 to 6 months.
   c. Participants in the earlier stages benefit most from **cognitive strategies** (e.g., listening to lectures and reading books without the expectation of actually engaging in exercise), whereas individuals in the later stages depend more on **behavioral techniques** (e.g., reminders to exercise and developing social support to help them establish and be able to maintain a regular exercise habit).

B. RECOGNIZING AND ACKNOWLEDGING INDIVIDUAL DIFFERENCES

There are **many ways to achieve a regular exercise or physical activity routine**. The recent Surgeon General's report on physical activity and health states that **moderate-intensity lifestyle activity (e.g., brisk walking, gardening) performed for a total of 30 minutes at least five times a week** produces important health benefits. Some participants may feel more comfortable using this type of **home-based approach** rather than an exercise facility where others might notice their appearance and skill level. Some participants may not perceive that they can achieve 30 minutes continuously, and they may not be aware that activity benefits can be achieved by accumulating shorter bouts. **Intermittent-activity prescriptions counteract the "all-or-none" thinking** (e.g., "I can't exercise for an hour so I might just as well not exercise at all") that leads to relapse.

C. DEALING WITH DIFFICULT CLIENTS

Despite the best efforts, some clients are difficult to work with. Issues related to interaction with the exercise professional must be resolved before exercise goals can be achieved.

1. The **dissatisfied client** is never pleased regardless of all efforts to please.
    a. The exercise professional must work hard at all times to remind the client that **the professional's goal is to assist in achieving exercise adherence**.
    b. If dissatisfaction remains after developing all possible options, **state the options, acknowledge that they may not be ideal, and ask the client for his or her preferred option**.
2. The **needy client** wants more support than can be given. Often, a primary goal of needy individuals is to gain attention. The exercise professional should:
    a. **Establish specific expectations** of what is possible.
    b. **Remain focused** on the exercise or physical activity issues and their behavioral skills.
    c. Remind the participant that the goal is health education and exercise adherence.
    d. Refer the client for additional help (e.g., professional counseling from a nutritionist or physician) if necessary.
3. The **hostile client** may try to elicit hostility in return. When faced with these clients, it is important to **maintain professionalism**.
    a. **Acknowledge** the client's anger.
    b. Try to **determine whether you should address the underlying issue** or ask the client what would make him or her feel less angry.
    c. If chronic hostility occurs, a **different exercise leader** may help to ameliorate the situation.
4. The **shy client** is usually pleasant but not talkative. Try asking probing and **open-ended questions** instead of those that just require yes/no answers.

VI. Problems Exceeding Your Level of Expertise

Referrals to other resources may be required when participants have **health problems** that may limit the types of exercise that can be performed.

A. Participants with **existing health problems** or perceived health limitations should be referred to a primary care physician for further evaluation or reassurance.

B. Participants with **psychological issues** (e.g., poor coping; difficulty managing stress, depression, or anxiety; chronic complaints of being overwhelmed) should be referred to a professional counselor or a physician for evaluation.
    1. **Symptoms of depression or anxiety** (*Table 5-1*) are serious. Participants with these symptoms should be referred to a physician or professional counselor as soon as possible.
    2. **Anxiousness before a fitness assessment** may be accompanied by high heart rate and rapid, shallow breathing. **Techniques for reducing pretest anxiety** include:
        a. Have the person sit quietly and do **deep-breathing exercises**.
        b. **Give thorough explanations**, and **allow practice** with unfamiliar equipment.
        c. **Schedule an additional practice session** on equipment to increase the participant's familiarity with staff, equipment, and setting.
    3. Individuals dealing with **life crises** may experience emotional difficulties that affect their exercise behavior. Examples of life crises include marital difficulty, divorce, unemployment, and financial problems. These individuals should be referred to a mental health professional as needed.

TABLE 5-1. Symptoms of Depression and Anxiety

Symptoms of Depression	Symptoms of Anxiety
Feeling sad or "down in the dumps" for more than 2 weeks.	Panic attacks (sudden episodes of fear and physiological arousal that occur for no apparent reason)
Withdrawal from social activities	
Tearfulness	Increased nervousness associated with going into crowded places like the mall or a gym
Excessive guilt	
Rapid weight loss or weight gain	
Feelings of fatigue	
Changing sleep patterns (e.g., early morning awakening)	Feeling "keyed up" or "on edge" most of the time
Expressions of wanting to be dead or wanting to die	

4. **Persons with substance abuse or eating disorders** should be referred to a physician or mental health professional.
5. **When making referrals, the exercise professional should be acquainted with the mental health professional and follow up with the participant after the referral.**

C. **SIGNS OF PSYCHOLOGICAL DISTRESS**
1. Significant disruption of normal lifestyle patterns in the participant or significant others.
2. Inability to work at a normal occupational level.
3. Inability to handle routine daily tasks.
4. Reduction in social support network.
5. Distorted perceptions of reality.

Review Test

DIRECTIONS: Carefully read all questions, and select the BEST single answer.

1. Theories are used in programs for
   A) Giving individuals an exercise prescription.
   B) Perceiving rewards of certain behaviors.
   C) Self-reevaluation.
   D) Providing a conceptual framework for behavioral assessment.

2. In which stage of motivational readiness is a person who is an irregular exerciser?
   A) Precontemplation.
   B) Contemplation.
   C) Preparation.
   D) Action.

3. Setting several short-term goals to attain a long-term goal to increase self-efficacy is an example of
   A) An application of cognitive-behavioral principles.
   B) An evaluation.
   C) A relationship to theory.
   D) An explanatory theory.

4. A limitation of psychological theories is
   A) They do not reinforce behavior.
   B) They leave out important elements (e.g., sociocultural factors).
   C) They make too many assumptions.
   D) They cannot evaluate programs.

5. The idea that intention is the most important determinant of behavior is a central component of the
   A) Relapse Prevention Model.
   B) Social Cognitive Theory.
   C) Theory of Planned Behavior.
   D) Transtheoretical Model.

6. In the Social Cognitive Theory, which three major dynamic interacting influences are postulated as determining behavioral change?
   A) Personal, behavioral, and environmental.
   B) Reinforcement, commitment, and social support.
   C) High-risk situations, social support, and perceived control.
   D) Stage of readiness, processes of change, and confidence.

7. A decisional balance sheet is used to
   A) Assess barriers and benefits for physical activity or exercise.
   B) Determine a person's self-efficacy.

   C) Determine a person's readiness to change behavior.
   D) All of the above.

8. An individual would not increase self-efficacy by
   A) Performance accomplishments.
   B) Vicarious experience.
   C) Verbal persuasion.
   D) Using a decisional balance sheet.

9. People in which stage are at the greatest risk of relapse?
   A) Precontemplation.
   B) Contemplation.
   C) Preparation.
   D) Action.

10. Which of the following strategies can help a person to maintain his or her physical activity?
    A) Schedule check-in appointments.
    B) Reduce barriers.
    C) Increase benefits.
    D) Educate regarding different types of exercise.
    E) All of the above.

11. Referrals to other sources may be required if someone
    A) Has health problems.
    B) Reports symptoms of depression.
    C) Has an eating disorder.
    D) All of the above.

12. Establishing specific expectations of what you are willing to do as a counselor and staying focused on exercise/physical activity issues and behavioral skills related to exercise are strategies for handling which type of client?
    A) A dissatisfied client.
    B) A needy client.
    C) A hostile client.
    D) A shy client.

13. Encouraging moderate-intensity activity and the accumulation of activity throughout the day are examples of
    A) Relapse prevention counseling.
    B) Using the stages of change.
    C) Allowing individuality in exercise choices.
    D) Addressing the individual's agenda.

14. Which of the following is an example of a behavioral process in the Transtheoretical Model?
    A) Consciousness raising.
    B) Stimulus control.

C)   Dramatic relief.

D)   Environmental reevaluation.

15. One mistake that health care providers and exercise promoters make is to
    A)   Assume that most individuals are ready to change their behavior.
    B)   Encourage the accumulation of moderate-intensity activity throughout the day.
    C)   Legitimize a client's concerns.
    D)   Use the five A's strategy for counseling.

16. The concept of shaping refers to
    A)   Using self-monitoring techniques (e.g., exercise logs).
    B)   Using visual prompts (e.g., packing a gym bag the night before) as reminders to exercise.
    C)   The process for establishing self-efficacy.
    D)   Setting intermediate goals that lead to a long-term goal.

17. Verbal encouragement, material incentives, self-praise, and use of specific contingency contracts are examples of
    A)   Shaping.
    B)   Reinforcement.
    C)   Antecedent control.
    D)   Setting goals.

18. The three functions of the Participant-Centered Education and Counseling Model include
    A)   Identifying high-risk situations, developing a plan for these situations, and eliminating "all-or-none" thinking.
    B)   Information gathering, developing a helping relationship, and participant education and counseling.
    C)   Exhibiting empathy, legitimizing a client's concerns, and forming a partnership.
    D)   Assessing, asking questions, and establishing a supportive relationship.

19. The Transtheoretical Model assumes that individuals
    A)   Move through the stages of behavioral change at a steady pace.
    B)   Only progress forward through the stages.
    C)   Move back and forth along the stage continuum.

D)   Tend to use behavioral processes during the earlier stages of change.

20. If an individual is in the action stage, he or she
    A)   Intends to start exercising in the next 6 months.
    B)   Participates in some exercise, but does so irregularly.
    C)   Has been physically active on a regular basis for less than 6 months.
    D)   Has been physically active on a regular basis for more than 6 months.

21. Which does NOT help to establish a supportive relationship?
    A)   Exhibit empathy.
    B)   Legitimize concerns.
    C)   Respect the person's abilities and efforts.
    D)   Address the agenda.

22. The five A's of counseling are
    A)   Address, Assess, Act, Assist, and Arrange follow-up.
    B)   Address, Assess, Advise, Assist, and Act.
    C)   Address, Assess, Advise, Assist, and Arrange follow-up.
    D)   Act, Assess, Advise, Assist, and Arrange follow-up.

23. Which of the following would assist anxious people before an exercise test?
    A)   Ask them to sit quietly in a chair for a few minutes.
    B)   Thoroughly explain the exercise test.
    C)   Familiarize them with the exercise equipment by brief practice.
    D)   All of the above

24. Which of the following are NOT symptoms of depression?
    A)   Hearing voices.
    B)   Change in sleep patterns.
    C)   Irritability.
    D)   All of the above.

25. Which of the following are symptoms of anxiety?
    A)   Panic attacks.
    B)   Increased nervousness.
    C)   Feelings of being "on edge."
    D)   All of the above.

ANSWERS AND EXPLANATIONS

1–D. Psychological theories are the foundation for the effective use of strategies and techniques of effective counseling and motivational skill-building for exercise adoption and maintenance. Theories provide a conceptual framework for assessment, development of programs or interventions, application of cognitive-behavioral or motivational principles, and evaluation of program effectiveness. Within the field of behavioral change, a theory is a set of assumptions that account for the relationships between certain variables and the behavior of interest.

2–C. The stages of motivational readiness describe five categories of readiness to change or maintain behavior. As applied to physical activity or exercise, they are precontemplation (stage 1: no physical activity or exercise, and no intention to start within the next 6 months), contemplation (stage 2: no physical activity or exercise, but an intention to start within the next 6 months), preparation (stage 3: participation in some physical activity or exercise, but not at levels meeting current and standard guidelines), action (stage 4: physical activity or exercise that meets standard guidelines for physical activity, but for less than 6 months), and maintenance (stage 5: exercise or activity for 6 months or longer).

3–A. Applications of cognitive-behavioral principles are the methods used within programs to improve motivational skills as suggested by the assessment. For example, setting several small short-term goals to attain a long-term goal is likely to increase self-efficacy as the person successfully reaches each short-term goal on the way to attaining the long-term goal.

4–B. A limitation of most psychological theories is that they have been developed to explain the behaviors of individuals or small groups. Therefore, these theories are limited in terms of understanding larger groups (e.g., communities), and they may leave out many important elements that might influence behavior (e.g., sociocultural elements). Despite these limitations, theories of behavioral change provide important tools to help change exercise behavior.

5–C. The Theory of Planned Behavior postulates that intention is the most important determinant of behavior. In turn, attitudes and subjective norms influence intention. Attitudes are determined by positive and negative beliefs about the outcome or process of performing the behavior. Subjective norms are influenced by perceptions about what others think or believe. The Theory of Planned Behavior extends the Theory of Reasoned Action by incorporating perceived behavioral control, which is determined by perceived power and control beliefs.

6–A. The Social Cognitive Theory is one of the most widely used and comprehensive theories of behavioral change. This theory is a dynamic model that asserts three major interacting influences: behavioral, personal, and environmental. The Social Cognitive Theory contains a number of different concepts of constructs that are implicated in the adoption and maintenance of healthy behavior and that are used for increasing and maintaining physical activity or exercise. They include observation learning, behavioral capability, outcome expectations, self-efficacy, self-control of performance, management of emotional arousal, and reinforcement.

7–A. Various assessments can be used to determine behavioral needs and strategies to encourage initiation, adherence, and return to participation if an individual has experienced a relapse. Assessing benefits and barriers entails using a decisional balance sheet. All of the perceived negative (e.g., lack of time) and positive (e.g., feeling more energetic) consequences for participating or not participating in exercise are written on a sheet of paper. This procedure can assist participants by reminding them of immediate as well as long-term positive consequences and by helping them to problem-solve negative consequences. Removing or resolving problem-solving barriers, one by one, can help with learning how to find time and enjoyment by decreasing the reasons for not being able to maintain a program of regular exercise. As a participant finds more reasons to become active and reduces the number of reasons for inactivity, the decisional balance tips in the positive direction and improves adherence.

8–D. Self-efficacy (confidence) is the degree to which individuals believe they can perform the desired behavior. It is possible to increase self-efficacy in four ways: performance accomplishments (e.g., setting a goal of walking 1 mile in 1 month by gradually increasing the weekly distance), vicarious experience (e.g., "This person is like me; if she can do it, then I probably can"), verbal persuasion (e.g., helping the person to see how he or she might understand the feasibility of a goal and a way to accomplish it), and physiologic states (e.g., getting the person to recognize and monitor the number of positive feelings that come from exercise). A decisional balance sheet would be used to assess benefits and barriers.

9–D. People in the action stage are at the greatest risk of relapse. Instruction about avoiding injury, exercise boredom, and burnout is important for those who have recently begun an exercise program. Providing social support and praise are the most important contributors to maintained activity. Planning for high-risk, relapse situations (e.g., vacations, sickness, bad weather, increased demands on time) is also important. The exercise professional can emphasize that a short lapse in activity can be a learning opportunity and is not failure. Planning can help to develop coping strategies and to eliminate the "all-or-none" thinking sometimes typical of people who have missed several exercise sessions and think they need to give it up.

10–A. After 6 months of regular activity, individuals are considered to be in the maintenance stage of exercise adoption. Some coping strategies have been developed, but the risk of dropping out remains. Scheduling check-in appointments can help the maintainer to stay motivated. Continued feedback is also important. If a maintainer is absent for several sessions, a prompt (e.g., a telephone call or letter noting the absence) can help to reestablish maintenance.

11–D. Referrals to other resources may be required when participants have health problems that may limit the types of exercise that can be performed. Existing health problems or perceived health limitations may be referred to a primary care physician for further evaluation and/or reassurance. Psychological issues (e.g., poor coping, difficulty managing stress, depression, anxiety, chronic complaints of being overwhelmed) should be referred for professional counseling and/or to a physician for evaluation. Symptoms of depression or anxiety are more serious and should be referred to a physician or professional counselor. Persons with eating disorders should be referred to a physician or mental health professional.

12–B. Despite the best efforts, working with some clients is difficult. Issues related to interaction with the exercise professional must be resolved before exercise goals can be achieved. The needy client wants more support than can be given. It is important, then, to establish specific expectations of what is possible and to remain focused on the exercise or physical activity issues

and behavioral skills related to those issues. Often, a primary goal of the needy individual is to gain attention. It is important to remember that the exercise professional is not a trained counselor, and in some cases, it may be appropriate to refer the client for additional help.

13–C. Recognizing and acknowledging individual differences is an important component of effective counseling. A regular exercise or physical activity routine can be achieved in many ways. Many participants may not perceive that they can achieve 30 minutes of continuous physical activity, and they may not be aware that activity benefits can be achieved through the accumulation of shorter bouts. Intermittent-activity prescriptions counteract the "all-or-none" type of thinking that often leads to relapse.

14–B. Key components of the Transtheoretical Model are the processes of behavioral change. These processes include five behavioral processes (counterconditioning, helping relationships, reinforcement management, self-liberation, stimulus control) and five cognitive processes (consciousness raising, dramatic relief, environmental reevaluation, self-reevaluation, social liberation).

15–A. Participants progress through various stages of change at varying rates and, in the process of changing, these participants move back and forth along the stage continuum. Different cognitive and behavioral processes or strategies are used during each stage. Discussing the benefits of physical activity and learning from previous attempts may assist those in the precontemplation stage. This group may not be aware of the risks associated with being sedentary, or they may have become discouraged by previous attempts to stay active and have feelings of failure. Multiple attempts may be required to succeed. The exercise professional should not assume that the participant in the precontemplation stage is ready for an exercise program.

16–D. Shaping is setting a series of intermediate goals that lead to a long-term goal. This is especially appropriate when applied to increasing frequency, intensity, duration, or types of activities. When initiating exercise programs in which the long-term goals may be too difficult for a novice, this strategy is particularly appropriate.

17–B. Reinforcement should be scheduled to occur both during and after exercise to offset any possible immediate negative consequences. Reinforcement can take the form of verbal encouragement, material incentives (based on contingency contracts), and natural reinforcements (e.g., stress relief, self-praise).

18–B. Effective counselors can use a three-function model of participant-centered education and counseling. The three functions of this model are information gathering, developing a helping relationship, and participant education and counseling.

19–C. The Transtheoretical Model of Change (Stages of Change or Motivational Readiness) incorporates constructs from other theories, including intention to change and processes (or strategies) of change. The basic concepts of this model are that people progress through five stages of change at varying rates and that, in the process of changing, they also move back and forth along the stage continuum. The model also holds that people use different cognitive and behavioral processes or strategies.

20–C. Stages of motivational readiness describe five categories of readiness to change or maintain behavior. As applied to physical activity or exercise, they are precontemplation (stage 1), contemplation (stage 2), preparation (stage 3), action (stage 4), and maintenance (stage 5). The action stage is when the person is engaged in physical activity or exercise that meets the ACSM recommendations for physical activity but has not maintained this program for 6 months or more.

21–D. Effective counselors can use a three-function model of participant-centered education and counseling. The three functions of this model are information gathering, developing a helping relationship, and participant education and counseling. To establish a supportive relationship, exhibit empathy by restating expressed emotion, legitimize concerns, respect abilities and positive efforts, support by providing rein-

forcement and follow-up, and partner by stating your willingness to work together.

22–C. Participant education and counseling is a multifactorial process that may involve a variety of situations and issues. For example, to counsel effectively about readiness to change, it is necessary to understand that waning motivation to exercise is universal. Effective counseling can assist a person who is experiencing a lapse (e.g., short break) to prevent it from turning into a relapse or collapse. During each counseling session, the five A's (Address the agenda, Assess, Advise, Assist, Arrange follow-up) should be used.

23–D. Anxiousness before a fitness assessment may be accompanied by a high heart rate and rapid, shallow breathing. This may be alleviated by having the person sit quietly and using deep-breathing exercises. Thorough explanations and practice on unfamiliar equipment can also reduce anxiety before exercise testing. Scheduling an additional practice session on equipment to increase familiarity with staff, equipment, and setting may assist those unable to reduce pretest anxiety.

24–A. Symptoms of depression or anxiety are serious and should be referred to a physician or professional counselor. Symptoms of depression include feeling sad or "down in the dumps" for more than a few weeks, tearfulness, withdrawal from social activities, excessive guilt, rapid weight loss or weight gain, feelings of fatigue, changing sleep patterns (e.g., early morning awakening), or expressions of wanting to be dead or to die.

25–D. Symptoms of anxiety include panic attacks (sudden episodes of fear and physiologic arousal that occur for no apparent reason), increased nervousness associated with going into crowded places (e.g., the mall, a gym), or feeling "keyed up" or "on edge" most of the time.

Health Appraisal and Fitness Testing

STEPHEN C. GLASS

I. Pretest Considerations

A. HEALTH APPRAISAL

Essential information is required before exercise testing to identify any necessary modifications of test protocols, risk factors for and/or contraindications to testing, and need for referral to a physician.

1. **Purpose**
   a. Safety
      Provides health and fitness professionals with information that can lead to **identification of individuals for whom exercise is contraindicated.**
   b. Risk Factor Identification
      1) Many medical conditions increase the health risk associated with physical activity or exercise testing.
      2) Health screening allows the health/fitness professional to **determine who may participate and who should be referred to a physician** before participation in exercise testing or physical activity.
   c. Exercise Prescription and Programming
      The information gathered allows health/-fitness professional to **develop specific exercise programs that are appropriate to the individual needs and goals of the client.**

2. **Health History**
   a. Present History
      1) Known disease and/or symptoms of disease.
      2) Activity level.
      3) Dietary behaviors (including caffeine and alcohol intake).
      4) Smoking/tobacco use.
      5) Medication use (including recreational drugs) and/or drug allergies.
   b. Past History
      1) Cardiorespiratory problems.
      2) Orthopedic problems.
      3) Recent illnesses/hospitalizations.

      4) Exercise history.
      5) Work history.
   c. Family History
      1) Onset of heart disease in first-degree relative before age 55 (men) or 65 (women).
      2) Other significant disorders, including diabetes, hyperlipidemia, stroke, and sudden death.
   d. Health Screening Questionnaire
      1) A preparticipation health screening tool, such as the **Physical Activity Readiness Questionnaire (PAR-Q)**, should be completed before exercise testing (*Figure 6-1*).
      2) To solicit reliable information, the questionnaire should be completed in a **quiet, private area.**
      3) **Review the responses** with the client to confirm the accuracy of the information and to determine the health risk status.

3. **Physical Assessment and Laboratory Tests**
   a. **Resting Heart Rate**
      After the client has been sitting quietly for 5 minutes, the pulse is palpated at the radial or carotid artery for 30 seconds. The normal resting heart rate is 60 to 100 bpm.
   b. **Resting Blood Pressure**
      1) Because blood pressure can fluctuate, accurate blood pressure assessment should be based on two or more measurements.
      2) Blood pressure should be measured with the client in both the supine and standing positions to screen for **postural hypotension.**
   c. **Lung Capacity**
      Tests of lung capacity assess airway patency and airflow volume and rate.
      1) **Forced Vital Capacity (FVC)**
         a) Is the volume of air expired following a maximal inspiration.
         b) Assesses the degree of restrictive pulmonary disease.

Physical Activity Readiness
Questionnaire - PAR-Q
(revised 1994)

PAR - Q & YOU

(A Questionnaire for People Aged 15 to 69)

Regular physical activity is fun and healthy, and increasingly more people are starting to become more active every day. Being more active is very safe for most people. However, some people should check with their doctor before they start becoming much more physically active.

If you are planning to become much more physically active than you are now, start by answering the seven questions in the box below. If you are between the ages of 15 and 69, the PAR-Q will tell you if you should check with your doctor before you start. If you are over 69 years of age, and you are not used to being very active, check with your doctor.

Common sense is your best guide when you answer these questions. Please read the questions carefully and answer each one honestly: check YES or NO.

YES	NO		
☐	☐	1.	Has your doctor ever said that you have a heart condition <u>and</u> that you should only do physical activity recommended by a doctor?
☐	☐	2.	Do you feel pain in your chest when you do physical activity?
☐	☐	3.	In the past month, have you had chest pain when you were not doing physical activity?
☐	☐	4.	Do you lose your balance because of dizziness or do you ever lose consciousness?
☐	☐	5.	Do you have a bone or joint problem that could be made worse by a change in your physical activity?
☐	☐	6.	Is your doctor currently prescribing drugs (for example, water pills) for your blood pressure or heart condition?
☐	☐	7.	Do you know of <u>any other reason</u> why you should not do physical activity?

If

you

answered

YES to one or more questions

Talk with your doctor by phone or in person BEFORE you start becoming much more physically active or BEFORE you have a fitness appraisal. Tell your doctor about the PAR-Q and which questions you answered YES.

- You may be able to do any activity you want—as long as you start slowly and build up gradually. Or, you may need to restrict your activities to those which are safe for you. Talk with your doctor about the kinds of activities you wish to participate in and follow his/her advice.
- Find out which community programs are safe and helpful for you.

NO to all questions

If you answered NO honestly to <u>all</u> PAR-Q questions, you can be reasonably sure that you can:

- start becoming much more physically active—begin slowly and build up gradually. This is the safest and easiest way to go.
- take part in a fitness appraisal—this is an excellent way to determine your basic fitness so that you can plan the best way for you to live actively.

DELAY BECOMING MUCH MORE ACTIVE:
- if you are not feeling well because of a temporary illness such as a cold or a fever—wait until you feel better; or
- if you are or may be pregnant—talk to your doctor before you start becoming more active.

Please note: if your health changes so that you then answer YES to any of the above questions, tell your fitness or health professional. Ask whether you should change your physical activity plan.

<u>Informed Use of the PAR-Q:</u> The Canadian Society for Exercise Physiology, Health Canada, and their agents assume no liability for persons who undertake physical activity, and if in doubt after completing this questionnaire, consult your doctor prior to physical activity.

You are encouraged to copy the PAR-Q but only if you use the entire form

NOTE: if the PAR-Q is being given to a person before he or she participates in physical activity program or a fitness appraisal, this section may be used for legal or administrative purposes.

I have read, understood and completed this questionnaire. Any questions I had were answered to my full satisfaction.

NAME _____

SIGNATURE _____ DATE _____

SIGNATURE OF PARENT _____ WITNESS _____
or GUARDIAN (for participants under the age of majority)

© Canadian Society for Exercise Physiology   Supported by: [🍁] Health Santé
Société canadienne de physiologie de l'exercice   Canada Canada

FIGURE 6-1. PAR-Q form. (Reprinted from the 1994 revised version of the Physical Activity Readiness Questionnaire [PAR-Q and YOU]. The PAR-Q and YOU is a copyrighted, preexercise screen owned by the Canadian Society for Exercise Physiology.)

2) **Forced Expiratory Capacity at 1 Second (FEV_1)**
  a) Is the proportion of the FVC expired in 1 second.
  b) Assesses the degree of airway obstruction.

3) **Maximal Voluntary Ventilation (MVV)**
  a) Is the maximal possible volume of airflow per minute.
  b) Represents the mechanical limit of pulmonary function.

d. Blood Tests
  Various blood tests may shed light on the client's current health status and help to guide exercise programming. Typically, blood samples are drawn following an overnight fast.

1) **Total Cholesterol (TC)**
  This is a measure of the total amount of cholesterol in the blood. It includes all cholesterol fractions.

2) **Low-Density Lipoprotein (LDL)**
  a) An LDL is a cholesterol-carrying protein that tends to deposit cholesterol on arterial walls, greatly accelerating atherosclerosis.
  b) The LDLs are also thought to act as free radicals and to damage cell walls. **High LDL levels mean increased risk.**

3) **High-Density Lipoprotein (HDL)**
   a) An HDL is a cholesterol-carrying protein that tends to remove cholesterol from the blood.
   b) The HDLs are also thought to remove cholesterol from cell walls, possibly reversing the progression of atherosclerosis. **High HDL levels are desirable.**
4) **TC:HDL Ratio**
   a) **This ratio is a useful index of dyslipidemia.**
   b) **This ratio may be significant (>4.3) even if both TC and HDL are within normal limits.**
5) **Fasting Glucose**
   a) This is a measure of blood glucose level without the influence of a meal.
   b) High levels are indicative of impaired glucose tolerance.

B. CONTRAINDICATIONS AND RISK STRATIFICATION

1. **Contraindications to Exercise Testing**
   Some clients have risk factors that outweigh the potential benefits derived from exercise testing *(Table 6-1)*.
   a. **Absolute contraindications** apply to clients for whom exercise testing should not be performed until the situation or condition has stabilized.
   b. **Relative contraindications** apply to clients who might be tested if the potential benefit from exercise testing outweighs the relative risk of testing.

2. **Risk Stratification**
   Clients can be initially classified into three risk strata for exercise testing: low risk, moderate risk, and high risk. Refer to Table 2-2 through 2-4 in *ACSM's Guidelines for Exercise Testing and Prescription*, 7th edition.
   a. Low Risk
      1) This category includes apparently healthy individuals (men younger than 45 years, women younger than 55 years) who are asymptomatic and have no more than one coronary risk factor for coronary artery disease (CAD) *(Table 6-2)*.
   b. Moderate Risk
      1) These clients(men aged 45 and older, women aged 55 and older) have signs or symptoms suggesting

TABLE 6-1. Contraindications to Exercise Testing

Absolute

A recent significant change in the resting electrocardiogram suggesting significant ischemia, recent myocardial infarction (within 2 days), or other acute cardiac event

Unstable angina

Uncontrolled cardiac arrhythmias causing symptoms or hemodynamic compromise

Severe symptomatic aortic stenosis

Uncontrolled symptomatic heart failure

Acute pulmonary embolus or pulmonary infarction

Acute myocarditis or pericarditis

Suspected or known dissecting aneurysm

Acute infections

Relative[a]

Left main coronary stenosis

Moderate stenotic valvular heart disease

Electrolyte abnormalities (e.g., hypokalemia, hypomagnesemia)

Severe arterial hypertension (systolic blood pressure of >200 mm Hg and/or diastolic blood pressure of >110 mm Hg) at rest

Tachyarrhythmias or bradyarrhythmias

Hypertrophic cardiomyopathy and other forms of outflow tract obstruction

Neuromuscular, musculoskeletal, or rheumatoid disorders that are exacerbated by exercise

High-degree atrioventricular block

Ventricular aneurysm

Uncontrolled metabolic disease (e.g., diabetes, thyrotoxicosis, myxedema)

Chronic infectious disease (e.g., mononucleosis, hepatitis, acquired immunodeficiency syndrome)

[a]Relative contraindications can be superseded if the benefits outweigh the risks of exercise. In some instances, these individuals can be exercised with caution and/or using low-level end points, especially if they are asymptomatic at rest.

(Modified from Gibbons RA, Balady GJ, Beasely JW, et al.: ACC/AHA guidelines for exercise testing. *J Am Coll Cardiol* 30:260–315, 1997.)

possible cardiopulmonary or metabolic disease and/or two or more risk factors for CAD.
   c. High Risk
      1) These clients have known cardiac, pulmonary, metabolic disease, or one or more signs and symptoms.
3. Following identification of a client's risk status, the health/fitness instructor or exercise specialist should make an informed decision regarding whether the individual should be tested or permitted to exercise according to the guidelines provided in Table 6-7 in the *Guidelines for Exercise Testing and Prescription*, 7th edition.

C. INFORMED CONSENT

1. **Purpose**
   a. Ethical Considerations
      1) A well-designed consent form provides the client with sufficient information to enable an **informed decision** about participation.

TABLE 6-2. Coronary Artery Disease Risk Factor Thresholds for Use with ACSM Risk Stratification

Risk Factors	Defining Criteria
Positive	
1. Family history	Myocardial infarction, coronary revascularization, or sudden death before 55 years of age in father or other male first-degree relative, or before 65 years of age in mother or other female first-degree relative
2. Cigarette smoking	Current cigarette smoker or those who quit within the previous 6 months
3. Hypertension	Systolic blood pressure of $\geq$140 mm Hg or diastolic blood pressure of $\geq$90 mm Hg, confirmed by measurements on at least two separate occasions, or on antihypertensive medication
4. Dyslipidemia	Low-density lipoprotein (LDL) cholesterol >130 mg $\cdot$ dL^{-1} (3.4 mmol $\cdot$ L^{-1}) or high-density lipoprotein (HDL) cholesterol <40 mg $\cdot$ dL^{-1} (1.03 mmol $\cdot$ L^{-1}) or on lipid-lowering medication. If total serum cholesterol is all that is available use >200 mg $\cdot$ dL^{-1} (5.2 mmol $\cdot$ L^{-1}) rather than low-density lipoprotein (LDL) >130 mg $\cdot$ dL^{-1}
5. Impaired fasting glucose	Fasting blood glucose $\geq$100 mg $\cdot$ dL^{-1} (5.6 mmol $\cdot$ L^{-1}) confirmed by measurements on at least two separate occasions
6. Obesity[a]	Body mass index of $\geq$30 kg $\cdot$ m^{-2} or waist girth of >102 cm for men and 88 cm for women or waist/hip ratio $\geq$0.95 for men and $\geq$0.86 for women
7. Sedentary lifestyle	Persons not participating in a regular exercise program or meeting the minimal physical activity recommendations[b] from the U.S. Surgeon General's report
Negative	
1. High serum HDL cholesterol[c]	>60 mg $\cdot$ dL^{-1} (1.6 mmol $\cdot$ L^{-1})

[a]Professional opinions vary regarding the most appropriate markers and thresholds for obesity; therefore, exercise professionals should use their own clinical judgment when evaluating this risk factor.

[b]Accumulating 30 minutes or more of moderate physical activity on most days of the week.

[c]It is common to sum risk factors in making clinical judgments. If high-density lipoprotein cholesterol (HDL) is high, subtract one risk factor from the sum of positive risk factors because high HDL levels decrease the risk of coronary artery disease.

Hypertension threshold based on National High Blood Pressure Education program. The Seventh Report of the Joint National Committee on Prevention, Detection, Evaluation, and Treatment of High Blood Pressure (JNC7). 2003. 03-5233. **Lipid thresholds** based on National Cholesterol Education Program. Third Report of the National Cholesterol Education Program (NCEP) Expert Panel on Detection, Evaluation, and Treatment of High Blood Cholesterol in Adults (Adult Treatment Panel III). NIH publication No. 02-5215, 2002. **Impaired FG threshold** based on Expert Committee on the Diagnosis and Classification of Diabetes Mellitus. Follow-up report on the diagnosis of diabetes mellitus. Diabetes Care 2003;26:3160–3167. **Obesity thresholds** based on Expert Panel on Detection, Evaluation, and Treatment of Overweight and Obesity in Adults. National Institutes of Health. Clinical guidelines on the identification, evaluation, and treatment of overweight and obesity in adults—the evidence report. Arch Int Med 1998;158:1855–1867. **Sedentary lifestyle thresholds** based on United States Department of Health and Human Services. Physical activity and health: a report of the Surgeon General. 1996.

(Adapted from Expert Panel on Detection, Evaluation, and Treatment of High Blood Cholesterol in Adults. Summary of the second report of the National Cholesterol Education Program (NCEP) expert panel on detection, evaluation, and treatment of high blood cholesterol in adults (Adult Treatment Panel II). *JAMA* 269:3015–3023, 1993.)

2) The consent form **details the expectations** of the client so that full participation is possible.

b. Legal Concerns
Although not a legal document, the use of a well-designed consent form provides written documentation that the client was made aware of the procedures, limitations, **risks** and discomforts, as well as the **benefits** of exercise.

2. **Limitations**
a. Informed consent **does not provide legal immunity** to a facility or individual in the event of injury to a client.
b. Informed consent **does provide evidence** that the client was made aware of the **purposes, procedures, and risks** associated with the test or exercise program.
c. Negligence, improper test administration, inadequate personnel qualifications, and insufficient safety procedures are **expressly not covered** by informed consent.

d. **Legal counsel** should be sought during development of the document.

3. **Content**
a. **Purpose**.
b. **Procedures** explained in lay terminology.
c. Potential **risks** and **discomforts**.
d. Expected **benefits**.
   1) To the participant.
   2) To society.
e. **Responsibilities** of the participant.
f. Provision of an **opportunity to ask questions** and have them answered.
g. **Confidentiality of results**.
h. **Right** of participant **to refuse or withdraw** from any aspect of the procedures.
i. **Signatures**.
   1) Participant.
   2) Test supervisor/administrator.
   3) Guardian for those younger than 18 years of age.
   4) Witness.
j. **Dates** of signatures.

4. **Administration**
   a. The consent form should be presented to the client in a **private, quiet setting**.
   b. The order of activities associated with completion of the document should be as follows:
      1) Private, quiet **reading** of the document.
      2) Private, **verbal explanation** of the contents of the document. with a verbally expressed **opportunity to ask questions** and have them answered.
      3) **Signing and dating** the document.
      4) **Presentation of a copy** of the signed document to the participant.

D. CLIENT PREPARATION

1. **Client teaching** includes a description of the test as well as specific and general instructions, such as:
   a. Avoid eating, smoking, and consuming alcohol or caffeine within 3 hours before testing.
   b. Avoid exercise or other strenuous physical activity on the day of the test.
   c. Get adequate sleep the night before the test.
   d. Wear comfortable, loose-fitting clothing.
2. **Preparing for electrocardiographic (ECG) monitoring** involves abrading the client's skin with a rough pad or sandpaper to remove dead skin cells, followed by cleansing with alcohol and scrubbing with gauze and then applying the ECG electrodes using the anatomical landmarks described in Chapter 12.

II. Fitness Testing: General Considerations

A. PURPOSE

1. **Education**
   A well-planned and implemented battery of fitness assessments provides information to current and potential clients about the various aspects of health-related fitness. The results of the fitness assessments provide a client with information useful for making possible lifestyle decisions.
2. **Exercise Prescription**
   Data collected via appropriate fitness assessments assists the health/fitness instructor in developing safe, effective programs of exercise based on the individual client's current fitness status.
3. **Evaluation of Progress**
   Baseline and follow-up testing provides evidence of progression toward fitness goals.

4. **Motivation**
   Fitness assessments provide information needed to develop reasonable, **attainable goals**. Progress toward or attainment of a goal is strong motivation for continued participation in an exercise program.
5. **Risk stratification**
   Results of fitness assessments can sometimes detect the presence of risk factors, which may influence both the exercise prescription and the subsequent assessments.

B. RISKS ASSOCIATED WITH EXERCISE TESTING

1. **Peak or Symptom-Limited Testing**
   a. The risk of death during or immediately after an exercise test is $\frac{1}{10,000}$.
   b. The risk of acute MI during or immediately after an exercise test is $\frac{1}{2,500}$.
   c. The risk of a complication requiring hospitalization is $\frac{1}{500}$.
2. **Submaximal Exercise Testing**
   The submaximal cycle ergometer test recommended by the ACSM has resulted in no reported deaths, MIs, or morbid events when care has been taken to ensure careful client screening, client compliance with appropriate pretest instructions, and appropriate supervision during the test.

C. SAFETY

To maximize safety, the following items should be assessed:
1. **Site**
   a. Emergency Plans
      1) Written, posted emergency **plans**.
      2) Posted emergency **numbers**.
      3) Regularly scheduled practices of responses to emergency situations, including a minimum of one **announced drill** and one **unannounced drill**.
   b. Room Layout
      The equipment and floor space should be arranged **to allow safe and expeditious exit** from the facility in an emergency.
2. **Equipment**
   a. Maintenance
      Develop a **written document that includes maintenance procedures** for all daily, weekly, and monthly activities **associated with maintaining** each piece of equipment.
   b. Positioning
      The equipment used for testing should be **positioned to ensure maximal visual supervision** of the client.

c. Cleanliness
Develop a **written document that includes cleaning procedures** for all daily, weekly, and monthly activities **associated with cleaning** each piece of equipment.

3. **Personnel**

a. **Certifications** (i.e., cardiopulmonary resuscitation, ACSM Health/Fitness Instructor, Exercise Specialist).

b. **Training** The personnel should be trained and standardized periodically.

D. TEST ORDER

When a battery of fitness assessments is administered to a client in a **single session**, the following order of tests is recommended:

1. **Resting measurements**
These include heart rate, blood pressure, and phlebotomy blood analysis.

2. **Body composition**
Some methods of assessing body composition are sensitive to the **hydration status**. Because some tests of cardiorespiratory or muscular fitness may have an acute effect on hydration, such assessments should be conducted before the body composition assessment.

3. **Cardiorespiratory Fitness**
Assessments of cardiorespiratory fitness often use **heart rate** as a predictive measurement. Assessing muscular fitness or flexibility can produce an increase in heart rate. Therefore, the cardiorespiratory assessment must be conducted before any other assessment that may affect the heart rate.

4. **Muscular Fitness**

a. When assessing both muscular and cardiorespiratory fitness in the same day, muscular fitness should be assessed after cardiorespiratory fitness.

b. Strenuous assessments of cardiorespiratory fitness should be followed by an **appropriate recovery period** before tests of muscular fitness are attempted.

5. **Flexibility**
Flexibility is most appropriately assessed when the body is **fully warmed** and when the subject has been given adequate time to stretch.

E. TEST TERMINATION

Clearly written instructions and regular practice will help to ensure that an assessment is conducted in a manner that is safe and that provides valid, useful information.

1. **Criteria for Stopping a Test**

a. Attainment of Desired Performance
The fitness professional must be familiar with the testing procedures to ensure **recognition of the desired end point** of the assessment.

b. Client or Equipment Complications
1) Signs and symptoms consistent with guidelines for test cessation (see Box 4-5 and 5-2, in *ACSM's Guidelines for Exercise Testing and Prescription*, 7th ed.).
2) Equipment failure.
3) Subject asks to stop.

2. **Procedures**

a. Nonlife-Threatening Situations
An active cool-down should be completed.

b. Life-Threatening Situations
The client should be removed from the testing equipment, and the site's emergency plan should be put into operation.

F. INTERPRETATION OF RESULTS

1. **Data Reduction**
Equations used to predict a fitness score should be appropriate both to the tests conducted and to the client.

2. **Normative data**

a. Selection
The norms against which results are compared should meet the following criteria:
1) Appropriate to the test administered.
2) Appropriate to the age, gender, and history of the client.

b. **Standard Error of the Estimate**
1) The standard error of the estimate is an indication of the error of the estimate compared with the actual measurement of the variable.
2) Knowledge of the standard error of the estimate associated with a test is critical to the appropriate interpretation of the results.
3) Reports to clients should clearly indicate the error associated with the testing.

3. **Repeated Assessment**

a. Methods
Follow-up assessment of any fitness component should **use the same test**, including procedures and protocols, as that used during the original assessment. It is therefore essential to keep precise records of all assessments.

b. Timing
Repeat testing should be conducted only **after sufficient time for alteration in**

the fitness component is assessed. The fitness professional should therefore be aware of the time course needed for physiologic adaptations.

   c. Interpretation of Significant Change
Care should be taken when interpreting small changes in fitness scores. Often, such changes are within the error of estimate of the procedures used.

G. BODY COMPOSITION ASSESSMENT

Body composition assessment examines the **relative proportions of fat versus fat-free (lean) tissue** in the body. The result is commonly reported as the **percentage body fat**, thus identifying the proportion of the total body mass composed of fat. **Fat-free mass** is then determined as the **balance of the total body mass**.

  1. **Hydrostatic (Underwater) Weighing**

    a. Principle
This method is based on **Archimedes's principle**—that a body immersed in water is buoyed by a counterforce equal to the weight of the water displaced. Because bone and muscle are more dense than water, and because fat is less dense than water, a person with more fat-free body mass weighs more in water than a person of the same weight with a greater percentage of body fat.

    b. Procedure

     1) The client is suspended from a scale in water and breathes out all of his or her air (**residual volume** can be indirectly measured or estimated and subtracted). While fully submerged in the water, the client then holds his or her breath for 5 seconds while weight is recorded.

     2) **Body density is then determined** through the following formula:

Body density = Weight in air/((Weight in air − Weight in Water)/Density of water) − Residual volume)

     3) Equations are then used to **convert body density into body fat percentage**. The two most common equations are:

%Fat = (457/Body density) − 414.2[1]
%Fat = (495/Body density) − 450[2]

---

[1]Equation from Brozek J, Grande F, Anderson J, Keys A: Densitometric analysis of body composition: Revision of some quantitative assumptions. *Ann NY Acad Sci* 110:113–140, 1963.
[2]Equation from Siri WE: Body composition from fluid spaces and density. *Univ Calif Donner Lab Med Phys Rep,* March 1956. Published with permission from University of California-Berkeley.

    c. Sources of Error

     1) Inaccurate measurement or estimation of lung residual volume.

     2) The great variability in bone density among individuals.

    d. Accuracy
Error is approximately 2-3% when procedures are performed correctly. Population-specific formulas can be found in *ACSM's Guidelines for Exercise Testing and Prescription,* 7th ed, Table 4-4.

  2. **Skinfold Measurements**

    a. Principle

     1) This technique assumes a relationship between subcutaneous fat and overall body fat, a predictable pattern of body fat distribution for men and for women, and a given fat-free density.

     2) **Age** is accounted for because of changes in body fat distribution with age. With aging, more fat is stored internally, thus altering the meaning of a given skinfold measure.

     3) **Body fat equations** are specific to age, gender, and ethnicity (*Table 6-3*)

    b. Procedure

     1) The **measurement technique** involves using the **thumb and index finger** to grasp a fold of skin **1 cm above** the site being measured (*Table 6-4*), placing the caliper jaws perpendicular to the fold and recording the measurement on the caliper.

     2) Hold the fold as the jaws compress, and take the measure after **1 to 2 seconds**.

     3) Rotate measures from one site to the next. Record two measurements at each site. If these two measurements vary by more than 1 cm, take a third measurement, and then average the two closest measurements.

    c. Sources of Error

     1) Improper site identification.
     2) Inaccurate calipers.
     3) Poor technique.
     4) A client who does not fit norms for standard equations (e.g., odd body fat distribution).

    d. Accuracy
Error is approximately 4% when performed correctly and the most suitable equation is used.

TABLE 6-3. Skinfold Prediction Equations

	Ethnicity	Gender	Age (years)	Equation
1	Black	Males	18–61	Db (g/cc) = 1.1120 − 0.00043499 (Σ7SKF chest, abdomen, thigh, triceps, subscapular, suprailiac, midaxillary) + 0.00000055 (Σ7SKF)^2 − 0.00028826 (age)
2	Black	Females	18–55	Db (g/cc) = 1.0970 − 0.00046971 (Σ7SKF chest, abdomen, thigh, triceps, subscapular, suprailiac, midaxillary) + 0.00000056 (Σ7SKF)^2 − 0.00012828 (age)
3	White	Males	18–61	Db (g/cc) = 1.109380 − 0.0008267 (Σ3SKF chest, abdomen, thigh) + 0.0000016 (Σ3SKF)^2 − 0.0002574 (age)
4	White	Females	18–55	Db (g/cc) = 1.0994921 − 0.0009929 (Σ3SKF triceps, suprailiac, thigh) + 0.0000023 (Σ3SKF)^2 − 0.0001392 (age)
5	Hispanic	Females	20–40	Db (g/cc) = 1.0970 − 0.00046971 (Σ3SKF chest, abdomen, thigh, triceps, subscapular, suprailiac, midaxillary) + 0.00000056 (Σ7SKF)^2 − 0.00012828 (age)
6	Black & white	Males	≤18	%BF = 0.735 (Σ2SKF triceps, calf) + 1.0
7	Black & white	Males (SKF, >35 mm)	≤18	%BF = 0.735 (Σ2SKF triceps, subscapular) + 1.6.
8	Black & white	Males (SKF, >35 mm)	≤18	%BF = 0.783 (Σ2SKF triceps, subscapular) − 0.008 (Σ2SKF)^2 + 1[a]
9	Black & white	Females	≤18	%BF = 0.610(Σ2SKF triceps, calf) + 5.1
10	Black & white	Females (SKF, >35 mm)	≤18	%BF = 0.546 (Σ2SKF triceps, subscapular) + 9.7
11	Black & white	Females (SKF, >35 mm)	≤18	%BF = 1.33 (Σ2SKF triceps, subscapular) − 0.013 (Σ2SKF)^2 − 2.5

[a]Intercept substitutions based on maturation and ethnicity for boys.

Age	Black	White
Prepubescent	−3.2	−1.7
Pubescent	−5.2	−3.4
Postpubescent	−6.8	−5.5

(Adapted from Heyward VH, Stolarcyzk LM: *Applied Body Composition Assessment*. Champaign, IL, Human Kinetics, 1996, pp 173–185.)

TABLE 6-4. Standardized Description of Skinfold Sites and Procedures

Skinfold Site

Abdominal	Vertical fold; 2 cm to the right side of the umbilicus
Triceps	Vertical fold; on the posterior midline of the upper arm, halfway between the acromion and olecranon processes, with the arm held freely to the side of the body
Biceps	Vertical fold; on the anterior aspect of the arm over the belly of the biceps muscle, 1 cm above the level used to mark the triceps site
Chest/pectoral	Diagonal fold; half the distance between the anterior axillary line and the nipple (men) or a third the distance between the anterior axillary line and the nipple (women)
Medial calf	Vertical fold; at the maximum circumference of the calf on the midline of its medial border
Midaxillary	Vertical fold; on the midaxillary line at the level of the xiphoid process of the sternum (an alternate method is a horizontal fold taken at the level of the xiphoid/sternal border in the midaxillary line)
Subscapular	Diagonal fold (45° angle); 1 to 2 cm below the inferior angle of the scapula
Suprailiac	Diagonal fold; in line with the natural angle of the iliac crest taken in the anterior axillary line immediately superior to the iliac crest
Thigh	Vertical fold; on the anterior midline of the thigh, midway between the proximal border of the patella and the inguinal crease (hip)

Procedures

- All measurements should be made on the right side of the body
- Caliper should be placed 1 cm away from the thumb and finger, perpendicular to the skinfold, and halfway between the crest and the base of the fold
- Pinch should be maintained while reading the caliper
- Wait 1 to 2 seconds (no longer) before reading caliper
- Take duplicate measures at each site and retest if duplicate measurements are not within 1 to 2 mm
- Rotate through measurement sites or allow time for skin to regain normal texture and thickness

(From *ACSM's Guidelines for Exercise Testing and Prescription*, 6th ed. Philadelphia, Lippincott Williams & Wilkins, 2000, p 65.)

3. **Anthropometry**
   a. Theoretical Basis
      1) Measurements of height, weight, and/or girth provide information about the relative distribution of body mass compared with "standard" distributions.
      2) The addition of anthropometric measurements to skinfold measurements may be used to predict "body fatness."
   b. Procedures
      Height and weight should be measured, and appropriate sites for the anthropometric measures are required.
   c. Sources of Error
      1) Inaccurate stance for assessing height.
      2) Unfamiliarity with the use of balance scales.
      3) Incorrect location of circumference site.
      4) Incorrect placement of the tape measure around the body segment to be measured.
      5) Inappropriate tension in the use of the tape measure.
   d. Accuracy
      Error is approximately 3% to 8% when performed correctly.
4. **Body Mass Index (BMI)**
   a. This basic weight-for-height ratio $(kg \cdot dL^{-1})$ can be quickly determined using a standard nomogram. The results are compared to a standard table to classify obesity according to a BMI value (*Table 6-5*)
   b. The BMI is commonly used in large population studies. It has been found to correlate with incidence of certain chronic diseases (e.g., hyperlipidemia).

TABLE 6-5. Classification of Disease Risk Based on Body Mass Index (BMI) and Waist Circumference*

	BMI (kg·m⁻²)	Disease Risk† Relative to Normal Weight and Waist Circumference	
		Men, ≤102 cm Women, ≤88 cm	Men, >102 cm Women, >88 cm
Underweight	<18.5	-	-
Normal	18.5–24.9	-	-
Overweight	25.0–29.9	Increased	High
Obesity, class			
I	30.0–34.9	High	Very high
II	35.0–39.9	Very high	Very high
III	≥40	Extremely high	Extremely high

*Modified from Expert Panel. Executive summary of the clinical guidelines on the identification, evaluation and treatment of overweight and obesity in adults. Arch Intern Med 1998;158:1855–1867.

†Disease risk for Type 2 diabetes, hypertension, and cardiovascular disease. Dashes (-) indicate that no additional risk at these levels of BMI was assigned. Increased waist circumference can also be a marker for increased risk even in persons of normal weight.

   c. **The BMI should not be used to assess an individual's body fat** during a fitness assessment, because it does not take into account fat-free density and skeletal mass.
5. **Waist-to-Hip Ratio (WHR)**
   A simple index of upper versus lower body fat distribution, WHR provides a predictor of disease risk related to fat distribution. First, waist circumference and hip circumference are measured. Then, WHR is calculated using a standard nomogram and is compared to available standards (*Table 6-6*).
6. **Bioelectrical Impedance Analysis**
   a. This quick, noninvasive method of measuring fat and fat-free body mass is relatively inexpensive and does not require a highly skilled technician.
   b. In the most common form, four electrodes are placed on the client's skin (typically two on the right hand and two on the right foot), and a high-frequency, low-level excitation current is sent through the body.
   c. Because electrical conductivity varies based on the fat content of tissue (fat-free tissue is a good conductor, whereas fat is not), the measured resistance to current flow correlates with body features.
   d. Sources of Error
      1) Inappropriate skin preparation.
      2) Inaccurate electrode placement.
      3) Lack of adherence to pretest diet/exercise recommendations.
      4) Use of inappropriate prediction equation.
      5) Inadequate hydration.
      6) Body temperature.
   e. Accuracy
      Error is 4% to 5% error when performed correctly.
7. **Near-Infrared Interactance**
   a. This technique, which is based on principles of light absorption and reflection, uses near-infrared spectroscopy to measure body composition.
      1) A fiberoptic probe is placed on a body site (e.g., biceps), and the infrared beam penetrates the skin.
      2) The measurement of reflected light is related to subcutaneous fat.
   b. Accuracy
      Error is 4% to 11% when performed appropriately.
8. **Dual-Energy X-Ray Absorptiometry**
   a. In this technique, an emitter passes photons at two different energies (one deep and one shallow) through body tissue, and

TABLE 6-6. Waist-To-Hip Circumference Ratio Standards for Men and Women

			Disease Risk Related to Obesity		
	Age	Low	Moderate	High	Very High
Men	20–29	<0.83	0.83–0.88	0.89–0.94	>0.94
	30–39	<0.84	0.84–0.91	0.92–0.96	>0.96
	40–49	<0.88	0.88–0.95	0.96–1.00	>1.00
	50–59	<0.90	0.90–0.96	0.97–1.02	>1.02
	60–69	<0.91	0.91–0.98	0.99–1.03	>1.03
Women	20–29	<0.71	0.71–0.77	0.78–0.82	>0.82
	30–39	<0.72	0.72–0.78	0.79–0.84	>0.84
	40–49	<0.73	0.73–0.79	0.80–0.87	>0.87
	50–59	<0.74	0.74–0.81	0.82–0.88	>0.88
	60–69	<0.76	0.76–0.83	0.84–0.90	>0.90

(With permission from Heyward VH, Stolarcyzk LM: *Applied Body Composition Assessment.* Champaign, IL, Human Kinetics, 1996, p 82.).

a scanner analyzes the energy that passes through the tissue.

b. A computer calculates fat, bone, and muscle tissue based on pixel strength.

H. CARDIORESPIRATORY FITNESS

1. **Purpose of Assessment**
   a. To measure variables such as heart rate, blood pressure, and oxygen uptake during exercise
   b. To evaluate the body's ability to absorb, distribute, and utilize oxygen.
   c. To help screen for CAD.
   d. To collect baseline and follow-up information for charting a client's fitness program progress to help motivate a client by establishing and meeting reasonable fitness goals.

2. **Basic Skills Needed to Assess Cardiorespiratory Fitness**
   a. Heart Rate Determination
      1) **Palpation**
         a) Heart rate can be determined by counting the number of pulses in a given period of time (10–30 seconds).
         b) The most common sites at which the pulse may be palpated include:
            (i) The radial artery.
            (ii) The carotid artery.
      2) **Auscultation**
         a) A stethoscope may be placed over the left aspect of the mid-sternum or just under the pectoralis major.
         b) Heart rate may be counted as the number of heart beats in a given period of time (10–30 seconds).

3) Electronic Monitoring
   a) Radiofrequency Transmitters
      (i) A chest strap with embedded electrodes is fastened around the chest just under the pectoral muscles.
      (ii) The electrodes sense the electrical current associated with the electrical activity of the heart to measure heart rate.
   b) Pulsatile Blood Flow Monitors
      (i) Sensors affixed to the ear lobe or finger sense the pulsing of blood.
      (ii) Some devices are currently not effective in monitoring exercise heart rate.

b. Blood Pressure Measurement
   Equipment for blood pressure measurement includes:
   1) **Sphygmomanometer.**
      A sphygmomanometer has three important components:
      a) A cloth cuff placed around the upper arm. Encased in the cuff is a bladder made of rubber or similar material.
      b) A diaphragmatic bulb and valve, which are used to increase or decrease the pressure in the cuff.
      c) A mercury column or aneroid (air pressure) manometer, which are used to indicate the pressure in the cuff.

2) **Stethoscope**

A stethoscope has two important components:

a) A diaphragm to focus sound waves.

b) Earpieces to direct the sound waves.

c. **Rating of Perceived Exertion (RPE)**

1) Provides the exercise professional with an indication of a subjective assessment of the relative intensity of the exercise.

2) Correlates well with such physiologic measures heart rate and percentage maximal oxygen uptake ($\dot{V}O_2$max).

3) Currently, two scales for assessing RPE are widely used:

a) Original Scale

(i) Ratings are from 6 to 20.

(ii) This scale was developed largely based on the linear response of $\dot{V}O_2$max and heart rate to changing exercise intensity.

b) Revised Scale

(i) Ratings are from 0 to 10.

(ii) The revised scale was based not only on the $\dot{V}O_2$max and heart rate responses to exercise but also on lactate accumulation and ventilation during exercise.

3. **Timing of Measurements During Assessments**

During most graded exercise tests, the following measurements are taken at the indicated times:

a. Heart Rate

1) During a 2-minute stage: every minute

2) During a 3-minute stage: at minutes 2 and 3, and then at every subsequent minute until steady state is achieved

b. Blood Pressure

Measured once during each stage, toward the end of the stage.

c. Rating of Perceived Exertion

Assessed once during each stage, toward the end of the stage.

d. Sequence of Measurements

For most graded exercise tests (with 3-minute stages), it is practical to take the measurements according to the following schedule:

1) At 2:00 minutes: heart rate.

2) At 2:15 minutes: RPE.

3) At 2:30 minutes: blood pressure.

4) At 3:00 minutes: heart rate.

4. **Equipment Calibration**

Accuracy of instrumentation is essential for valid assessments of cardiorespiratory endurance and all other areas of health-related fitness. All equipment should be calibrated at regular intervals. A regular schedule for equipment calibration should be established for all testing equipment.

a. **Cycle Ergometer**

Workload ($kg \cdot m \cdot min^{-1}$) is determined by **resistance × distance flywheel traveled per revolution ÷ revolutions per minute**.

1) Resistance

a) On most mechanically braked ergometers, calibration requires identification of the attachment of the resistance pendulum to the resistance belt.

b) The zero mark on the resistance indicator is checked and adjusted as required.

c) A known weight is hung from the point at which the resistance belt is attached to the pendulum.

d) The resistance should be checked at each resistance that might be used during testing.

e) Any discrepancies in the resistance markings are noted on a new scale, which is fastened over the original resistance markings.

2) Distance per Revolution

The distance the flywheel travels per revolution of the pedal must be accurately determined by measuring the circumference of the flywheel, then determining the number of flywheel revolutions per pedal revolution.

3) Revolutions Pedaled per Minute (rpm)

a) Because the workload on a cycle ergometer is expressed in $kg \cdot m \cdot min^{-1}$, it is necessary to check the accuracy of the device used to determine the rpm.

b) A mechanical or electronic metronome may be checked for accuracy using an accurate clock or stopwatch.

b. Treadmill Calibration

1) Speed

Calibrating the speed of a motorized treadmill requires knowledge of both the length of the treadmill belt and the number of revolutions of the belt per minute.

    a)   The length of the belt may be measured using a long cloth tape or a rolling measuring device.

    b)   The treadmill rpm is determined by marking a fixed point on the belt and a corresponding point on the treadmill frame or other fixed object, then measuring the time needed for a fixed number of revolutions (e.g., 20 for slower speeds, 50 for higher speeds).

  2)   Grade

    a)   The grade of a treadmill is expressed as the relationship of rise to run.

      (i)   The **run** is the distance between two fixed points on the floor or other flat surface.

      (ii)   The **rise** is the difference between two perpendicular distances measured from the belt surface to the floor.

    b)   Treadmill grade is determined by dividing the rise by the run and expressing the result as a percentage.

5.   **Protocol Selection**

Test selection is influenced by the purpose and goals of the exercise test and by characteristics of the client being tested.

  a.   **Maximal Testing**

    1)   A maximal exercise test can be most effective in detecting CAD and accurately measuring $\dot{V}O_2$max (using on-line measurements of expired gases or estimated using prediction equations).

    2)   The choice of maximal testing should be based on the reason for the exercise test (e.g., CAD screening, functional capacity measurement).

    3)   Maximal testing is expensive, and guidelines for testing various populations and age groups should be followed (*Table 6-7*)

  b.   **Submaximal Testing**

    1)   Submaximal exercise tests are used extensively to assess fitness, to evaluate changes in fitness following a training program, and to provide an estimate of $\dot{V}O_2$max for establishing an initial training program.

    2)   Submaximal testing estimates $\dot{V}O_2$max based on the assumed linear relationship between heart rate and $\dot{V}O_2$max. Heart rate is measured at multiple workloads during the test, and $\dot{V}O_2$max at an estimated maximum

TABLE 6-7. ACSM Recommendations for A) Medical Examination and Exercise Testing Prior to Exercise Participation and B) Medical Supervision of Submaximal and Maximal Exercise Testing

	Risk Strata[a]		
	Low Risk	Moderate Risk	High Risk
A.			
Moderate Exercise[b]	Not necessary[c]	Not necessary	Recommended
Vigorous Exercise[d]	Not necessary	Recommended	Recommended
B.			
Submaximal Exercise Test	Not necessary	Not necessary	Recommended[e]
Maximal Exercise Test	Not necessary	Recommended[e]	Recommended

[a] See section I.B.2. in this chapter

[b] Moderate Exercise = 40-59% of $\dot{V}O_2R$

[c] Not necessary reflects the notion that a medical examination, exercise test, and medical supervision would not be essential; however, they should not be viewed as inappropriate

[d] Vigorous Exercise Intensity ≥ 60% $\dot{V}O_2R$

[e] When medical supervision is recommended, the physician should be in proximity and readily available should there be an emergent need.

(Modified from Table 2-1 from *Guidelines for Exercise Testing and Prescription,* 7th ed. Baltimore: Lippincott Williams & Wilkins, 2005)

heart rate (220 − Age) is calculated (*Figure 6-2*)

3) **Submaximal testing is based on several assumptions**:
   a) Measurements are made while the client is **in steady state**.
   b) A linear relationship exists between heart rate and $\dot{V}O_2$.
   c) Maximal heart rate is similar for all individuals in a given age group.
   d) Mechanical efficiency is the same for all clients.

c. Discontinuous and Continuous Protocols
   1) In a **discontinuous test protocol**, the test is momentarily stopped. Measurements are obtained, and the test is then resumed. Discontinuous protocols are generally used only in special circumstances because of the lengthy time such a test requires. Examples include:
      a) Individuals being tested using arm ergometry, stopping for blood pressure measurement.
      b) Clients with claudication who develop leg pain and need rest periods.

   2) **A continuous test protocol**, which is the most common form, involves multiple stages of increasing work intensity with no stoppages.

d. Protocol Selection for Overweight Clients
   1) During weight-bearing exercise, a client's absolute oxygen costs are directly proportional to his or her body mass.
   2) In some cases, weight-supported exercise (e.g., cycle ergometry) is preferred for an overweight client to minimize orthopedic stress and to reduce the risk of injury.

e. Protocol Selection for Children
   1) **Physical fitness testing** is common in school-based physical education programs to evaluate skill-related fitness and, most importantly, health-related fitness (*Tables 6-8 and 6-9*).
   2) **Clinical exercise testing** is also performed to screen for preexisting cardiorespiratory disease in children.
   3) **Challenges** involved in testing children include the difficulty of assessing changes in physical fitness as a result of training or maturation.
   4) **Contraindications** to exercise testing in children include:
      a) Acute inflammatory disease.
      b) MI.
      c) Pulmonary disease.
      d) Renal disease.
      e) Hepatitis.
      f) Uncontrolled congestive heart failure.
      g) Severe systemic hypertension.
      h) Use of any medication that affects the cardiovascular response to exercise.

f. Protocol Selection for the Elderly
   1) Exercise testing in the elderly must take into account **age-related changes** in cardiovascular and other

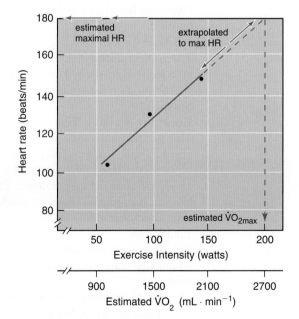

FIGURE 6-2. Heart rate (HR) obtained from at least two (more are preferable) submaximal exercise intensities may be extrapolated to the age-predicted maximal HR. A vertical line to the intensity scale estimates maximal exercise intensity, from which an estimated maximum oxygen uptake ($\dot{V}O_2$max) can be calculated.

TABLE 6-8. Field Tests for Children

Health Fitness Component	Field Test
Cardiorespiratory fitness	1-mile walk/run
Muscular fitness	Curl-up test
	Pull-ups/push-up test
Flexibility	Sit and reach test
Body composition	Body mass index or skinfolds

(From *ACSM's Guidelines for Exercise Testing and Prescription*, 7th ed. Baltimore, Lippincott Williams & Wilkins, 2005, p 241.)

TABLE 6-9. Protocols Suitable for Graded Exercise Testing of Children

Modified Balke Treadmill Protocol

Subject	Speed (mph)	Initial Grade (%)	Increment (%)	Stage Duration (min)
Poorly fit	3.00	6	2	2
Sedentary	3.25	6	2	2
Active	5.00	0	2.5	2
Athlete	5.25	0	2.5	2

The McMaster Cycle Test

Height (cm)	Initial Load (W)	Increments (W)	Step Duration (min)
<120	12.5	12.5	2
120–139.9	12.5	25	2
140–159.9	25	25	2
≥160	25	50 (boys)	2
		25 (girls)	

(Adapted from Skinner J: *Exercise Testing and Exercise Prescription for Special Cases,* 2nd ed. Philadelphia, Lea & Febiger, 1993.)

physiological variables. These variables include:

   a)   Maximal heart rate.

   b)   Maximal cardiac output.

   c) $\dot{V}O_2$max.

   d)   Resting and exercise blood pressure.

   e)   Residual volume.

   f)   Vital capacity.

   g)   Reaction time.

   h)   Muscular strength.

   i)   Bone mass.

   j)   Flexibility.

   k)   Glucose tolerance.

   l)   Body fat percentage.

2)   Other factors to consider include the great **variations in physiological status** in elderly clients caused by differing levels of activity and the presence of underlying disease.

3)   Modifications to standard test protocols may be needed for severely deconditioned clients or those with physical limitations.

4)   Given the longer adaptation time to a workload in elderly compared to younger adults, a **prolonged warm-up phase is recommended**.

g. Protocol Selection for Clients with Cardiorespiratory Disorders

  1)   Exercise testing may help to differentiate exercise-induced breathlessness from dyspnea caused by cardiorespiratory disease.

  2)   Oxygen uptake, ventilation, and oxygen saturation should be measured during exercise testing, because desaturation is possible during exercise.

3)   Test protocol selection should be individualized, because each client will respond differently. Protocols should be adjusted to achieve a test duration of 8 to 12 minutes.

6. **Modes of Exercise Testing**

a. **Field Tests**

These tests can be administered with minimal equipment and in clients with varying conditions.

  1)   **Cooper 12-Minute Test**

The subject must cover the greatest distance possible during the 12-minute test period. The $\dot{V}O_2$max is estimated based on the distance covered.

  2)   **1.5-Mile Test**

The subject must cover 1.5 miles as rapidly as possible. The $\dot{V}O_2$max is estimated on the basis of this time.

  3)   **Rockport Walking Test**

This submaximal test requires the client to walk 1 mile as fast as possible, with the heart rate measured for 15 seconds immediately posttest. The $\dot{V}O_2$max is predicted based on gender, time, and heart rate.

  4)   Limitations

Although these tests are easy to administer, they have certain limitations:

    a)   An individual's motivation may influence his or her test performance and, thus, the accuracy of the test.

    b)   Clients unaccustomed to the test may pace themselves inappropriately, which may affect results.

   c) Because the client is not monitored (heart rate, blood pressure, symptoms), those who are at risk or older should not be tested using this method.

b. **Nuclear/Radionuclide Imaging**

In these exercise tests, radioactive substances are injected into the bloodstream to visualize aspects of the circulatory system more closely. This technique helps to increase test sensitivity and specificity.

1) **Perfusion Imaging**

   a) During the last minute of a standard stress test, thallium-201 is injected into the bloodstream. Thallium-201 enters myocardial cells in proportion to the amount of blood flow to those cells and emits energy detectable with a scintillation counter.

   b) Images of the myocardium can be constructed immediately following a stress test and 4 to 24 hours later.

     (i) Areas with little or no perfusion immediately following a test indicate areas of ischemia.

     (ii) Any "cold spots" remaining 4 to 24 hours later indicate necrotic tissue.

   c) Areas of reversible ischemia will reperfuse, and cold spots will disappear in later testing.

   d) **Single-photon emission computed tomography (SPECT)** enhances sensitivity and also allows for multidimensional viewing.

2) **Ventriculography**

To visualize the resting and exercise cardiac functions related to cardiac output, ejection fraction, and wall motion, a test such as a **multiple-gated acquisition study (MUGA)** is performed.

   a) Technetium-99m is injected into the bloodstream, where it attaches to red blood cells.

   b) Areas where the blood pools (e.g., ventricles) are visual-

ized by the technetium emissions.

   c) Changes in ejection fraction or wall motion abnormalities may be indicative of a failing heart or compromised blood flow through the coronary circulation.

c. **Exercise Echocardiography**

This technique uses ECG monitoring to identify the cardiac cycle, along with high-frequency sound waves to evaluate cardiac wall motion and pump function. Measurements can be made during or immediately after stationary cycle ergometry.

d. Pharmacologic Testing

1) In some instances, a client is not able to complete an exercise stress test because of muscular limitations, neurologic disability, peripheral vascular disease, or other conditions that prevent a person from achieving a sufficient work intensity to provide an accurate cardiovascular assessment.

2) **Two common tests** are used that do not involve exercise but, rather, drug-induced changes in cardiovascular work.

   a) **Dipyridamole (Persantine) Perfusion Imaging**

     (i) Infusion of dipyridamole causes vasodilation of normal coronary arteries, with little effect on narrowed arteries.

     (ii) Dipyridamole is often used in conjunction with a nuclear imaging agent (e.g., thallium) and a nuclear imaging technique (e.g., thallium scanning, SPECT).

     (iii) Arteries are visualized before and after drug administration, and the findings are compared.

   b) **Dobutamine Testing**

     (i) Dobutamine infusion elevates heart rate and increases myocardial oxygen demand.

     (ii) When used in concert with echocardiography, dobutamine testing can elicit abnormalities of heart wall motion.

e. **Holter ECG Monitoring**
   1) This test is used to track ECG abnormalities during the course of a day.
   2) Generally, a single-lead ECG is connected to a battery pack and a recorder.
   3) The ECG monitoring is done continuously for up to 24 hours and is recorded. The client records his or her activities during the day as well as any symptoms experienced during these activities.
   4) The ECG tracings are reviewed and compared with the client's activity log to identify precipitating events for ECG abnormalities.

I. **MUSCULAR FITNESS**
   1. **Muscular Strength Assessment**
      a. Purposes
         1) To determine maximum strength to create a prudent strength-training program.
         2) To monitor progress and revise the strength-training program.
         3) To determine physical strength for performing standardized work tasks (e.g., preemployment screenings).
      b. **Resistance Training Methods**
         1) In **isotonic (free-weight) training**, the weight is held constant through the range of motion (ROM), but speed can vary with client movement.
         2) In **isokinetic training**, the speed of movement is kept constant through the ROM, but force can vary with client movement.
         3) In **variable-resistance training**, the weight is altered using mechanical assistance to compensate for changes in the muscle's ability to generate force because of changes in the lever system.
         4) In **isometric (static) training**, the joint angle remains constant while force is exerted.
      c. Strength-Testing Devices
         1) **Cable Tensiometer**
            This device measures static strength by measuring force exerted while pulling on a steel cable. Various limbs can be tested, and varying the length of the cables can assess different joint angles.
            a) Advantages
               (i) It can assess strength for almost all major muscle groups.
               (ii) Results are reliable.
            b) Disadvantages
               (i) Strength is assessed statically.
               (ii) Results may not apply to dynamic movements in demonstrating strength.
         2) **Dynamometer**
            This is a more portable static strength-testing device that generally tests leg, back, and forearm strength.
            a) Advantages
               (i) Portable.
               (ii) Less cumbersome than cable tensiometers.
               (iii) Numerous clients can be tested quickly.
            b) Disadvantages
               (i) Only a limited number of muscle groups can be tested.
               (ii) Reliability is questionable.
         3) **Strain Gauge**
            a) Thin electroconductive material is placed over machined metal parts and connected to an electrical source. As force is exerted, the gauge is bent or deformed, altering its electrical conductivity. Measurement of the change in conductivity reflects the amount of force generated.
            b) For example, a strain gauge is installed on the crank arm of a cycle ergometer pedal. As the cyclist pushes on the crank (pedals), the arm bends, changing the strain gauge's conductivity and allowing measurement of force.
      d. **One-Repetition Maximum (1-RM) Testing**
         1) Assesses the maximum amount of weight that can be lifted one time for a given exercise.
         2) Begins with a weight that the client can lift easily. Following a successful lift, the client rests for 2 to 3 minutes. Then, 5 to 10 pounds of weight are added, and the client lifts again.

3) Generally, four to six trials are needed to determine the 1-RM.
4) Advantages
   a) Easy to administer
   b) Multiple muscle groups can be tested.
   c) The same equipment used for testing can often be used for training.
   d) Provides a measure of dynamic strength, which is most applicable to real-world settings.
5) Disadvantages
   a) In unconditioned clients, posttest muscle soreness is likely.
   b) Strength is limited by the weakest point in the ROM.
   c) The tester needs to take into account the skill involved with each lift and ensure the client can safely and effectively perform the lifts.
6) Submaximal Tests to Estimate Strength
   a) Submaximal lifts to fatigue are commonly used to estimate the 1-RM.
   b) The weight used for the submaximal assessment must be carefully selected so that the client performs from 2 to 14 repetitions before fatigue.
e. Equipment
   Common equipment includes:
   1) Free weights (e.g., barbells, dumbbells), which require the lifter to determine the planes of movement
   2) Variable-resistance machines, for which the plane and range of movement are limited by the machine and the resistance is increased by adding additional plates of weight to the stack being lifted.
   3) Isokinetic machines, which limit movement to a constant velocity.
   4) Isometric equipment (e.g., handgrip dynamometers), which measure strength at a constant joint angle.
f. Safety
   To reduce the risk of injury during assessments of muscular strength, address the following items:
   1) One or more properly trained spotters should assist the lifter.

2) Proper form should be demonstrated by the exercise professional and be required of the lifter.
3) The lifter should be coached to breathe during both concentric (exhale) and eccentric (inhale) movements.
4) Adequate rest should be provided between lifting attempts.
g. Special Considerations
   1) Muscle force varies over joint ROM because of changes in joint angle. Therefore, dynamic muscle strength testing (1-RM) is not useful for establishing strength throughout the ROM.
   2) Acceleration and inertia can both influence the performance of a dynamic strength test. Therefore, dynamic strength testing should be standardized with regard to velocity.
   3) Body position must be stabilized to isolate the muscle group being tested.

2. **Muscular Endurance Assessment**
   These techniques assess the client's ability to exert a submaximal force repeatedly.
   a. **Static Endurance**
      1) A submaximal force is held for as long as possible. Time is measured as an index of endurance performance.
      2) The same devices used to assess static strength can be used in this technique. In addition, measuring the drop in force with time will give an index of fatigue/muscular endurance.
   b. **Dynamic Endurance**
      1) Maximum repetitions completed at a set percentage of 1-RM and/or body weight, taking into account the size of the muscle mass being assessed (e.g., chest endurance, 50% of 1-RM or 60% of body weight; biceps endurance, 50% of 1-RM or 15% of body weight).
      2) **Isokinetic endurance** measures the number of repetitions completed above 50% of maximal torque.
      3) **Calisthenic tests** include sit-ups, push-ups, and pull-ups. The number of repetitions is assessed with the client lifting his or her own body weight.

4) Clients who are not physically fit may be able to complete only a few repetitions. Thus, these tests may be more useful for assessing strength than for assessing endurance.

3. **Flexibility Assessment**

a. Definition

1) Flexibility is the **functional range of motion (ROM) about a joint**.

2) Flexibility is specific to each joint and, therefore, can vary from one joint to another.

3) The functional ROM refers to **the ability to move the joint without incurring pain** or a limit to performance.

b. Rationale for Assessment

1) Inadequate flexibility is associated with decreased performance of activities of independent living and decreased ability to engage in specific physical movements.

2) Flexibility can decrease quickly with chronic disuse or improve significantly with appropriate exercise intervention.

c. Procedure

1) Depending on the joint, **flexion, extension, rotation, abduction, adduction, supination, pronation, or deviation can be assessed** (*Table 6-10 and Figure 6-3*).

2) The client should **warm up** before flexibility testing by lightly exercising the joint to be tested. This promotes a more accurate measure of flexibility and reduces the risk of injury.

3) Measurements are taken with the limb starting in an anatomically neutral position to improve reliability.

4) **Repeated measurements** of flexibility are essential to ensure accurate assessment of ROM.

d. Measurement Devices

1) Portable and cost-effective **goniometers** consist of two arms that intersect at a disk that can measure 360° of movement. One arm is held on the stationary portion of the limb; the other moves with the portion of the joint that moves.

2) **Inclinometers/fleximeters** are either handheld or attached to a limb, head, or trunk to measure ROM. These

TABLE 6-10. Range of Motion of the Major Joints

Join	Motion	Average Ranges (°)
Spinal		
Cervical	Flexion	0–60
	Extension	0–75
	Lateral flexion	0–45
	Rotation	0–80
Thoracic	Flexion	0–50
	Rotation	0–30
Lumbar	Flexion	0–60
	Extension	0–25
	Lateral flexion	0–25
Upper Extremity		
Shoulder	Flexion	0–180
	Extension	0–50
	Abduction	0–180
	Adduction	0–50
	Internal rotation	0–90
	External rotation	0–90
Elbow	Flexion	0–140
Forearm	Supination	0–80
	Pronation	0–80
Wrist	Flexion	0–60
	Extension	0–60
	Ulnar deviation	0–30
	Radial deviation	0–20
Thumb	Abduction	0–60
	Flexion	
	Carpal-metacarpal	0–15
	Metacarpal-phalangeal	0–50
	Interphalangeal	0–80
	Extension	
	Carpal-metacarpal	0–20
	Metacarpal-phalangeal	0–5
	Interphalangeal	0–20
Fingers	Flexion	
	Metacarpal-phalangeal	0–90
	Proximal Interphalangeal	0–100
	Distal Interphalangeal	0–80
	Extension	
	Metacarpal-phalangeal	0–45
Lower Extremity		
Hip	Flexion	0–100
	Extension	0–30
	Abduction	0–40
	Adduction	0–20
	Internal rotation	0–40
	External rotation	0–50
Knee	Flexion	0–150
Ankle	Dorsiflexion	0–20
	Plantarflexion	0–40
Subtalar	Inversion	0–30
	Eversion	0–20

devices, which have a high measurement reliability, are excellent to use when a goniometer is not feasible.

3) **Tape measures** can accurately measure lateral trunk flexion and lumbar flexion as well as changes in ROM in the carpometacarpal and interphalangeal joints.

Hip Flexibility Screening

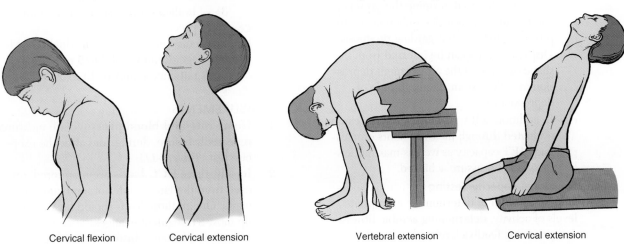

Internal rotation

External rotation

Straight leg raising

Combined flexion and extension

Neck and Trunk Flexibility Screening

Cervical flexion

Cervical extension

Vertebral extension

Cervical extension

FIGURE 6-3. Top: Hip flexibility screening. *Internal rotation* involves flexing the hip and knee and moving the leg as far to the side as possible by rolling the thigh. *External rotation* involves moving the leg as far as possible past the midline by rolling the thigh outward. *Straight leg raising* consists of keeping the contralateral lower extremity in full extension while lifting the other extremity without bending the knee. Note the limited hamstring flexibility. In the *combined test of hip flexion and extension,* one bent hip and knee are brought as close to the chest as possible, while allowing the other limb to drop over the edge of the table into extension (Thomas Test for hip extension). Bottom: Neck and trunk flexibility screening. In *cervical flexion,* the chin should touch the chest. *Cervical extension* involves bending the head as far as possible posteriorly. In *vertebral flexion,* with the hips and knees bent, the trunk should touch the anterior thighs. *Vertebral extension* involves backward movement of the trunk as far posterior as possible without hip extension. (Modified from *ACSM's Resource Manual for Guidelines for Exercise Testing and Prescription,* 4th ed. Baltimore, Lippincott Williams & Wilkins, 2001, pp 385–386.)

III. Clinical Exercise Testing

A. INDICATIONS

1. **Predischarge Exercise Testing Following MI**

   a. This testing is done to determine minimal standards of functional capacity and to **evaluate the client's ability to perform activities of daily living**.

   b. This testing is also conducted to evaluate the **effectiveness of medications** and the client's hemodynamic response to exercise.

   c. This testing can reassure the client (and family members) of his or her capacity for physical work.

2. **Postdischarge Exercise Testing Following MI or Cardiac Surgery**

   a. Testing can demonstrate the **degree of improvement since discharge**. Maximal testing is usually conducted 3 to 6 weeks after the event.

   b. Results are used to design an exercise program, to identify signs or symptoms, and to aid decisions on medication adjustments.

3. **Diagnostic Testing and Determination of Disease Severity and Prognosis**

   a. Maximal testing with measures of heart rate, blood pressure, and ECG is the most cost-effective screening tool for detecting signs and symptoms of heart disease.

   b. Individuals diagnosed with heart disease are also tested to determine the presence and extent of myocardial ischemia and to provide information regarding prognosis.

   c. Disease severity can be inferred from the shape or slope of the ST-segment depression as well as from the magnitude of depression.

   d. In addition, left ventricular function can be evaluated through measurements of maximal MET capacity as well as maximal systolic blood pressure achieved.

4. **Functional Capacity Testing**
   Testing is useful in determining appropriate levels of activity, determining aerobic fitness, and providing feedback related to fitness improvements as part of a training program.

B. EXERCISE TEST MODALITIES AND PROTOCOLS

1. **Treadmill**
   In this common test modality, the client walks or runs at a predetermined pace on a treadmill whose grade can be adjusted. By raising the grade of the treadmill, the tester increases stress on the client. Both ECG and blood pressure readings evaluate the effects of this stress.

   a. In the **Bruce protocol**, work rate is increased in 3-MET increments in 3-minute stages by gradually increasing both the grade and speed of the treadmill. Although this protocol is widely used, it may not be appropriate for less-fit individuals.

   b. For clients who can complete only a submaximal protocol, the **modified Bruce protocol** may be used. This involves gradually increasing the grade while maintaining a constant low speed (1.7 mph).

   c. A variation of the Bruce protocol is the **ramp protocol**, which uses both grade and speed increases, but at a slower pace than in the Bruce protocol, to increase the work rate.

   d. Other treadmill protocols include the **Balke-Ware, Naughton** (both of which are most appropriate for less-fit clients), and **Ellestad** (appropriate for fit clients).

2. **Cycle Ergometer**

   a. Cycle ergometry has several advantages over the treadmill:

      1) It keeps the upper body stable, ensuring more accurate ECG and blood pressure measurements.

      2) It supports the client's body weight, making it more appropriate for clients with poor balance.

      3) It allows work rate to be set more precisely.

   b. Protocols can be easily individualized. Most use stage durations of 2 to 5 minutes and work rate increments of 15 to 50 W.

C. MEASUREMENTS

1. **Heart rate and blood pressure** are measured repeatedly before, during, and after the exercise test (*Table 6-11*).

2. Ideally, three **ECG leads** are monitored, one each from the lateral, inferior, and anterior views. One of those leads should be V_5 to pick up most ST-segment changes.

3. Monitoring for any **clinical signs** (e.g., changes in gait, skin color, or responsiveness) that may develop during the test helps to identify test termination criteria and enhances client safety.

4. The client's subjective report of **ratings of perceived exertion (RPE)** reflects his or her perception of work effort during testing.

TABLE 6-11. Sequence of Measures for Heart Rate, Blood Pressure, Rating of Perceived Exertion (RPE), and Electrocardiogram (ECG) During Exercise Testing

Pretest
1. 12-Lead ECG in supine and exercise postures
2. Blood pressure measurements in the supine position and exercise posture

Exercise[a]
1. 12-Lead ECG recorded during last 15 seconds of every stage and at peak exercise (3-lead ECG observed/recorded every minute on monitor)
2. Blood pressure measurements should be obtained during the last minute of each stage[b]
3. Rating scales: RPE at the end of each stage, other scales if applicable

Posttest
1. 12-Lead ECG immediately after exercise, then every 1 to 2 minutes for at least 5 minutes to allow any exercise-induced changes to return to baseline
2. Blood pressure measurements should be obtained immediately after exercise, then every 1 to 2 minutes until stabilized near baseline level
3. Symptomatic ratings should be obtained using appropriate scales as long as symptoms persist after exercise

[a]In addition, these referenced variables should be assessed and recorded whenever adverse symptoms or abnormal ECG changes occur.

[b]An unchanged or decreasing systolic blood pressure with increasing workloads should be retaken (verified immediately).

(From *ACSM's Guidelines for Exercise Testing and Prescription,* 7th ed. Baltimore, Lippincott Williams & Wilkins, 2005.)

   a. The RPE can help to determine the test end point as well as information to be used in a future exercise prescription.
   b. The client is instructed to report his or her perception of effort during the last minute of each work stage, generally using a scale of 1 to 10 or 6 to 20.
5. **Perceptual scales** (e.g., 1–4, with 1 representing minimal discomfort and 4 severe discomfort) allow the client to express his or her degree of perceived angina or dyspnea during testing. This can be done nonverbally with hand signals (*Figure 6-4*).

D. INDICATIONS FOR TERMINATING AN EXERCISE TEST ARE CLASSIFIED AS ABSOLUTE OR RELATIVE (*TABLE 6-12*).

E. POSTEXERCISE PERIOD

1. **Active recovery,** involving walking or riding the cycle ergometer with a light load for 3 to 6 minutes, helps to maintain venous return and prevents blood pooling, hypotensive response, and compromised cardiac output.
2. Heart rate, ECG, and blood pressure are monitored, and the client is instructed to lie supine until the ST-segment changes return to baseline and the heart rate falls below 100 bpm.

F. INTERPRETATION OF RESULTS

1. The value of a stress test depends on proper test performance, careful client monitoring, and understanding the sensitivity and specificity of the test to make informed decisions regarding further testing or exercise prescription.
2. **Prognostic implications** are based on sensitivity and specificity.
   a. **Sensitivity** refers to the percentage of cases in which exercise testing accurately identifies the presence of CAD.
      1) **Current sensitivity** for detecting CAD using the exercise stress test **is approximately 70%**.
      2) **Sensitivity is enhanced by the following factors**:
         a) The client exercises to near-maximal levels of exertion.
         b) Multiple-lead ECG is used.

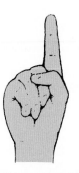 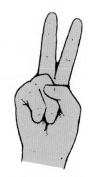

1 ONSET OF DISCOMFORT
You notice chest sensation.

2 MODERATE DISCOMFORT
You feel the pain increasing.

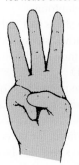 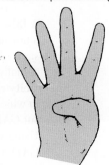

3 MODERATELY SEVERE
The discomfort would cause you to rest or take nitroglycerin.

4 SEVERE DISCOMFORT

FIGURE 6-4. Nonverbal rating scale for exertional chest discomfort. The scale is particularly useful with gas exchange techniques. A rating of 3 is the appropriate end point. (Reprinted with permission from *ACSM's Resource Manual for Guidelines for Exercise Testing and Prescription,* 4th ed. Baltimore, Lippincott Williams & Wilkins, 2001, p 292.)

TABLE 6-12. Indications for Terminating Exercise Testing

Absolute Indications

Drop in systolic blood pressure of 10 mm Hg or greater from baseline blood pressure despite an increase in workload, when accompanied by other evidence of ischemia

Moderate to severe angina

Increasing nervous system symptoms (e.g., ataxia, dizziness, near syncope)

Signs of poor perfusion (e.g., cyanosis, pallor)

Technical difficulties monitoring the electrocardiogram or systolic blood pressure

Subject's desire to stop

Sustained ventricular tachycardia

ST-segment elevation ($\geq$10 mm) in leads without diagnostic Q waves (other than V$_1$ or aVR).

Relative Indications

Drop in systolic blood pressure of 10 mm Hg or greater from baseline blood pressure despite an increase in workload, in the absence of other evidence of ischemia

ST-segment or QRS changes, such as excessive ST-segment depression (>2 mm horizontal or down-sloping ST-segment depression) or marked axis shift

Arrhythmias other than sustained ventricular tachycardia, including multifocal PVCs, triplets of PVCs, supraventricular tachycardia, heart block, or bradyarrhythmias

Fatigue, shortness of breath, wheezing, leg cramps, or claudication

Development of bundle-branch block or intraventricular conduction delay that cannot be distinguished from ventricular tachycardia

Increasing chest pain

Hypertensive response[a]

[a] Systolic blood pressure of more than 250 mm Hg and/or a diastolic blood pressure of more than 115 mm Hg.

(Reprinted with permission from Gibbons RA, Balady GJ, Beasely JW, et al.: ACC/AHA guidelines for exercise testing. *J Am Coll Cardiol* 30:260–315, 1997.)

c) Other criteria besides ECG are assessed (e.g., blood pressure response, symptoms)

3) A **false-negative** stress test indicates a normal (or negative) stress test (no signs of CAD) in individuals who actually have CAD

b. **Specificity** refers to the percentage of cases in which the exercise test accurately rules out CAD.

1) Using standard criteria for detecting CAD, the exercise stress test has an approximately 84% specificity. That is, 84% of healthy people tested show no signs or symptoms of CAD.

2) A **false-positive** stress test indicates CAD in individuals who actually do not have CAD (*Table 6-13*)

IV. Assessing Fitness in Other Populations

A. CHILDREN

1. Purpose
   a. Assessment of health status.
   b. Comparison with criterion-referenced standards.
   c. Determination of change resulting from exercise programs.

2. Considerations
   a. In performing laboratory assessments of cardiovascular function, a **treadmill is preferable to a cycle ergometer**.
   b. Inexperience, local muscle fatigue, inability to maintain cadence, and/or the short attention span of children make it difficult for many children to complete a cycle ergometer test.
   c. Closure of the epiphyseal plates is not complete until after puberty. Therefore, it is **not recommended that children perform maximal tests for muscular strength**.

3. Modifications
   a. **Treadmill Tests**
      Keep speed constant, adjusting only the grade.
   b. **Cycle Ergometer Tests**
      Adjustments to the ergometer, including modifications to the handlebars, seat post, and pedal crank arms are often required to fit the smaller anatomy.

4. Protocols
   Recommended field tests for assessing health-related physical fitness in children include a

TABLE 6-13. Causes of False-Negative and False-Positive Tests

False Positive	False Negative
Resting repolarization abnormalities	Failure to reach ischemic threshold secondary to medications
Cardiac hypertrophy	
Accelerated conduction defects	Monitoring an insufficient number of leads to detect ECG changes
Digitalis	
Nonischemic cardiomyopathy	
Hypokalemia	Angiographically significant disease compensated by collateral circulation
Vasoregulatory abnormalities	
Mitral valve prolapse	
Pericardial disease	Muscoloskeletal limitations preceding cardiac abnormalities
Coronary spasm in absence of CAD	
Anemia	
Female gender	

(From *ACSM's Resource Manual for Guidelines for Exercise Testing and Prescription*, 4th ed. Baltimore, Lippincott Williams & Wilkins, 2001, p 373.)

1- or 0.5-mile run/walk, BMI, pull-ups, sit-ups, push-ups, and sit-and-reach test.

B. OLDER ADULTS

1. Purpose

Fitness testing is conducted in older adults for the same reasons as in younger adults:

a. Exercise prescription.

b. Evaluation of progress.

c. Motivation.

d. Education.

2. General Considerations

a. Adults of any specified age will vary widely in their physiologic response to exercise testing.

b. Deconditioning and disease often accompany aging. These factors must be taken into account in selecting appropriate fitness test protocols.

c. Adaptation to a specific workload is often prolonged in older adults. Therefore, a prolonged warm-up, followed by small increments in workload, is recommended.

3. Modifications

Test stages in graded exercise tests should be prolonged, lasting at least 3 minutes, to allow the participant to reach steady state.

4. Protocols

a. Choose protocols that account for musculoskeletal and aerobic impairments (*Table 6-14*).

b. Most protocols have 1- to 2-MET increments, with stages lasting from 2 to 5 minutes

TABLE 6-14.

Functional Class	Clinical Status	O₂ Cost ml/kg/min	METS	Bicycle Ergometer For 70 kg body weight Kpm/min (watts)	Bruce 3 min stages Mph/%GR	Ramp Per 30 sec Mph/%GR	Bruce Ramp Per min Mph/%GR	Balke-Ware %Grade at 3.3 mph 1 min stages	USAFSAM Mph/%GR	"Slow" USAFSAM Mph/%GR	Modified Balke Mph/%GR	ACIP Mph/%GR	Mod. Naughton (CHF) Mph/%GR	METS
Normal and I — Healthy, dependent on age, activity		73.5	21		5.5 / 20		5.8 / 20							21
		70	20				5.6 / 19							20
		66.5	19											19
		63	18		5.0 / 18		5.3 / 18							18
		59.5	17				5.0 / 18							17
		56.0	16				4.8 / 17	26, 25						16
		52.5	15	1500 (246)			4.5 / 16	24, 23, 22				3.4 / 24.0		15
		49.0	14		4.2 / 16	3.0 / 25.0; 3.0 / 24.0	4.2 / 16	21, 20	3.3 / 25		3.0 / 25	3.1 / 24.0	3.0 / 25	14
		45.5	13	1350 (221)		3.0 / 23.0; 3.0 / 22.0	4.1 / 15	19, 18			3.0 / 22.5	3.0 / 21.0	3.0 / 22.5	13
		42.0	12	1200 (197)		3.0 / 21.0; 3.0 / 20.0	3.8 / 14	17, 16	3.3 / 20		3.0 / 20		3.0 / 20	12
		38.5	11	1050 (172)		3.0 / 19.0; 3.0 / 18.0	3.4 / 14	15, 14			3.0 / 17.5	3.0 / 17.5	3.0 / 17.5	11
	Sedentary Healthy	35.0	10	900 (148)	3.4 / 14	3.0 / 17.0; 3.0 / 16.0	3.1 / 13	13, 12	3.3 / 15		3.0 / 15	3.0 / 14.0	3.0 / 15	10
		31.5	9	750 (123)		3.0 / 15.0; 3.0 / 14.0	2.8 / 12	11, 10		2 / 25	3.0 / 12.5		3.0 / 12.5	9
		28.0	8	600 (98)		3.0 / 13.0; 3.0 / 12.0	2.5 / 12	9, 8	3.3 / 10	2 / 20	3.0 / 10	3.0 / 10.5	3.0 / 10	8
	Limited	24.5	7		2.5 / 12	3.0 / 11.0; 3.0 / 10.0	2.3 / 11; 2.1 / 10	7, 6		2 / 15	3.0 / 7.5	3.0 / 7.0	3.0 / 7.5	7
II	Symptomatic	21.0	6	450 (74)		3.0 / 9.0; 3.0 / 8.0	1.7 / 10	5, 4	3.3 / 5	2 / 10	3.0 / 5	3.0 / 3.0	2.0 / 10.5	6
		17.5	5		1.7 / 10	3.0 / 7.0; 3.0 / 6.0	1.3 / 5	3, 2		2 / 5	3.0 / 2.5	2.5 / 2.0	2.0 / 7.0	5
III		14.0	4	300 (49)		3.0 / 5.0; 3.0 / 4.0	1.0 / 0	1	3.3 / 0	2 / 0	3.0 / 0	2.0 / 0.0	2.0 / 3.5	4
		10.5	3	150 (24)		3.0 / 3.0; 3.0 / 2.0; 3.0 / 1.0; 3.0 / 0			2.0 / 0		2.0 / 0		1.5 / 0	3
		7.0	2			2.5 / 0; 1.5 / 0							1.0 / 0	2
IV		3.5	1			1.0 / 0; 0.5 / 0								1

Review Test

DIRECTIONS: Carefully read all questions, and select the BEST single answer.

1. A client's health screening should be administered before
   A) Any contact with the client.
   B) Any physical activity by the client at your facility.
   C) Fitness assessment or programming.
   D) The initial "walk-through" showing of a facility.

2. A well-designed consent document developed in consultation with a qualified legal professional provides your facility with
   A) Documentation of a good-faith effort to educate your clients.
   B) Legal documentation of a client's understanding of assessment procedures.
   C) Legal immunity against lawsuits.
   D) No legal benefit.

3. Relative contraindications for exercise testing are conditions for which
   A) A physician should be present during the testing procedures.
   B) Exercise testing should not be performed until the condition improves.
   C) Exercise testing will not provide accurate assessment of health-related fitness.
   D) Professional judgment about the risks and benefits of testing should determine whether to conduct an assessment.

4. A male client is 42 years old. His father died of a heart attack at age 62. He has a consistent resting blood pressure (measured over 6 weeks) of 132/86 mm Hg and a total serum cholesterol of 5.4 mmol/L. Based on his CAD risk stratification, which of the following activities is appropriate?
   A) Maximal assessment of cardiorespiratory fitness without a physician supervising.
   B) Submaximal assessment of cardiorespiratory fitness without a physician supervising.
   C) Vigorous exercise without a previous medical assessment.
   D) Vigorous exercise without a previous physician-supervised exercise test.

5. During calibration of a treadmill, the belt length was found to be 5.5 m. It took 1 minute and 40 seconds for the belt to travel 20 revolutions. What is the treadmill speed?
   A) 4 m/min.
   B) 66 m/min.
   C) 79 m/min.
   D) 110 m/min.

6. Which of the following would most appropriately assess a previously sedentary, 40-year-old female client's muscular strength?
   A) Using a 30-pound (18-kg) barbell to perform biceps curls to fatigue.
   B) Holding a handgrip dynamometer at 15 pounds (7 kg) to fatigue.
   C) Performing modified curl-ups to fatigue.
   D) Using a 5-pound (2.2-kg) dumbbell to perform multiple sets of biceps curls to fatigue.

7. Flexibility is a measure of the
   A) Disease-free ROM about a joint.
   B) Effort-free ROM about a joint.
   C) Habitually used ROM about a joint.
   D) Pain-free ROM about a joint.

8. Which of the following is a FALSE statement regarding informed consent?
   A) Informed consent is not a legal document.
   B) Informed consent does not provide legal immunity to a facility or individual in the event of injury to a client.
   C) Negligence, improper test administration, inadequate personnel qualifications, and insufficient safety procedures are all items expressly covered by the informed consent.
   D) Informed consent does not relieve the facility or individual of the responsibility to do everything possible to ensure the safety of the client.

9. Which of the following statements about underwater weighing is TRUE?
   A) It can divide the body into bone, muscle, and fat components.
   B) It assumes standard densities for bone, muscle, and fat.
   C) It can divide the body into visceral and subcutaneous fat components.
   D) It is a direct method of assessing body composition.

10. Which of the following criteria would NOT classify a client as having "increased risk"?
    A) Signs and/or symptoms of cardiopulmonary disease.
    B) Signs and/or symptoms of metabolic disease.
    C) Two or more major risk factors for CAD.
    D) Male older than 40 years with a history of clinical depression.

11. A client must be given specific instructions for the days preceding a fitness assessment. Which of the following is NOT a necessary instruction to a client for a fitness assessment?
    A) Men and women should avoid liquids for 12 hours before the test.
    B) Clients should be instructed to avoid alcohol, tobacco products, or caffeine at least 3 hours before the test.
    C) Clients should avoid strenuous exercise or physical activity on the day of the test.
    D) Men and women should be instructed to get an adequate amount of sleep the night before the assessment.

12. Hydrodensitometry (hydrostatic weighing, underwater weighing) has several sources of error. Which of the following is NOT a common source of error when using this technique to determine body composition?
    A) Measurement of the vital capacity of the lungs.
    B) Interindividual variability in the amount of air in the gastrointestinal tract.
    C) Interindividual variability in the density of the individual lean tissue compartment.
    D) Measurement of the residual volume.

13. The definition of cardiorespiratory fitness is
    A) The maximal force that a muscle or muscle group can generate in a single effort.
    B) The coordinated capacity of the heart, blood vessels, respiratory system, and tissue metabolic systems to take in, deliver, and use oxygen.
    C) The ability to sustain a held maximal force or to continue repeated submaximal contractions.
    D) The functional ROM about a joint.

14. Which of the following formulae is used for determining workload on a bicycle ergometer?
    A) Belt length × resistance × grade.
    B) Belt length × resistance × revolutions pedaled per minute.
    C) Resistance × distance flywheel traveled per revolution × revolutions per minute.
    D) Resistance × distance flywheel traveled per revolution.

15. Adults age physiologically at individual rates. Therefore, adults of any specified age will vary widely in their physiologic responses to exercise testing. Special consideration should be given to older adults when giving a fitness test, because
    A) Age is often accompanied by deconditioning and disease.
    B) Age predisposes older adults to clinical depression and neurologic diseases.
    C) Older adults cannot be physically stressed beyond 75% of age-adjusted maximum.
    D) Older adults are not as motivated to exercise as those who are younger.

16. A client with a functional capacity of 7 MET, an ejection fraction of 37%, and an ST-segment depression of 1 mm below baseline on exertion
    A) Should not exercise until his or her ejection fraction is >50%.
    B) Is considered to be at low risk.
    C) Is considered to be at moderate risk.
    D) Is considered to be at high risk.

17. The most accurate screening method for signs and symptoms of CAD is a
    A) Maximal exercise test with a 12-lead ECG.
    B) Submaximal exercise test with a 12-lead ECG.
    C) Discontinuous protocol, stopping at 85% of maximal heart rate.
    D) Continuous protocol, stopping at 85% of maximal heart rate.

18. What is the best test to help determine ejection fraction at rest and during exercise?
    A) Angiography.
    B) Thallium stress test.
    C) Single-proton emission computer tomography.
    D) MUGA (blood pool imagery) study.

19. A "cold spot" detected in the inferior portion of the left ventricle during a stress test that resolves 3 hours later most likely indicates
    A) An old inferior MI.
    B) A MI that is healing.
    C) Reversible myocardial ischemia.
    D) The need for multiple bypass surgery.

20. What is the best test of cardiovascular function for a client who is obese, has claudication in the legs, and has limited mobility because of neurologic damage from uncontrolled diabetes?
    A) Dipyridamole or dobutamine testing and assessment of cardiovascular variables.
    B) Discontinuous treadmill exercise test.
    C) Resting echocardiography.
    D) Continuous submaximal cycle ergometer test.

21. Although 12-lead testing is the optimal ECG configuration, if only one lead can be used, which one should it be?
    A) Lead II.
    B) Lead AV_L.
    C) Lead V_5.
    D) Lead V_1.

22. Which of the following is an indication for terminating an exercise test?
    A) The client requests test termination.
    B) The respiratory exchange rate exceeds 0.95.
    C) The maximal heart rate exceeds 200 bpm.
    D) The RPE exceeds 17 on the standard scale.

23. Given the sensitivity of the exercise ECG, stress testing conducted on 100 cardiac rehabilitation clients with documented CAD would be expected to produce what results?
    A) All 100 clients show ECG indicators of CAD.
    B) Approximately 50 clients show ECG indicators of CAD.
    C) Approximately 30 clients would show ECG indicators of CAD.
    D) Approximately 70 clients would show ECG indicators of CAD.

24. What action should you take for a 55-year-old client who has three risk factors for heart disease and complains of fatigue on exertion?
    A) Conduct a submaximal stress test without the presence of a physician.
    B) Conduct a maximal diagnostic stress test in the presence of a physician.
    C) Use a questionnaire to evaluate activity, and do not conduct a test.
    D) Start the client exercising slowly, and test after 6 weeks.

25. For a client taking a β-blocker who has lowered resting blood pressure and heart rate, which of the following statements is TRUE?
    A) A submaximal test will provide the best estimate of the client's fitness.
    B) A submaximal test may underestimate the client's fitness.
    C) A submaximal test may overestimate the client's fitness.
    D) The client should be tested only when not taking the medication.

26. Two individuals have the same body weight, gender, ethnic background, and skinfold measurement results. One is 25 years old; the other is 45 years.

Given this scenario, which of the following statements is TRUE?
    A) They both have the same percentage of body fat.
    B) The 25-year-old individual is fatter.
    C) The 45-year-old individual is fatter.
    D) Who is fatter cannot be determined from the information given.

27. Lead V_1 is located at the
    A) Fifth intercostal space, left sternal border.
    B) Midclavicular line, fourth intercostal space.
    C) Fourth intercostal space, right sternal border.
    D) Midclavicular line, lateral to the xiphoid process.

28. Following termination of a stress test, a 12-lead ECG is
    A) Monitored immediately, then every 1 to 2 minutes until exercise-induced changes are at baseline.
    B) Monitored immediately, then at 2 and 5 minutes after the test.
    C) Monitored immediately only.
    D) Monitored and recorded only if any signs or symptoms arise during recovery.

29. For a client who has a contraindication to exercise testing but could benefit greatly from the information gained through testing, which of the following statements is TRUE?
    A) The contraindication is considered to be a relative contraindication.
    B) The contraindication is considered to be an absolute contraindication.
    C) The client should not be tested until the contraindication is resolved.
    D) A submaximal test is the only test that the client should complete.

30. A client who has a measured FVC of 3.5 L and can expel 3.1 L within 1 second has
    A) An obstructive defect.
    B) A restrictive defect.
    C) An FEV_1 of 3.1.
    D) An FEV_1 of 89%.

ANSWERS AND EXPLANATIONS

1-B. A client should not be allowed to engage in any physical activity, including fitness assessment, at your facility before his or her health risk status has been determined. Informational meetings or "walk-throughs" of the facility that do not incorporate physical activity do not require health screening.

2-A. An appropriately prepared consent form is a written document that provides evidence that you made a good-faith effort to inform your client about the procedures, risks, and benefits of the activities in which he or she will participate. The document does not provide legal immunity against lawsuits.

3-D.   Identification of risk conditions for exercise testing includes familiarization with those conditions that may increase risk but not necessarily preclude fitness assessment. Such conditions are called relative contraindications. Conditions that preclude testing until they have stabilized are absolute contraindications.

4-C.   The client has only one risk factor, hypercholesterolemia. He is classified as Low Risk and further medical examination and exercise testing is not necessary prior to initiation of exercise training.

5-B.   The belt length is 5.5 m. Twenty revolutions equals 110 meters total distance (20 revolutions × 5.5 meters per revolution). This distance was traveled in 100 seconds (60 seconds + 40 seconds), resulting in a speed of 1.1 m/s (110 meters per 100 seconds). Converting this to meters per min results in a treadmill speed of 66 m/min.

6-A.   Muscular strength is assessed most appropriately via either a determination of 1-RM or through lifting a submaximal weight that a client can lift, at most, 2 to 14 times. A weight of 30 pounds (18 kg) for a previously sedentary middle-aged woman is probably an adequate weight to allow 2 to 14 repetitions. The held handgrip exercise, modified curl-ups, and 5-pound dumbbell exercise meet the criteria for muscular endurance assessments.

7-D.   The ROM may be limited by pain. This decreases the function of the joint. Therefore, flexibility is limited by painful actions. Disease status and effort can affect the ROM. The ROM habitually used is not necessarily an indication of the complete ROM through which an individual can move.

8-C.   Negligence, improper test administration, inadequate personnel qualifications, and insufficient safety procedures are all items that are expressly NOT covered by informed consent. Informed consent is also not a legal document. It does not provide legal immunity to a facility or an individual in the event of injury to a client, and it does not relieve the facility or the individual of the responsibility to do everything possible to ensure the safety of the client.

9-B.   Underwater weighing is based on the concept that the human body can be divided into a fat component and a fat-free component. Fat is expressed relative to body weight (this includes all fat). This is an indirect method of measurement, because fat is not actually separated by dissection.

10-D.   Signs and/or symptoms of cardiopulmonary disease, signs and/or symptoms of metabolic disease, and two or more major risk factors for CAD are all indications of an increased risk for development of CAD. Known disease is the fourth condition that places a client into the increased risk category.

11-A.   The client should wear appropriate, comfortable, loose-fitting clothing; be adequately hydrated; avoid alcohol, tobacco, caffeine, and food for at least 3 hours before the test; avoid strenuous exercise or physical activity on the day of the test; and get adequate sleep the night before the test.

12-A.   It is the measurement of residual volume of air in the lungs and not the vital capacity of the lungs that is a source of error. Residual volume is difficult to directly measure and is often estimated using vital capacity.

13-B.   The coordinated capacity of the heart, blood vessels, respiratory system, and tissue metabolic systems to take in, deliver, and use oxygen is the definition of cardiorespiratory fitness. The maximal force that a muscle or muscle group can generate in a single effort is the definition of muscular strength. The ability to sustain a held maximal force or to continue repeated submaximal contractions is the definition of muscular endurance. The functional ROM about a joint is the definition of flexibility.

14-C.   To determine the workload on a bicycle ergometer, you must know the resistance against the flywheel, the distance the flywheel travels per revolution, and the number of revolutions per minute.

15-A.   Fitness testing is conducted in older adults for the same reasons as in younger adults, including exercise prescription, evaluation of progress, motivation, and education. Age is often accompanied by deconditioning and disease, and these factors must be considered when selecting appropriate fitness test protocols. In addition, adaptation to a specific workload is often prolonged in older adults (a prolonged warm-up followed by small increments in workload is recommended). Test stages in graded exercise tests should be prolonged, lasting at least 3 minutes, to allow the participant to reach a steady state. An appropriate test protocol should be selected to accommodate these special needs.

16-C. Individuals at moderate risk have signs or symptoms that suggest possible cardiopulmonary or metabolic disease and/or two or more risk factors. Other moderate-risk criteria include functional capacity of less than 6 to 8 MET at 3 weeks after a clinical event; shock or congestive heart failure during a recent MI, moderate left ventricular dysfunction (ejection fraction, 31%–49%); exercise-induced ST-segment depression of 1 to 2 mm below baseline, and reversible ischemic defects.

17-A. A maximal stress test requires the heart to work at its peak capacity. If heart disease is present, then signs and/or symptoms should be detected. A submaximal test may not stress the heart sufficiently to allow detection of ischemia.

18-D. A MUGA study may be performed to assess resting and exercise cardiac function related to cardiac output, ejection fraction, and wall motion. In this test, technetium-99m is injected into the bloodstream, where it attaches to red blood cells. Areas where the blood pools (e.g., ventricles) are visualized by the technetium emissions.

19-C. During a standard stress test, a client is connected to an intravenous line. During the last minute of exercise, thallium-201 is injected into the bloodstream. Thallium enters myocardial cells in proportion to the amount of blood flow to those cells, and it emits energy detectable with a scintillation counter. Images of the myocardium can be constructed immediately following a stress test and then 4 to 24 hours later. Areas with little or no perfusion immediately following a test indicate areas of ischemia. Persistence of these cold spots for 4 to 24 hours later indicates necrotic tissue. Areas of reversible ischemia will reperfuse, and cold spots will disappear in later testing.

20-A. In some instances, clients are not able to complete a stress test because of muscular limitations, neurologic disability, peripheral vascular disease, or other conditions that prevent them from achieving a sufficient work intensity to provide an accurate cardiovascular assessment.

21-C. During the test, three leads should be monitored, one each from the lateral, inferior, and anterior views. Research has shown that one of these leads should be V_5, because it will pick up most ST-segment changes.

22-A. Criteria are classified as absolute or relative indications. These criteria are based both on measured physiological responses and on symptoms displayed by the client. Under any test condition, however, the test must be stopped if the client requests that it be stopped.

23-D. Sensitivity refers to the percentage of cases in which exercise testing accurately identifies the presence of CAD. The exercise ECG is not completely sensitive to detecting CAD, but it is the most cost-effective first-line screening tool. Current sensitivity for detecting CAD using the exercise stress test is approximately 70%.

24-B. A maximal exercise test can be most effective in detecting CAD as well as allowing the technician to measure maximal oxygen uptake ($\dot{V}O_2max$). Therefore, when screening for CAD, a maximal diagnostic stress test (ECG, physician supervision) is recommended.

25-C. Submaximal testing estimates $\dot{V}O_2max$ based on the assumed linear relationship between heart rate and $\dot{V}O_2$. Heart rate is measured at multiple workloads during the test, and $\dot{V}O_2max$ at an estimated maximal heart rate is calculated. Submaximal testing is based on several assumptions:

- Measurements are done while the client is at steady state.

- The relationship between heart rate and $\dot{V}O_2max$ is linear.

- Maximal heart rate is similar for any given age.

- A β-blocker will change the reliability of the assumption, showing a lower heart rate for a given workload and, thus, predicting a higher achievable workload and $\dot{V}O_2max$.

26-C. Age is accounted for in skinfold equations because of the changes in body fat distribution with age. With aging, more fat is stored internally, altering the meaning of a given skinfold measure. Thus, the same skinfold for an older man indicates a higher relative body fat than a younger man of equivalent size and sum of skinfold.

27-C. The position for lead V_1 is located by palpation along the intercostal spaces to the fourth space; the electrode is placed along the right sternal border.

28-A. The 12-lead ECG should be recorded immediately after exercise and then every 1 to 2 minutes for either 5 minutes or until exercise-induced ECG changes are at baseline.

29-A. Relative contraindications include clients who might be tested if the potential benefit from exer-

cise testing outweighs the relative risk. Absolute contraindications refer to individuals who should not undergo exercise testing until the situation or condition has stabilized.

30-D. The FEV_1 is calculated as

(Volume expired in 1 second/FVC) × 100

An obstructive defect is indicated by an FEV_1 of less than 70%; a restrictive defect is indicated by a FVC of less than 70% of that predicted.

Safety, Injury Prevention, and Emergency Care

CHAPTER 7

FREDERICK S. DANIELS

I. General Considerations

A. All forms of exercise, from clinical testing to supervised exercise and from cardiac rehabilitation to general fitness programs, entail some risk *(Table 7-1)*.

B. Every clinical exercise physiologist, exercise specialist, and health/fitness instructor must understand the risks associated with exercise testing and training, be able to implement preventive measures, and know how to respond in case of injury or medical emergency.

C. Every clinical testing and exercise program must have an **emergency response system** to respond to injuries and medical emergencies.

II. Risks of Participation in Exercise

A. PHYSICAL DEMANDS
At higher intensities, the potential exists for either **injury** or an **emergency situation** that requires a correct and timely response.

B. BENEFITS SHOULD OUTWEIGH RISKS
The fitness instructor must create as safe an environment as possible by:
1. **Understanding the risks.**
2. Being able to **implement preventive** measures.
3. Having **knowledge regarding the appropriate care of injuries.**
4. **Creating, practicing, and implementing emergency plans** in the event of a medical emergency.

C. POTENTIAL SOURCES OF RISK
1. **Exercise Equipment**
   Exercise equipment can **malfunction**, be **used incorrectly**, or be in **disrepair** or **poor condition**.

2. **Environment**
   The exercise environment must be **clean** and properly **maintained**.
3. **Staff**
   Staff must be **properly trained**, act in a **responsible and safe** manner, and **design safe exercise programs**.
4. **Medical History**
   The exercise professional must **know the client's medical history, medication use, and restrictions**.
5. **Individual Factors**
   a. **Age**.
   b. **Level of exercise experience**.
   c. **Medical history**.
   d. **Lack of experience and familiarity** with equipment.
   e. **Lack of knowledge** about proper principles of exercise.

D. PREVENTION STRATEGIES FOR STAFF AND CLIENTS
1. Think about safety.
2. Exercise intelligently.
3. Purchase good equipment and supplies.
4. Use proper technique.
5. Follow the rules.
6. Train staff on a regular basis.
7. In a group exercise setting, staff should understand the following:
   a. Exercise space for each client (e.g., size of the room, number of participants).
   b. Temperature and humidity of the space.
   c. Fitness level and special needs of participants.
   d. Proper flooring to match group activity.
   e. Appropriate warm-up and cool-down.

TABLE 7-1. Possible Medical Complications of Exercise

Cardiovascular Complications	Metabolic Complications	Endocrine Complications	Traumatic Injuries
Cardiac arrest	Volume depletion	Amenorrhea	Bruises
Ischemia	Dehydration	Complications in those with	Strains and sprains
Angina	Rhabdomyolysis	diabetes	Muscle and tendon tears and
Myocardial infarction	Renal failure	Hypoglycemia	ruptures
Arrhythmias	Electrolyte disturbances	Hyperglycemia	Fractures
Supraventricular tachycardia		Retinal hemorrhage	Contusions and lacerations
Atrial fibrillation	**Thermal Complications**	Osteoporosis	Bleeding
Ventricular tachycardia	Hyperthermia		Crush injuries
Ventricular fibrillation	Heat rash	**Neurologic Complications**	Blunt trauma
Bradyarrhythmias	Heat cramps	Dizziness	Internal organ injury
Bundle branch blocks	Heat syncope	Syncope (fainting)	Splenic rupture
Atrioventricular nodal blocks	Heat exhaustion	Cerebral vascular accident	Myocardial contusion
Congestive heart failure	Heat stroke	(stroke)	Drowning
Hypertension	Hypothermia	Insomnia	Head injuries
Hypotension	Frostbite		Eye injuries
Aneurysm rupture		**Musculoskeletal Complications**	Death
Underlying medical conditions	**Pulmonary Complications**	Mechanical injuries	
predisposing to increased	Exercise-induced asthma	Back injuries	
complications	Bronchospasm	Stress fractures	
Hypertrophic cardiomy-	Pulmonary embolism	Carpal tunnel syndrome	
opathy	Pulmonary edema	Joint pain/injury	
Coronary artery anomalies	Pneumothorax	Muscle cramps/spasms	
Idiopathic left ventricular	Exercise-induced anaphylaxis	Tendonitis	
hypertrophy	Exacerbation of underlying	Exacerbation of musculoskeletal	
Marfan syndrome	pulmonary disease	diseases	
Aortic stenosis			
Right ventricular dysplasia	**Gastrointestinal Complications**	**Overuse Complications**	
Congenital heart defects	Vomiting	Overuse syndromes	
Myocarditis	Cramps	Overtraining	
Pericarditis	Diarrhea	Overexercising	
Amyloidosis		Shin splints	
Sarcoidosis		Plantar fasciitis	
Long QT syndrome			
Sickle-cell trait			

(From *ACSM's Resource Manual for Guidelines for Exercise Testing and Prescription*, 4th ed. Baltimore, Lippincott Williams & Wilkins, 2001, p 502.)

III. Safety in the Facility

A. AREAS OF SAFETY

1. **Specific Areas of Safety**
   a. Building design.
   b. Physical plant.
   c. Fixtures.
   d. Furniture.
   e. Equipment.
   f. Program design.
   g. Staff training.
2. **Americans with Disabilities Act (ADA)**
   a. The ADA lists specific standards that enhance safety and access for both **disabled and nondisabled** exercisers.
   b. The ADA is especially important for fitness facilities because of the **variety of individuals that may participate** in exercise programs.
3. **ACSM Health/Fitness Facility Standards for Safety**
   a. Ability to respond in a timely manner to any reasonable foreseeable emergency.
   b. Appropriate signage alerting clients of risk.
   c. Conformity with all relevant laws, regulations, and published standards.

B. CREATION OF A SAFE ENVIRONMENT

1. This is a primary responsibility in all fitness facilities.
2. Managers and staff must **meet a standard of care for safety** in developing and operating facilities and equipment by **looking beyond obvious safety parameters**.
3. Environmental factors (e.g., temperature, humidity, altitude, pollution) must be monitored and controlled, because performance and health can be affected by these conditions.
   a. High temperature can lead to dehydration, heat exhaustion, and even heat stroke.
   b. Low temperature can lead to dehydration, reduced coordination, chills, and potentially, frostbite.
   c. High humidity can reduce the body's ability to control core temperature and can lead to heat exhaustion.

d. Exposure to high altitude can lead to headaches, nausea, and altitude sickness.

e. In addition to affecting performance negatively, pollution can lead to wheezing, coughing, and irritation of the eyes and mouth.

C. EQUIPMENT

1. Includes pieces used for **testing cardiovascular, strength, flexibility, rehabilitation, pool, locker room, and emergency equipment.**

2. **Criteria for equipment selection include:**
   a. Proper anatomic position.
   b. Ability to adjust to different body sizes.
   c. Quality of design and materials.
   d. Durability.
   e. Repair history.
   f. Cost.

3. **Test the equipment** before purchase, and follow the manufacturer's instructions for installation.

4. **Inspect the equipment** regularly for cleanliness, disrepair, and proper functioning to allow early recognition of problems.

5. **Other safety considerations include:**
   a. All **electrical plugs** should be secured and grounded.
   b. Treadmills should have easily accessible **emergency cutoff switches.**
   c. **Safety instructions** should be mounted on all equipment.
   d. Machines should **restrict joint movements beyond the normal range of motion.**

D. FURNITURE AND FIXTURES

1. **Locker room and reception furniture** are used frequently and should be selected for **ergonomics and safety.**

2. **Inspection, routine maintenance, and cleaning** are equally important with furniture.

3. Lighting should be bright enough to see instructions and records clearly and should create a positive, motivating atmosphere.

E. SURFACES

1. Proper surfaces must be provided to **prevent slips and falls.**

2. Selection of surfaces **should meet minimal standards** for the activity being carried out and should **comply with the ADA.**

3. Maintenance includes:
   a. Proper cleaning and disinfecting.
   b. Removal of oil and dust.

c. Inspection for cracks, holes, exposed seams, and warping.

F. SUPPLIES AND SMALL EQUIPMENT

1. This category of equipment includes heart rate (HR) monitors, blood pressure (BP) units, stopwatches, skinfold calipers, exercise gloves, etc.

2. **Equipment must be in proper working order and calibrated.**

3. Devices that do not function correctly may provide incorrect information and precipitate an unsafe situation.

G. ROUTINE AND REQUIRED MAINTENANCE AND REPAIRS

1. **Help to ensure that equipment, furniture, and physical plant function safely and according to specifications.**

2. **Increase the life of the equipment.**

3. **Reduce the risk of a mechanical problem.**

4. **A routine maintenance schedule** for exercise equipment should be in place.

5. A procedure for reporting problems and a repair process that reduces downtime include **documentation of the problem, repair history, and resolution of the problem** (*Figure 7-1*)

H. MAINTENANCE AND HOUSEKEEPING

1. Contribute to safety by presenting a clean environment.

2. Help to maintain proper equipment functioning.

3. Slippery surfaces, dirty equipment and furniture, poorly maintained ventilation, and equipment in disrepair increase the risk of accidents.

4. Equipment and fixtures must be **regularly cleaned and disinfected.**
   a. **Written standards** must outline clearly the procedure for routine cleaning and maintenance.
   b. Solutions and materials must be safe for the skin and **hypoallergenic.**
   c. The professional staff should have a role in the cleaning and maintenance of exercise equipment. **Knowledge of procedures and chemical safety is critical.**

IV. Weight Room Safety

A. WEIGHTS

The use of weights—either machine or free weights (e.g., dumbbells, barbells)—increases risk of injury because of the amount of weight used, improper technique, fatigue, and improper behavior.

Fitness Equipment Repair Chart

Date	Equipment	Serial No.	Problem	Date repaired	Order No.	Cost

FIGURE 7-1. An example of a repair log for fitness equipment. (From *ACSM's Resource Manual for Guidelines for Exercise Testing and Prescription,* 4th ed. Philadelphia, Lippincott Williams & Wilkins, 2001, p 646)

B. METHODS TO INCREASE SAFETY

1. **Spotting**: A second person assists in the initial lift, correcting the lifter's technique and lifting the weight to safety if the lifter is unable to handle the weight.

2. **Buddy system**: Exercise with a partner who can offer encouragement and motivation, knowledge of correct technique, and assistance if a problem develops.

3. **Speed of movement**: Movements should be controlled with a slow, smooth pace (4 seconds up and 4 seconds down).

4. **Replacing weights**: A safe environment requires returning weights to their proper place after exercise.

5. **Placement of equipment**: Adequate space between machines and weight benches is important for safety.

6. **Equipment inspection and routine maintenance**.

V. Testing and Evaluation Area

This area must be safely organized and similarly prepared for emergencies. Equipment should include:

A. Sphygmomanometer, stethoscope, mouth guard for cardiopulmonary resuscitation (CPR), first-aid kit, automated defibrillator.

B. Telephone to activate the public emergency medical system (EMS).

1. Should have **posted, written procedures to activate the EMS** (e.g., 911).

2. Should include the following instructions:
    a. **Identify** yourself, your location, and the phone number.
    b. **Provide** a clear and succinct **explanation** of the problem.
    c. **Offer medical history and medications** (if known).
    d. **Provide vital signs and state of consciousness**.
    e. **Explain the treatment actions** taken and their results.

C. BACK BOARD AND NECK BOARD

A back board and neck board are not required in the testing area, but they should be immediately accessible.

D. EMERGENCY EQUIPMENT

1. **Emergency equipment must be**:
    a. Clearly marked.
    b. Readily accessible at all times.
    c. Calibrated and maintained regularly.

2. **Necessary emergency equipment includes**:
    a. Telephones with the numbers of the EMS or 911, physicians, cardiac code team (clinical setting), police, and fire.
    b. First-aid kits.
    c. First-responder bloodborne pathogen kits (infection control kit).
    d. Latex gloves.
    e. CPR mouthpieces.
    f. Resuscitation bags (clinical setting).
    g. Back board.
    h. Splints.
    i. Defibrillator (clinical facility) or automatic external defibrillator (AED) (fitness facility).
    j. Emergency drugs and materials (e.g., epinephrine, dextrose, blood glucose meter) in the clinical setting.

3. Staff should know how to use, and routinely practice the use of emergency equipment.

VI. Safety During Exercise Testing and Training

A. CLIENT/PATIENT SAFETY

1. **Monitoring for Signs of Fatigue and Distress**
    During exercise testing, the clinical exercise specialist monitors the patient's HR and rhythm (on an electrocardiogram [ECG]), BP, respiration, and other parameters for signs of fatigue and/or distress.
    a. **Manifestations of cardiac or pulmonary distress** necessitate stopping the test immediately and, possibly, initiating the emergency response system (see Chapter 6, Table 6-12).
    b. **Less severe manifestations** (e.g., light-headedness, muscular fatigue, intermittent premature ventricular contractions, wheezing) may not necessitate immediate test termination.

2. **Indications for stopping an exercise session** include those listed in Chapter 6, Table 6-2, as well as the following:
    a. **Signs of confusion or inability to concentrate**.
    b. **Dizziness**.
    c. Convulsions.
    d. **Physical injury**.
    e. **Nausea**.

B. STAFF SAFETY

1. Fitness/clinical exercise staff must demonstrate professional competence with all programs and use of exercise or testing areas.

2. Safety of the fitness/clinical exercise staff can be maximized by following federal Occupational Safety and Health Administration (OSHA) standards.
   a. **Wash hands thoroughly** before working with a client or patient.
   b. **Wear gloves and other protective clothing** (when necessary) when any possibility of exposure to bloodborne pathogens exists.
   c. **Keep cords out of the path** of both staff and clients/patients to eliminate the possibility of trips or falls.
   d. **Keep long hair and loose clothing from catching on equipment.**

VII. Medications and Safety

Various medications can affect a patient's response to exercise testing or training. For a full review, please refer to Appendix A in *ACSM's Guidelines for Exercise Testing and Prescription,* 7th ed.

VIII. Safety Plans

A. Clearly outline procedures for maintaining a safe environment and reducing the risk of accidents.

B. **APPROPRIATE SAFETY PLANS INCLUDE:**
   1. **Fire**
      a. Procedures for **evacuation.**
      b. Regular **inspection of fire extinguishers.**
   2. **Power Failure**
      a. Procedures that **reduce the risk of power outages and electrical malfunction.**
      b. Procedures for **evacuation** and **contacting the authorities.**
   3. **Flood**
      a. Procedures to **reduce the risk of flooding** in areas such as the pool, shower, and whirlpool.
      b. Procedures for **cleanup and salvage.**
   4. **Earthquake**
      a. Procedures for **evacuation.**
      b. Procedures for **safety of equipment and persons** in the facility.
   5. **Bloodborne Pathogens/Hazardous Waste**
      a. OSHA has specific **standards** that must be **posted** and closely adhered to when applicable.
      b. All staff must be **familiar** with and trained in these procedures.
   6. **Staff Certification in First Aid and CPR**
   7. **Posted Information**
      a. Clearly visible signs should be posted for fire extinguishers, first-aid kits, CPR mouth shields, and for activating the EMS (911).

   b. Emergency procedures should be posted adjacent to all phones to assist in enacting the emergency plan.

IX. Proper Documentation

Events should be recorded. This includes **written policies** and procedures, **rules,** patient and client **rights,** as well as the **benefits and risks** of exercise programs. Such documents offers important **protections against liability and negligence** for both facilities and professional staff. **Liability insurance and legal assistance is recommended as well.**

A. **PARTICIPANT AGREEMENTS**
   1. Participant agreements define the **risks** of an exercise program, exact **type** of exercise program, exact **costs,** and **who shares the risk and responsibility** for the member's exercise (*Figure 7-2*)
   2. An **attorney** should assist in creating these forms.

B. **INFORMED CONSENT**
   Informed consent provides **detailed explanation** of the test or exercise program, including:
   1. Potential **benefits and risks.**
   2. **Purpose** of the test or exercise program.
   3. **Client responsibilities.**
   4. **Opportunity** for the member to ask **questions.**

C. **WAIVERS**
   1. Waivers **allow clients to circumvent** a policy or rule but **place the risk** for this directly **on the client.**
   2. Waivers offer a form of **protection** for both the **instructor** and the **facility.**

D. **INCIDENT REPORTS**
   1. Incident reports are a record of an incident or event that involves **unusual circumstances,** such as a participant not following club policies or rules, or some other **unusual incident.**
   2. These reports should include:
      a. **Detailed documentation** of the entire incident.
      b. Names of **involved clients and witnesses.**
      c. All **actions by staff** to resolve the problem or emergency situation.
      d. Any **follow-up action** required and/or taken.

X. Emergency Management

Safe and effective management of an emergency situation will ensure the best care and protection for clients, staff, and facility.

SAMPLE

PARTICIPANT'S RELEASE AND AGREEMENT

I, the undersigned, hereby agree to participate in an exercise class and/or program ("Program") offered by the XYZ Health Club. I understand that there are inherent risks in participating in a program of strenuous exercise. I warrant and represent that I am in acceptable health and that I may participate in the Program. I agree that I have been honest in my statements regarding my health and medical history and if there are any medical or health conditions or problems, I further agree to obtain a physician's clearance before participating in the Program. If restrictions exist, I will inform XYZ Health Club at the time and allow XYZ Health Club staff to contact my physician for additional information.

I agree that XYZ Health Club shall not be liable or responsible for any injuries to me or illnesses resulting from my participation in the Program and I expressly release and discharge XYZ Health Club and it employees, agents, and assigns, from all claims, actions or judgements which I or my heirs, executors, administrators or assigns may have or claim to have against XYZ Health Club, and/or its employees, agents or assigns for all injuries, illnesses or other damage which may occur in connection with my participtation in the Program. This release shall be binding upon my heirs, executors, administrators, and assigns.

I have read this release and agreement and I understand all of its terms. I execute it voluntarily and with full knowledge of its significance.

Signature: _____   Date: _____

Print name: _____

Witness: _____   Date: _____

FIGURE 7-2. A sample of a participant's release and agreement.

A. EMERGENCY PLAN

1. **An emergency plan is mandatory** in all testing and exercise areas.
2. **The emergency plan must specify** the following:
    a. The specific responsibilities of each staff member.
    b. The methods to activate the emergency procedures.
    c. The required equipment.
    d. Predetermined contacts for emergency response and specific information to forward to appropriate medical personnel.
    e. A map of emergency exits, emergency equipment locations, phones, fire alarms, and fire extinguishers.
    f. Step-by-step actions to take for each common medical emergency, nonmedical emergency (e.g., flood, power outage, fire), and disaster (natural or man-made).
3. **All emergency incidents must be documented** with dates, times, actions, people involved, and outcomes.
4. **The plan should be practiced**, with both announced and unannounced drills, on a quarterly basis.

B. STAFF ROLE

The professional staff role during an emergency should include:
1. **Control the situation** by implementing the emergency plan and taking charge.
2. **Maintain order and calm**, especially regarding the victim.
3. **Activate the EMS**, if necessary.
4. Assure that **proper documentation** of the event occurs.

C. STAFF TRAINING

All staff, including nonclinical staff, should be trained in the emergency plan:
1. Staff training includes **in-services, safety plans, and emergency procedures**.
2. **In-services with physicians, nurses, and paramedics** are especially recommended.

3. Review and update **emergency plans** as necessary, including regularly scheduled drills.

4. Exercise staff should have training in the proper use of emergency equipment.

5. CPR and first aid **certification should be current** in all staff. Basic life support is mandatory, and advanced cardiac life support is recommended for clinical staff.

6. Staff should be fully trained to recognize:

   a. **Absolute and relative contraindications** to exercise.

   b. **Absolute and relative reasons for terminating an exercise test or exercise session**.

7. A physician should be present or nearby in every clinical exercise test setting to assist with or manage emergencies.

XI. General Emergency Response Guidelines

A. CONTACTS

1. Activating the EMS

a. This may entail calling a paramedic/ambulance group or an emergency medical team within the facility.

b. **Information to communicate includes**:

   1) **Patient's location**.

   2) **Patient's status**, including vital signs.

   3) Symptoms and actions that led to the emergency.

   4) Actions of the exercise staff in caring for the patient after the onset of symptoms.

2. Communicating with a Physician or Other Appropriate Medical Professional

a. Report the signs and symptoms associated with the emergency, as well as the patient's status before the start of the test.

b. State the patient's current vital signs and symptoms.

c. Ask for recommendations.

3. Contacting the Patient's Family Physician

The patient's family physician should be contacted, particularly if a physician is not present at the facility.

a. Indicate to the family physician that a medical emergency has occurred with one of his or her patients.

b. Be prepared to report the symptoms associated with the emergency as well as the patient's status before the start of the test.

c. Present vital signs and present symptoms.

d. Ask for recommendations.

4. Contacting the Patient's Family

a. Explain the situation in whatever detail the family needs.

b. Indicate if the patient has been transported to a hospital or emergency department and how the family can find that location.

c. Assist the family in any other way possible.

B. INITIAL ACTIONS

1. **Initial monitoring** during a medical emergency should include:

   a. **HR** through palpation or ECG.

   b. **Heart rhythm** through ECG.

   c. **BP**.

   d. **Respiration**.

   e. **Physical signs of complications**, including:

      1) **Loss of balance**.

      2) **Convulsions/seizure**.

      3) **Shivering**.

      4) **Cold, clammy skin**.

      5) **Verbal and nonverbal expression of pain**.

   f. **Blood glucose level** in patients with diabetes.

2. **First aid procedures** should be initiated as indicated (*Table 7-2*)

3. **After the patient is stabilized**, he or she should be transported to a facility (e.g., hospital, medical center, physician's office) or department (e.g., emergency room) for appropriate treatment.

C. FOLLOW-UP ACTIONS

After an emergency incident, follow-up with the patient serves several purposes.

1. **It clarifies the patient's current medical status**, aiding in understanding the causes of the emergency.

2. **It provides more information regarding the consequences of the staff's actions** to help determine whether the response to the emergency was effective.

3. **It allows the staff to finalize the incident report**, with a final analysis of the patient's status (which may not be known until days after the incident).

D. DOCUMENTATION

1. Careful documentation of an emergency event provides important information for the safety of the patient, management of the program, and protection of the staff and facility.

2. **Information should include**:

   a. **Time line of events**.

   b. Names of **All people involved**, including witnesses.

TABLE 7-2. Possible Medical Emergencies and Suggested First Aid

Problem	First Aid
Heat cramps	Replace lost fluids; replace sodium and potassium lost through excessive sweating.
Heat exhaustion and heat stroke	Move victim to a shaded area; have victim lie down with his or her feet elevated above the level of the heart.
	Remove excess clothing
	Cool victim with sips of cool fluid; sprinkle water on him or her and on the facial area; rub an ice pack over major vessels in armpits, groin, and neck areas.
	Victim should seek immediate medical attention and be given intravenous fluids as soon as possible.
Fainting (syncope)	Leave the victim lying down; turn victim on his or her side if vomiting occurs.
	Maintain an open airway.
	Loosen any tight clothing.
	Take blood pressure and pulse if possible.
	Seek medical attention, because this is a potentially life-threatening situation and the cause of fainting must be determined.
Hypoglycemia (symptoms include diaphoresis, pallor, tremor, tachycardia, palpitation, visual disturbances, mental confusion, weakness, light-headedness, fatigue, headache, memory loss, seizure, and coma)	May become life-threatening; seek medical attention to treat cause.
	Give oral glucose solutions (e.g., Kool-Aid with sugar, nondiet soft drinks, juice, milk); if patient is able to ingest solids, gelatin sweetened with sugar, mild chocolate, or fruit may be given.
Hyperglycemia (symptoms include dehydration, hypotension, reflex tachycardia, osmotic diuresis, impaired consciousness, nausea, vomiting, abdominal pain, hyperventilation, acetone odor on breath)	May be life-threatening if it leads to diabetic ketoacidosis
	Seek immediate medical attention.
	Rehydrate with intravenous normal saline.
	Correct electrolyte loss (K^+).
	Administer insulin.
Sprains/strains	No weight bearing on affected extremity.
	Loosen shoes; apply a pillow or blanket-type splint around the affected extremity.
	Elevate the affected extremity.
	Apply a bag of crushed ice to the affected area.
	Seek medical attention if pain or swelling persists.
Simple/compound fractures	Immobilize the affected extremity.
	Splint the affected extremity to prevent further injury to the bone or soft tissue.
	Use anything at hand as a splint.
	Do not attempt to reduce any dislocation in the field unless there is danger of losing life or limb.
	Seek immediate medical attention.
	Protect the victim from further injury.
Bronchospasm	Maintain an open airway.
	Give bronchodilators via nebulizer if prescribed for patient.
	Give oxygen by nasal cannula if available.
Hypotension/shock	Lay the victim down with his or her feet elevated.
	Maintain an open airway.
	Monitor vital signs (pulse, blood pressure).
	Call for immediate advanced life support measures, because this is a life-threatening emergency that requires intensive monitoring of vital signs and administration of intravenous fluids and drugs to maintain adequate tissue perfusion during evaluation to determine the cause (e.g., hypovolemia, cardiogenic shock, sepsis).
Bleeding	Apply direct pressure over the site to stop the bleeding.
Lacerations	Protect the wound from contamination and infection.
Incisions	May need to seek medical attention; victim may need stitches or tetanus shot.
Puncture wounds	If bleeding is severe, elevate the injured part of the body in addition to direct pressure, and if an artery is severed, apply direct pressure over the main artery to the affected limb and seek immediate medical attention.
Abrasions	
Contusions	

(With permission from Strauss WE, et al. Emergency plans and procedures for an exercise facility. In *ACSM's Resource Manual for Guidelines for Exercise Testing and Prescription*, 2nd ed. Philadelphia, Lea & Febiger, 1993, p 373.)

c. **Actions taken by the staff** to resolve the emergency situation.
d. **All communications** with medical personnel, family, and other staff.
e. Follow-up actions.

XII. Injury Prevention

A. PREPARTICIPATION SCREENING
Preparticipation screening may uncover medical and physical risks to exercise.

B. IMPROVED FITNESS
1. **Musculoskeletal fitness** may reduce risk of injury.
2. **Physiologic fitness** may help to prevent many chronic medical conditions.
3. All **four components of fitness** are important and should be a part of all fitness programs.
   a. **Conditioning should be well balanced among cardiovascular, flexibility, strength, and endurance** as well as throughout the muscle groups and major joints.
   b. The **progression** of exercise training should be gradual.
   c. **Flexibility** is an important component of fitness and may contribute to injury prevention.
   d. **Warm-up and cool-down**
      1) Prepare the body for exercise and safely return the body to a resting state.
      2) May prevent complications (e.g., musculoskeletal injury, cardiac crisis, dizziness) that can result from immediate changes in exercise intensity.
   e. **Rest**
      1) Is an important part of conditioning.
      2) Can facilitate recovery from the stress of exercise.
      3) Can reduce the risk of injury.
      4) Includes rest between exercises and exercise sessions as well as that prescribed for acute injury.

C. PROPER INSTRUCTION
Proper instruction assists in preventing injuries and avoiding emergency situations.

D. EXERCISE CLOTHING AND EQUIPMENT
1. Gloves, helmets, protective glasses, and so on are important to safety during certain modes of exercise.

2. Clothing should fit properly and be layered to maintain warmth (in cold environments) or be appropriate for hot/humid environments.
3. Shoes must be appropriate for the exercise or sport.

E. HYDRATION
1. Hydration is not always appropriately driven by thirst.
2. Hydrate regularly during exercise.

XIII. Contraindications to Exercise testing and Training

For certain individuals, the risks for complications during exercise testing and training outweigh the potential benefits.

A. **Identifying a client's/patient's contraindications** to exercise testing and training (*Table 6-1*) involves:
   1. **Reviewing the medical history**.
   2. **Assessing cardiac risk**.
   3. **Evaluating physical examination findings**.
   4. **Evaluating laboratory test results**.

B. A client/patient with **absolute contraindications** should not undergo exercise testing or training until those conditions are stabilized.

C. A client/patient with **relative contraindications** may undergo exercise testing and training only after careful analysis of his or her risk-to-benefit ratio.

D. In some cases, clinical exercise testing may still be performed for a patient with contraindications to guide drug therapy.

XIV. Musculoskeletal Injuries

The incidence of exercise-related injury has been reported to be as high as 80% in participants and instructors (*Table 7-3*)

A. RISK FACTORS
1. **Extrinsic Factors**
   a. Excessive load.
   b. Training errors.
      1) Poor technique.
      2) Excessive stress on joints.
      3) Spine not in a neutral position.
   c. Adverse environmental conditions.

TABLE 7-3. General Injury Classifications

Injury	Major Signs and Symptoms
Muscle	
Acute	
Contusions	Soft-tissue hemorrhage, hematoma, ecchymosis, movement restriction
Strains	Hemorrhage, local tenderness, loss of strength/ROM
Tendon injuries	Loss of strength/ROM; palpable defect
Muscle cramps/spasms	Involuntary muscle contraction; muscle pain
Acute-onset muscle soreness	Muscle pain, fatigue; resolves when exercise has ceased
Delayed-onset muscle soreness	Muscle stiffness 24 to 48 hours after exercise; tenderness and pain.
Chronic	
Myositis/fasciitis	Local swelling and tenderness
Tendinitis	Gradual onset, diffuse or localized tenderness and swelling, pain
Tenosynovitis	Crepitus, diffuse swelling, pain
Bursitis	Swelling, pain, some loss of function
Joint	
Acute	
Sprains	Swelling, pain, joint instability, loss of function
Acute joint synovitis	Pain during motion, swelling, pain
Subluxation/dislocation	Loss of limb function, deformity, swelling, point tenderness
Chronic	
Osteochondrosis	Joint locking, swelling, pain, disability
Osteoarthritis	Pain, articular crepitus, stiffness, reduced ROM
Capsulitis/synovitis	Joint edema, reduced ROM, joint crepitus
Bone	
Periostitis	Pain over bone, especially under pressure
Acute fracture	Deformity, bone point tenderness, swelling and ecchymosis
Stress fracture	Vague pain that persists when attempting activity; local tenderness

ROM, range of motion.

   d. Faulty equipment.
   e. Overtraining (overuse) signs and symptoms.
      1) Chronic soreness.
      2) Fatigue.
      3) Changes in menstrual cycle.
      4) Lack of desire to rest.

2. Intrinsic Factors
   a. Fitness level.
   b. Body composition.
   c. Anatomic abnormalities.
   d. Gender.
   e. Age.
   f. Past injury.
   g. Disease.
   h. Restricted range of motion.
   i. Muscle weakness and imbalance.
   j. Not performing warm-up and stretching exercises.

B. BASIC PRINCIPLES OF CARE
  1. Objectives are to **decrease pain, reduce swelling, and prevent further injury**.
  2. Objectives usually can be met by:
   a. **"RICES"**: Rest, Ice, Compression, Elevation, and Stabilization.
      1) **Rest** prevents further injury and ensures initiation of the healing process.
      2) **Ice** reduces swelling, bleeding, inflammation, and pain.
      3) **Compression** reduces swelling and bleeding.
      4) **Elevation** decreases blood flow and controls edema.
      5) **Stabilization** reduces muscle spasm in the injured area by assisting in the relaxation of associated muscles.
   b. Heat
      1) Is used to relieve pain and muscle spasms.
      2) Should not be applied during the acute inflammatory phase.
   c. Splints or Casts
      1) May be used to immobilize the area and improve healing.
      2) Immobilization is used primarily for fractures and severe sprains.
   d. Medications
      1) May be used to reduce swelling and inflammation.
      2) May be used to treat the pain associated with swelling.
   e. Care of Low Back Injury
      1) Neutral spine during exercise (pain-free).
      2) Aerobic exercise.

3) Unloaded flexion/extension of spine (cat stretch).
4) Hip and knee flexion and extension.
5) Lunges.
6) Single leg extension holds.
7) Abdominal curl-ups.
8) Horizontal isometric side support.
9) Low weight, high repetitions to emphasize endurance strength.

XV. Other Medical Emergencies and Associated Treatment

Serious complications rarely occur during an exercise session. When complications do occur, however, the exercise staff must be prepared to take appropriate action. (Refer to *Tables 7-2* and *7-4*.)

A. HEAT EXHAUSTION/HEAT STROKE
1. Replace fluids.
2. Have the client lie down.
3. Elevate the feet.
4. Remove excess clothing.
5. Cool with water (externally).
6. Seek immediate attention.

B. FAINTING
1. Place the client in the supine position, with the feet above the head if possible.
2. Maintain an open airway.
3. Loosen tight clothing.
4. Take BP and HR if possible.
5. Seek medical attention if the client remains unconscious.

C. SIMPLE/COMPOUND FRACTURES
1. Immobilize and splint the extremity.
2. Seek immediate medical attention.

D. SEIZURE
1. Do not touch the person during convulsions.
2. Attempt to ensure safety by seeing that the client does not injure herself or himself.
3. Seek medical attention.

E. BLEEDING
1. Follow precautions regarding bloodborne pathogens.
2. Apply direct pressure over the site to stop the bleeding.
3. Protect the wound from contamination.
4. Elevate the injured area if the bleeding is severe.
5. Seek medical attention if stitches may be required.

F. CARDIAC ARREST
Incidence is 0.4 in 10,000 clinical exercise tests.
1. Signs and Symptoms
a. Rapid onset of fatigue.
b. Ventricular tachycardia.
c. Ventricular fibrillation.
d. Bradycardia.
2. Response
a. **If the patient is breathing and has a pulse**:
1) Call the EMS immediately.
2) Place the client/patient in the recovery position (prone, with one knee and hip slightly flexed) with the head to one side to avoid airway obstruction. **Do not** attempt this position with patients who have suspected cervical spine injury.
3) Stay with the client/patient, and continue to monitor his or her vital signs.
b. **If the client/patient is suspected of not breathing or having a pulse**:
1) Assess breathing and pulse.
2) Call the EMS.
3) Perform CPR, or use an AED.
4) Assist the medical staff or EMS in caring for the patient.

G. MYOCARDIAL INFARCTION (MI)
An MI is ischemic myocardial necrosis resulting from an abrupt reduction in blood flow to the myocardium. Reduced blood flow often results from arterial plaque buildup that occludes the coronary arteries.
1. Signs and Symptoms
a. Visceral pain described as pressure or aching that radiates down the left arm, chest, back, or jaw.
b. Gastrointestinal upset.
c. Dyspnea/shortness of breath.
d. Shock.
e. Ventricular fibrillation.
f. Bradycardia.
g. Cool, clammy skin.
2. Response
a. Terminate exercise immediately, and monitor HR and BP.
b. Call the EMS immediately.
c. Assess the client/patient carefully to determine if an MI is occurring; **prompt diagnosis is critical**.
d. Relieve client/patient distress.
e. Assist as needed with administration of thrombolytic agents to reperfuse occluded arteries.

TABLE 7-4. Acute Responses for Common Injuries/Emergencies

Injury/Emergency	Signs/Symptoms	Acute Care
Closed skin wounds (blisters, corns)	Pain, swelling, infection	Clean with antiseptic soap; apply sterile dressing, antibiotic ointment.
Open skin wounds (lacerations, abrasions)	Pain, redness, bleeding, swelling, headache, mild fever	Apply pressure to stop bleeding; clean with soap or sterile saline; apply sterile dressing; refer to physician for stitches or tetanus shot.
Contusions (bruises)	Swelling, localized pain, loss of function if severe	RICES; apply padding for protection if necessary.
Strains[a]		
Grade I	Pain, localized tenderness, tightness	RICES.
Grade II	Loss of function, hemorrhage	RICES; refer for physician evaluation if victim has impaired function.
Grade III	Palpable defect	Immobilization; RICES; immediate referral to physician.
Sprains[a]		
Grade I	Pain, point tenderness, strength loss, edema	RICES.
Grade II	Hemorrhage, measurable laxity	RICES; physician evaluation.
Grade III	Palpable or observable defect	Immobilization; RICES; physician evaluation.
Fractures		
Stress	Pain, point tenderness	Physician evaluation; rest.
Simple	Swelling, disability, pain	Immobilize with splint; physician evaluation; radiography.
Compound	Bleeding, swelling, pain, disability	Immobilize; control bleeding; apply sterile dressing; immediate physician evaluation.
Dizziness/syncope	Disoriented, confused, pale skin color	Determine responsiveness; place the victim supine, with his or her legs elevated; administer fluids if conscious; begin emergency breathing or compressions as needed.
Hypoglycemia (low blood sugar)	Pale skin color, skin moist and sweaty, tachycardia, hunger, double vision	Administer sugar if conscious; if unconscious, place sugar granules under tongue; if recovery requires more than 1 or 2 minutes, activate the EMS.
Hyperglycemia (high blood sugar)	Confused, nauseous, headache, breath has a sweet and fruity order, thirsty, abdominal pain and vomiting, hyperventilation.	Activate the EMS; administer fluids if conscious; turn head to side if vomiting
Hypothermia	Shivering, but may stop with extreme drops in core temperature; loss of coordination; muscle stiffness, lethargy	Activate the EMS, and transport to hospital; remove wet clothing, and replace with dry, warm clothing.
Hyperthermia		
Heat cramps	Involuntary, isolated muscle spasms	Administer fluids; apply direct pressure to spasm and release; massage cramping area with ice.
Heat syncope	Weakness, fatigue, hypotension, pale skin, syncope	Move to cool area; place supine, with legs elevated; administer fluids if conscious; check blood pressure.
Heat exhaustion	Profuse sweating, cold and clammy skin, multiple muscle spasms, headache, nausea, loss of consciousness, dizziness, tachycardia, low blood pressure	Move to cool area; place supine, with feet elevated,; administer fluids, monitor body temperature; refer for physician evaluation.
Heat stroke	Hot and dry skin, but can be sweating; dyspnea; confusion; often unconscious	Activate the EMS, and transport to hospital immediately; remove clothing, dowse with cool water; wrap in cool, wet sheets; administer fluids if conscious.
Angina (pain, pressure or tingling in the chest, neck, jaw, arm, and/or back)	Pain, sweating, denial of medical problem, nausea, shortness of breath	Stop activity, and place in seated or supine position (whichever position is most comfortable); activate the EMS if pain is not relieved; if unresponsive, check breathing and pulse; begin CPR if necessary.
Dyspnea, labored breathing	Hyperventilation, dizziness, wheezing, coughing, loss of coordination	Maintain an open airway; administer bronchodilator if prescribed; try pursed-lip breathing; if no relief, activate the EMS and transport.

[a]Signs and symptoms for each grade include those for the grade below the one listed (i.e., signs and symptoms of grade II also include those of grade I, and signs and symptoms of grade III include those of grades I and II).

CPR, cardiopulmonary resuscitation; EMS, emergency medical system; RICES, rest, ice, compression, elevation, stabilization

f.   Administer pain-relief medications as ordered by the physician.

g.   Stay with the client/patient, and continue to monitor his or her vital signs.

h.   Be prepared to begin CPR, or employ the AED.

H.   HYPERGLYCEMIA

Hyperglycemia is an abnormally high blood glucose level (>200 mg/dL) that can impair function and, if severe, can become an emergency situation (diabetic ketoacidosis).

1.   **Signs and Symptoms**
   a.   Confusion.
   b.   Headache.
   c.   Sweet, fruity breath odor.
   d.   Thirst.
   e.   Nausea and vomiting.
   f.   Reflex tachycardia.
   g.   Abdominal pain.
   h.   Hyperventilation.

2.   **Response**
   a.   Call the EMS.
   b.   Rehydrate and correct electrolyte loss through fluid administration.
   c.   Administer insulin.
   d.   Turn the client's/patient's head to one side if he or she is vomiting.

I.   TRANSIENT ISCHEMIC ATTACK

Transient ischemic attacks are sudden, brief ischemic attacks that usually involve the carotid or vertebral arteries in the neck.

1.   **Signs and Symptoms**
   a.   Pain in jaw or neck
   b.   Slight paralysis of one side (hemiparesis).
   c.   Difficulty speaking (aphasia).
   d.   Burning or tingling sensation in extremities.
   e.   Fatigue.

2.   **Response**
   a.   Stop exercise immediately.
   b.   Have the client/patient sit or lie down.
   c.   Administer prescribed medication if available.
   d.   Contact the physician.
   e.   If pain and other symptoms continue beyond 30 minutes, call the EMS.

J.   CORONARY THROMBOSIS

Coronary thrombosis is coronary occlusion by a thrombus (a clot of lipid-rich atherosclerotic plaque). Symptoms are caused by the rupture of these plaque deposits within the coronary arteries.

1.   **Signs and Symptoms**
   a.   Pain described as pressure or aching that radiates down the left arm, chest, or back.

b.   Gastrointestinal upset.
   c.   Dyspnea.
   d.   Shock.
   e.   Ventricular fibrillation.
   f.   Bradycardia.
   g.   Cool, clammy skin.

2.   **Response**
   a.   Call the EMS immediately.
   b.   Relieve patient distress.
   c.   Provide pain relief as prescribed by the physician.
   d.   Administer thrombolytic agents as ordered by the physician.
   e.   Stay with the patient, and continue monitoring his or her vital signs.

K.   INTERNAL CARDIAC DEFIBRILLATOR DISCHARGE

An internal cardiac defibrillator may dysfunction and discharge when it should not.

1.   **Signs and Symptoms**
   a.   Severe, sudden chest pain.
   b.   Dyspnea.
   c.   Muscle contractions in the chest or abdomen associated with discharge.
   d.   Loss of consciousness.
   e.   Ventricular fibrillation.
   f.   Cardiac arrest.

2.   **Response**
   a.   Call the EMS or physician immediately.
   b.   Place the patient in the recovery position, with the head turned to one side.
   c.   Stay with the patient, and monitor his or her vital signs.
   d.   **If the patient is not breathing or does not have a palpable pulse:**
      1)   Assess breathing and pulse.
      2)   Perform CPR, or use an AED. However, avoid pressure or contact within the area of defibrillator application.

L.   SERIOUS ARRHYTHMIAS

1.   Various arrhythmias can develop during exercise testing and training. Those considered to be serious and that require emergency attention include:
   a.   **Ventricular fibrillation.**
   b.   **Ventricular tachycardia.**
   c.   **Atrial fibrillation.**
   d.   **Torsades de pointes.**
   e.   **Bradycardia.**

2.   The most severe arrhythmias (atrial fibrillation, ventricular fibrillation) **can result in an MI** and require defibrillation to control.

M. HYPOGLYCEMIA

Actual blood glucose levels that elicit hypoglycemic symptoms are highly individualized. Generally, however, levels of less than 50 mg/dL may be problematic.

1. **Signs and Symptoms**
   a. Tremors.
   b. Tachycardia.
   c. Diaphoresis.
   d. Visual disturbances.
   e. Confusion.
   f. Headache.
   g. Fatigue.
   h. Light-headedness.
   i. Seizures.
2. **Response to a Hypoglycemic Emergency**
   a. Contact the EMS immediately.
   b. Give the client/patient an **oral glucose solution** (e.g., orange juice, nondiet soft drink).
   c. Keep the client/patient comfortable and safe.

N. BRONCHOSPASM

Bronchospasm is an obstruction of the airway caused by spasm of airway smooth muscle, edema of airway mucosa, increased mucus secretion, or injury.

1. **Signs and symptoms**
   a. Dyspnea.
   b. Hyperventilation.
   c. Coughing.
   d. Wheezing.
   e. Chest tightness.
2. **Response**
   a. Maintain an open airway.
   b. Administer a bronchodilator if prescribed by a physician.
   c. Administer oxygen if available.

d. Replace fluids and electrolytes.
e. Keep the client/patient calm to reduce his or her anxiety.

O. HYPOTENSION/SHOCK

1. **Signs and Symptoms**
   a. Chills.
   b. Loss of consciousness.
   c. Bradycardia.
   d. Dizziness.
   e. Confusion.
2. **Response**
   a. Have the client/patient lie supine with the feet elevated.
   b. Maintain an open airway.
   c. Monitor vital signs.
   d. Call the EMS.

XVI. Common Category I Medications Administered in Medical Emergencies

A. **Epinephrine** is an endogenous catecholamine that optimizes blood flow to the heart and brain by increasing aortic diastolic pressure and preferentially shunting blood to the internal carotid artery (enhancing cerebral blood flow).

B. **Lidocaine** is an antiarrhythmic agent that decreases automaticity in the ventricular myocardium and raises the fibrillation threshold.

C. **Oxygen** ensures adequate arterial oxygen content and greatly enhances tissue oxygenation.

D. **Atropine** is a parasympathetic blocking agent used in the treatment of bradyarrhythmias.

Review Test

DIRECTIONS: Carefully read all questions, and select the BEST single answer.

1. The clinical exercise physiologist shares a responsibility to
   A) Implement measures to stop disease.
   B) Make patients look healthy.
   C) Implement preventive measures to reduce the risk of medical emergencies.
   D) Develop a plan to reduce the physical demands of exercise testing.

2. Which of the following is NOT considered to be a benefit of follow-up in an emergency situation?
   A) It provides information regarding the patient's current status, which may help to determine the cause of the emergency.
   B) It provides statistics that will help to justify the emergency response program.
   C) It allows the staff to finalize the incident report.
   D) It provides information to determine the consequences of the staff's actions.

3. Which of the following actions involving termination of exercise testing is correct?
   A) Immediately terminate the test if muscular fatigue occurs.
   B) Initiate the test termination process when cardiac complications occur.
   C) Initiate the test termination process when intermittent premature ventricular contractions are detected on ECG.
   D) Immediately terminate the test when intermittent premature ventricular contractions are detected on ECG.

4. Safety procedures for clinical staff help protect them from
   A) Bloodborne pathogens.
   B) Theft.
   C) Violent patients.
   D) Work-related injuries.

5. The treatment modality RICES includes all of the following EXCEPT
   A) Covering.
   B) Ice.
   C) Stabilization.
   D) Rest.

6. Which of the following statements about emergency equipment is MOST important?
   A) Each piece of equipment should be painted a specific color for easy identification.
   B) Use of emergency equipment should be practiced routinely.

C) Emergency equipment should include pencils, not pens.
D) Emergency equipment should be kept clean at all times.

7. Identifying a patient's risk of complications is important. Which of the following is NOT considered to be a common aspect of the risk identification process?
   A) Laboratory results.
   B) Assessment of cardiac risk.
   C) Review of medical history.
   D) Assessment of work history.

8. Symptoms of hyperglycemia include all of the following EXCEPT
   A) Tremor.
   B) Confusion.
   C) Bradycardia.
   D) Slurred speech.

9. Emergency procedures and safety include which of the following?
   A) Injury prevention.
   B) Basic principles for exercise training.
   C) Metabolic injuries.
   D) Emergency consequences.

10. Category 1 medications include all of the following EXCEPT
    A) Lidocaine.
    B) Oxygen.
    C) Xylocaine.
    D) Epinephrine.

11. The emergency response system (EMS) is:
    A) The combination of the ambulance and the emergency room.
    B) Critical for the staff to be able to respond adequately to an emergency.
    C) The protocol used to practice safety plans.
    D) Required by most health departments.

12. In developing an emergency plan, program administrators must take into account all of the following factors EXCEPT
    A) Type of flooring.
    B) Type of electrical wiring.
    C) Ventilation, temperature, and humidity.
    D) Types of exercise equipment.

13. Documentation in the context of emergency response commonly refers to
    A) Records of each exercise session.
    B) Records of attendance.
    C) Records of all emergency situations.
    D) Manuals for all emergency equipment.

14. A patient who exhibits tachycardia, diaphoresis, light-headedness, and visual disturbances may be experiencing
    A) Hypoglycemia.
    B) Congestive heart failure.
    C) Hyperglycemia.
    D) Hypotension.

15. Which of the following is NOT part of an emergency plan?
    A) The plan should list the schedule of each staff member so that they can all be accounted for during an emergency.
    B) The plan must be written.
    C) The plan should outline each specific action.
    D) The staff should be prepared and trained in the plan.

16. The physician's role in an emergency plan is
    A) Not important, because most facilities are hospital-based and the emergency room is nearby.
    B) Not significant, because a physician is not necessary when testing is conducted.
    C) An agency that certifies a managed care organization.
    D) Critical, because the physician must be present and can handle any emergency situation.

17. What is OSHA?
    A) A state agency that licenses medical facilities.
    B) A federal agency that sets standards for staff and patient safety.
    C) An agency that certifies a managed care organization.
    D) A state agency that inspects emergency protocols within medical facilities.

18. The preparation of professional staff should include training in
    A) Advanced basic life support and ENT.
    B) CPR and basic life support.
    C) CPR and EMS.
    D) Advanced cardiac life support and ENT.

19. Which of the following is NOT considered to be an absolute contraindication to exercise testing?
    A) Unstable angina.
    B) Psychosis.
    C) Suspected myocarditis.
    D) Moderate valvular heart disease.

20. Which of the following manifestations would be an indication for stopping an exercise test?
    A) Low cholesterol (<125 mol).
    B) Diastolic BP greater than 105 mm Hg.
    C) Intermittent premature ventricular contractions.
    D) Low blood sugar (<100 mg/dL).

21. Serious complications during an exercise session
    A) Occur more often with women.
    B) Rarely occur.
    C) Occur at a rate of 1 in 3,000 hours of exercise.
    D) Occur more often during the late hours because of client fatigue.

22. The exercise staff's role when an injury or emergency occurs should be to:
    A) Control the situation by implementing the emergency plan and taking charge.
    B) Find someone to implement the emergency plan.
    C) Get everyone out of the facility to avoid chaos.
    D) Hope that an emergency contact is available to help with the situation.

23. In preventing injuries, hydration is very important, because
    A) It controls breathing and the Valsalva maneuver.
    B) It helps to regulate carbohydrate utilization during cardiovascular exercise.
    C) It helps to regulate body temperature and electrolyte balance.
    D) It helps to prevent blood pooling during the cool-down.

24. What U.S. legislation is critical for operators of fitness facilities to understand and adhere to regarding safety?
    A) The Americans with Handicaps Act.
    B) The Civil Rights Act of 1966.
    C) The Health Portability Act of 1996.
    D) The Americans with Disabilities Act.

25. What is the most appropriate action in assisting a person suffering from a seizure?
    A) Hold the person down so that he or she does not hurt himself or herself.
    B) Do not touch the person, but be sure that he or she is in a safe area.
    C) Place a wedge in the person's mouth so that he or she does not swallow the tongue.
    D) Ignore the person, and allow the seizure to pass.

26. One of the **first** actions that a fitness instructor should consider in preventing injury is to
    A) Teach the client how to warm-up and cool-down.
    B) Instruct the client on safety procedures when using the facility.
    C) Conduct a preparticipation screening.
    D) Instruct the client on how to use the exercise equipment safely.

27. How should a fitness instructor advise a client with regard to progression of the exercise program?
    A) The progression should be gradual and slow.
    B) The progression should be at specific increments based on a calendar schedule (e.g., add 10% every 2 weeks).
    C) Be aggressive in increasing the program to increase fitness.
    D) Progress the program only when the client feels ready.

28. How can exercise equipment add to the risk of participation?
    A) Because it is expensive.
    B) Because it is hard to move.
    C) Because it is used incorrectly.
    D) Because of the time one waits to use it.

29. Prevention strategies of staff and clients must include
    A) Following the rules.
    B) Keeping the facility clean.
    C) Hiring good front-desk staff.
    D) Developing clever, unique programs.

30. An equipment maintenance plan should include
    A) A floor plan.
    B) A client advisory statement.
    C) A document that records maintenance and repair history.
    D) Temperature and humidity readings.

31. In cleaning the facility and equipment, what must an operator be aware of?
    A) That signs are written clearly.
    B) That surfaces are brightly colored.
    C) That solutions and cleaning materials are safe for the skin and hypoallergenic.
    D) That disinfectants smell pleasant.

32. Which of the following are symptoms of hypoglycemia?
    A) Hypotension.
    B) Cold, clammy skin.
    C) Tachycardia and slurred speech.
    D) Bronchospasms and hyperventilation.

33. RICES refers to
    A) Relaxation, Ice, Compression, Energy, and Stabilization.
    B) Relaxation, Incremental heat, Care for injury, Energy, and Standardization.
    C) Rest, Ice, Common sense, Energy, and Standardization.
    D) Rest, Ice, Compression, Elevation, and Stabilization.

34. Complaints of pain in the chest with associated pain radiating down the left arm may be signs of
    A) Cardiac crisis.
    B) Hypotension.
    C) Seizure.
    D) Heartburn.

35. Beyond the general safety parameters, such as keeping equipment in good repair, a facility must create a safe environment for any individual, especially
    A) Guest clients.
    B) Staff.
    C) Health care providers.
    D) Special populations.

36. Weight room safety should include
    A) A phone.
    B) Lifting gloves and back belts.
    C) Male trainers to help with spotting.
    D) Safe passageways and use of the buddy system.

37. Fire, bloodborne pathogens, and power outage should all be included in
    A) Facility insurance.
    B) Safety plans.
    C) Maintenance plans.
    D) Testing by the facility and staff.

38. The potential benefits and risks of an exercise test should be written in what document?
    A) Description of services.
    B) Safety plan.
    C) Informed consent.
    D) Exercise waivers.

39. Documentation offers important
    A) Liability and negligence protection.
    B) Liability and risk protection.
    C) Safety and communication programs.
    D) Billing and classification tools.

40. Emergency procedures should be
    A) Given to all clients when they join.
    B) Put away in a safe place.
    C) Posted under each phone.
    D) Posted above each fire extinguisher.

41. Which of the following is NOT a principle of low back care?
    A) Abdominal curl-ups/
    B) Unloaded flexion/extension of the spine.
    C) Neutral spine during all exercises.
    D) Controlled leg press or squat with light weights.

42. What is the fitness instructor's primary responsibility in conducting an exercise test?
    A) Maintaining a safe environment by not putting the client in danger.
    B) Making sure that the data collected are accurate.
    C) Completing the test.
    D) Encouragement and support.

43. What are some of the risks for musculoskeletal injury?
    A) Poor signage in the facility.
    B) Extrinsic factors—intensity, terrain, equipment.
    C) Intrinsic factors—frequency, attitude, gender.
    D) Membership type.

44. Chronic soreness and fatigue are symptoms of
    A) Hyperglycemia.
    B) Strain.
    C) Overuse injury.
    D) Hypoglycemia.

45. Exercise clothing
    A) Creates an important fashion statement.
    B) Should be bright so that you are easily seen in an aerobics class.
    C) Has only one rule: be comfortable.
    D) Must be safe and performs appropriately, like the exercise equipment.

ANSWERS AND EXPLANATIONS

1–C. The clinical exercise physiologist must understand the risks of exercise while realizing the benefits. If the benefits clearly outweigh the risks, preventive measures should be implemented to reduce that risk. The clinical exercise physiologist cannot eradicate or cure disease; he or she can only work to help prevent or reduce the symptoms of disease. The clinical exercise physiologist is concerned with the patient's health, not with the patient's appearance.

2–B. The follow-up is an important function following an incident. Justification of a program has no relevance when investigating an incident. The primary concern should be the health status of the patient and the cause of the emergency. The patient's present status is, indeed, part of the follow-up, because it will provide medical information that can help to determine the cause of injury. Also, information from the patient can help to piece together the specific actions of the incident. In addition, this follow-up information will help staff members to complete their report, because they may learn new and helpful information that should be included. The final report with the follow-up information will assist program administrators in determining the consequences of their actions.

3–C. Intermittent premature ventricular contractions (PVCs) are not a serious concern, so the tester can begin the test termination process instead of terminating the test immediately. Muscular fatigue and intermittent PVCs do not require immediate termination of the test; initiating the test termination process is appropriate. Cardiac complications are considered to be very serious and require immediate termination, not merely initiation of the test termination process.

4–A. Because of the importance of infection control, bloodborne pathogens must be a concern for all staff, and OSHA regulations help to protect both patients and staff. Theft and violent patients may be concerns but are not part of any emergency plan. The plan may include injuries in general but not work-related injuries specifically.

5–A. Covering is not part of RICES. Compression is the "C" component.

6–B. Routine practice in using emergency equipment is an important part of the emergency plan to ensure that staff members know how to use the equipment correctly in an emergency situation. Identification of equipment through tagging, not color, is important. Whether to use pens or pencils is irrelevant, and although equipment should be kept clean, this is not an essential part of emergency equipment protocol.

7–D. Work history is not a relevant part of the identification process. Work history most likely will not provide any meaningful information regarding the risk of medical emergencies. The review of medical history is very important and can identify significant cardiac risk factors. Assessment of laboratory results may indicate signs of potential cardiac or pulmonary risk, which could contraindicate exercise testing. Assessment of cardiac risk is critical to the determination of potential complications and clearly is part of the identification process.

8–C. Tachycardia, not bradycardia, is a possible sign of hyperglycemia. Elevated blood sugar overloads the endocrine system; tremors, confusion, and slurred speech are common responses to this overload.

9–A. Injury prevention often is overlooked, but it is an important part of a facility's emergency procedures and safety program. All clinical exercise physiologists should understand how to avoid emergencies. Basic principles for exercise training are important for general day-to-day operations but not for emergency procedures.

10–C. Xylocaine, though similar to lidocaine, is not an antiarrhythmic agent, as lidocaine is. Thus, xylocaine cannot help to stabilize the heart in a cardiac crisis. Oxygen often is overlooked as a drug, but it helps to keep tissues alive. Epinephrine optimizes blood flow to the heart and brain and is an important category 1 medication.

11–B. The emergency response system is designed to help the staff adequately handle emergencies. The ambulance and emergency room as well as the protocols used to practice safety procedures may be a part of an emergency response plan, but they are not part of the emergency response system. Health departments do not regulate emergency response systems.

12–D. Flooring and electrical wiring are important factors in the risk of accidents. Environmental factors can increase the risk of crises; for example, poor air quality, high temperatures, and high humidity can cause pulmonary difficulties and increase the risk of heat exhaustion.

13–C. Documentation of every aspect of an emergency situation is an important component of any emergency response system. Records of exercise sessions and attendance may be important for standard operations but are not important for emergency response. Equipment manuals should be on file but are not considered to be documentation in this context.

14–A. Common signs and symptoms of hypoglycemia include tachycardia, diaphoresis, light-headedness, and visual disturbances. Congestive heart failure and hypotension do not produce tachycardia. Hyperglycemia does not produce diaphoresis.

15–A. Accounting for staff in an emergency is not essential. Writing down the plan is essential so that the staff can read it as part of their training as well as have a document to refer to during an emergency. Delineating specific actions by each staff member in an emergency situation and training the staff in these actions obviously are integral parts of any emergency plan.

16–C. Communication with the physician is very important during a medical crisis, and exercise staff should have a ready means of communicating with a physician in the event of an emergency. A physician should be nearby, but not necessarily in the room, during any exercise test.

17–B. OSHA is a federal agency that sets safety standards for staff and patients. The National Committee for Quality Assurance (NCQA) is an accreditation agency that inspects and certifies MCOs.

18–B. CPR and basic life support are important certifications in the care of medical emergencies. There is no advanced basic life support certification. Both EMS and ENT are not appropriate emergency care training for exercise staff.

19–D. Individuals with moderate valvular heart disease are able to function under the stress of exercise, especially if they are under the care of a cardiac specialist and receive permission to undergo an exercise test. Unstable angina may lead to a significant cardiac crisis when exercise is introduced, so it is considered to be an absolute contraindication with exercise. Psychosis is a significant emotional distress and can lead to difficulties in completing the exercise test, so it is considered to be an absolute contraindication. Myocarditis is an absolute contraindication of exercise testing, because inflammation of the heart's muscular walls can cause severe cardiac complications with the increased stroke volume and HR associated with the stress of exercise.

20–D. Low blood sugar may indicate a lack of glucose for muscle activity. Low blood sugar also leads to hypoglycemia, which can bring about light-headedness, tachycardia, and confusion, suggesting that the exercise session be stopped. Low cholesterol should have little or no effect on the exerciser. As long as the diastolic BP does not change significantly (by more than 20 mm Hg) during the test, 105 mm Hg is not considered to be a contraindication to exercise. Intermittent PVCs do not pose a danger to an exerciser, so the test should not be halted.

21–B. Medical complications and injury can and do occur in an exercise setting. Fortunately, however, serious complications rarely occur. No data suggest that women suffer more serious complications with exercise than men. Also, no data support the statements that serious complications occur late in the day and that serious complications occurs at a rate significantly lower than 1 in 3,000 hours of exercise. In truth, this rate is closer to 1 in 3,000,000 hours of exercise.

22–A. One of the exercise staff's responsibilities when an injury or emergency occurs is to control the situation by implementing the emergency plan and taking charge. Staff should make sure the proper actions are taken to ensure the safety and care of injured clients. One of those actions is to instruct the people around him or her to help implement the plan. It is inappropriate for the staff to sit back and let someone else implement the plan or hope that an emergency contact can take control of the situation. Controlling the situation and instructing those around the staff is the primary role, and getting people out of the facility may only happen under certain situations.

23–C. Hydration is one of the most important principles of exercise. Two of the effects of hydration are regulating body temperature and electrolyte balance. If either is out of balance because of dehydration (lack of appropriate hydration), it can lead to nausea, light-headedness, and heat exhaustion. Hydration does not affect breathing, carbohydrate utilization, or blood pooling.

24–D. The ADA protects individuals with any disability from discrimination of access. Fitness facilities must provide free and easy access to all disabled individuals throughout the facility. The Americans with Handicaps Act does not exist, and the Civil Rights Act was enacted in 1964, not in 1966. The Health Portability Act involves employees with health insurance and is not related to safety.

25–B. Most people undergoing seizures display convulsing actions. With a convulsing seizure, the safest action is to not touch the person and to let the convulsion pass. Any action can cause potential danger to you and the victim. It is not safe to hold the person down or try to wedge anything into the victim's mouth.

26–C. Before starting a fitness program, it is important to understand the client's medical history and risk of a crisis during exercise. A preparticipation screening can help to establish this understanding and prevent injury or crisis. Teaching the warm-up and cool-down prevents injury, but it is not the first thing that you do. The same argument applies to teaching safety procedures and safe use of the equipment.

27–A. It is always safest to advise clients to progress in a fitness program gradually and slowly. This advice also increases the chance for program success and increased motivation. Using the calendar method does not take into account individual effects in adjusting to exercise. Clients may not be ready to progress when the calendar indicates that it is time to do so, just as clients do not always know when to increase or may not be aggressive enough. Always taking an aggressive approach increases the risk of injury, because the increase may be too much too soon.

28–C. Using exercise equipment incorrectly can place excess stress on muscles and joints and increase the risk of injury, which adds to the risk of participation. The expense and ability to move exercise equipment have no bearing on the risk of participation. The time that one waits also does not add to the risk, unless the client uses the equipment incorrectly.

29–A. Prevention strategies refer to the risk of injury. One of the critical aspects in preventing injuries is to follow the rules, which are made to prevent problems. Keeping the facility clean and hiring good front-desk staff are important and can help to prevent problems, but they are not considered to be prevention strategies. Unique programs are designed to attract clients, not to prevent risk.

30–C. The maintenance plan ensures that the exercise equipment is functioning properly and safely. Records that document maintenance and repairs are important in tracking when to maintain equipment and to make sure that repairs are conducted and completed. A floor plan is not necessary in a maintenance plan. Temperature and humidity readings should be included in a program plan (when necessary) but not a maintenance plan. A client advisory statement does not exist.

31–C. When cleaning a facility, it is very important that the solutions used do not cause skin problems or allergic reactions. A safe facility must avoid these problems. Cleaning a facility usually does not involve signs or require particular colors of surfaces. A pleasant smell is nice to have, but this does not prevent problems or allergic reactions.

32–C. Hypoglycemia, or low blood sugar, has many symptoms, which include tachycardia and slurred speech. Hypoglycemia may increase BP, but it does not cause hypotension or low BP. Bronchospasms and cold, clammy skin are not symptoms of hypoglycemia.

33–D. RICES refers to Rest (let the injury heal without stress), Ice (reduces swelling and promotes healing), Compression (reduces swelling), Elevation (reduces swelling), and Stabilization (reduces muscle spasm by assisting in relaxation of associated muscles). Energy, incremental heat, standardization, and common sense do not decrease swelling, promote healing, reduce muscle spasm, or reduce the stress to the injury.

34–A. Symptoms of a cardiac crisis (e.g., heart failure, heart attack) include pain in the chest and pain radiating down the left arm. Hypertension, not hypotension, is a possible cause of a cardiac crisis. A seizure and heartburn are not associated with a cardiac crisis.

35–D. A safe environment is very important, and this fact is most important to many of the special populations that may have difficulty negotiating their way around a facility because of injury, disability, or age. Health care providers, staff, and guest clients are important, but in most cases, they do not require special attention regarding safety.

36–D. The weight room can be a dangerous place if safety is not a priority. Dumbbells, plates, and bars can fall or be thrown and cause injury. Safe passageways reduce the risk of a client getting hit by an exercising client. The buddy system helps with spotting and instruction, which reduces the risk of injury. A phone can cause distractions. Lifting gloves and belts may be helpful to clients in easing the burden of lifting, but they are not critical for safety. Female trainers can be just as effective as male trainers in spotting.

37–B. Safety plans help to educate and guide staff in developing and maintaining a safe facility. The safety plan should include procedures for a fire, a power outage, and the exposure to bloodborne pathogens. Facility insurance addresses fire and, possibly, power outages, but it does not address bloodborne pathogens. Maintenance plans address the repair and maintenance of the equipment, but they do not address any of the three factors listed in the question. Testing by staff may involve bloodborne pathogens, but this has no involvement in fires or power outages.

38–C. Informed consent is a document that a client reads, or that is read to a client by a staff member, that explains the exercise test to be conducted in detail along with the potential benefits and risks, the purpose of the test, and the client's responsibilities. The informed consent does not explain the services. The safety plan is designed to create a safe exercise environment and does not discuss potential benefits or risks. Exercise waivers place the total responsibility of exercise on the client and may list the risks, but they do not discuss the benefits.

39–A. Documentation provides a record of events and a written description of the rules, rights, and risks of the program. These documents are designed to ensure the safety of both the clients and the staff. They also are designed to protect the facility and staff from liability or negligence issues, because they promote safety and reduce the risk of injury. Documentation does not protect against risk, but it provides tools to help reduce it. Program design or policies are written into documents, but they are not the programs. Documentation also may be tools for billing and classification, but it is not necessarily as important as computer software or the management of the data needed for both of these programs.

40–C. Emergency procedures should be easy to find so that the staff can act quickly to handle the emergency, not spend time looking for the procedures. The procedures should be placed by the phones, because they often are used in an emergency to dial 911 and to initiate emergency help. Emergency procedures should not be given to clients, because they should not be involved in enacting them. Only the staff should implement the emergency procedures. Placing the procedures in a safe place does not make them easy to find when they are needed. By the phones is a better place than by the fire extinguishers to put the emergency procedures, because unlike a fire extinguisher, a phone is used in almost all emergencies.

41–D. Leg press and squats with any type of weight adds compression to the spine, which can have significant adverse effects in the care of a low back injury. It is very important to increase flexibility and muscular strength without excessive load or compression. Abdominal curl-ups, unloaded flexion/extension of the spine (cat stretch), and maintaining a neutral spine during exercise are principles that do not place unnecessary load or compression on the spine and serve to increase both the flexibility and strength of supporting structures.

42–A. Safety is the most important responsibility for a fitness instructor. A fitness instructor must never endanger anyone. Accurate data are good to obtain, but this is secondary to safety. Completing the test and encouragement also are goals, but not the top priority, of the fitness instructor.

43–B. Included with the many risks for musculoskeletal injury are extrinsic or outside factors. If intensity is too high, one could overstress joints and muscles. Rough or uneven terrain can lead to falls. Poorly designed or maintained equipment can cause breakdowns or incorrect positioning, which in turn can cause injury. Signage usually does not lead to injury, and membership type is not a factor in musculoskeletal injury. Although intrinsic factors are included in the risks, frequency is not an intrinsic factor, so this answer is incorrect.

44–C. Chronic soreness, fatigue, lack of desire to rest, and changes in menstrual cycle are all symptoms of an overuse injury. Overtraining is another term used for this condition, which often occurs in individuals who are training for competition or who become obsessed with fitness training. Hyperglycemia and hypoglycemia are related to blood glucose levels and do not exhibit chronic soreness. A strain may show as a symptom; how-ever, fatigue usually is not associated with this condition.

45–D. Exercise clothing also is exercise equipment, and like the exercise machines that one uses, it is critical that exercise clothing be safe and per-form adequately. If not, then the risk of injury is increased. Fashion statements do not mean that the clothes are safe and perform appropriately. Bright clothing is not important in an aerobics class. Although comfort is important, safety and importance are more important and critical.

8 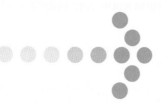 Exercise Programming

JOHN W. WYGAND AND KATHLEEN M. CAHILL

I. Introduction

A. PURPOSE OF EXERCISE PROGRAMS
1. Enhancement of physical **fitness for daily activities**, recreation, or competitive athletic endeavors.
2. Primary or secondary **disease prevention**.

B. ACSM/CENTERS FOR DISEASE CONTROL AND PREVENTION RECOMMENDATIONS
1. All adults should accumulate 30 minutes of physical activity on most (preferably all) days of the week.
2. Health benefits can be accrued with moderate amounts of physical activity (e.g., 30 min of walking, or 15 min of jogging), but greater benefits may be realized from greater amounts of physical activity.

C. The ACSM recommends a target range of 150 to 400 kcal of energy expenditure per day.
1. The lower end of this range (1,000 kcal/week) is associated with a significant health benefit.
2. Based on a dose-response relationship, individuals should be encouraged to move toward the upper end of the recommended range as their fitness improves.
3. Weekly caloric expenditure in excess of **2,000 kcal per week** has been shown to be successful for short- and long term weight control as well as for primary and secondary prevention of chronic disease.

D. Components of a comprehensive exercise program include:
1. **Warm-up.**
2. **Cardiovascular endurance (aerobic) exercise stimulus.**
3. **Resistance exercise.**
4. **Flexibility training.**
5. **Cool-down.**

II. Essential Components of an Exercise Prescription

A. Development of a systematic, individualized exercise prescription depends on the thoughtful, scientific integration of five essential components into a structured exercise program:
1. **Mode.**
2. **Frequency.**
3. **Intensity.**
4. **Duration.**
5. **Progression.**

B. These essential components are applied in an exercise program regardless of the participant's age, health status, or fitness level.

C. Consideration of the **limitations, needs**, and **goals** of each individual will result in a more individualized, safer, and effective exercise program.

D. The following data obtained from a graded exercise test provide the basis for the exercise prescription:
1. **Heart rate (HR).**
2. **Blood pressure (BP).**
3. **Rating of perceived exertion (RPE).**
4. **Functional capacity.**

III. Cardiovascular Endurance Exercise

A. The ability to take in, deliver, and use oxygen is dependent on the function of the circulatory systems and cellular metabolic capacities.

B. The amount of expected improvement in cardiovascular endurance fitness is directly related to the frequency, intensity, duration, and mode of exercise.

C. Maximal oxygen uptake ($\dot{V}O_{2max}$) is genetically limited and may increase between 5% and 30% with training.

D. MODE

Mode is the type of exercise.

1. Cardiovascular endurance exercise is most effective when **large muscle groups** are engaged in **continuous, rhythmic** (aerobic) activity.

2. Various activities, such as walking, jogging, cycling, rowing, stair climbing, aerobic dance ("aerobics"), water exercise, and cross-country skiing, may be incorporated to increase enjoyment and improve compliance.

3. The potential for musculoskeletal injury increases when excessive weight-bearing activity is performed.

4. Comfortable, supportive walking or running shoes are important.

5. Selection of mode should be based on the desired outcomes, focusing on the exercises most likely to **sustain participation** (adherence and compliance) and enjoyment.

6. Cardiovascular endurance exercise requires the involvement of large muscle groups in activity performed in a rhythmic fashion over a prolonged duration.

7. **Stair Climbing**
   a. Necessary equipment is commonly found in fitness centers.
   b. An upright posture is important to avoid low back trauma.
   c. Weak quadriceps and gluteals may cause dependence on handrails for support, reducing the intensity of the exercise.

8. **Aerobics** is typically a group activity.
   a. Intensity is usually controlled by music and choreographed movement patterns.
   b. The HR is not an accurate indicator of intensity when arm movement is vigorously added to the routine.
   c. The RPE is an appropriate indicator of intensity.
   d. **High-Impact Aerobics**
      1) Involve movement patterns in which both feet leave the floor simultaneously.
      2) May require significant energy expenditure.
      3) Increase the potential for musculoskeletal injury.
   e. **Low-Impact Aerobics**
      1) Involve movement patterns in which one foot remains in contact with the floor at all times.
      2) Produce low-impact forces and low incidence of musculoskeletal injury.
      3) Are appropriate for highly fit individuals.
      4) Can be increased in intensity by using greater horizontal displacement during movement.
   f. **Step Aerobics**
      1) Involve choreographed movement patterns performed on and off bench steps varying in height from 4 to 12 inches.
      2) Have an energy cost that ranges from 6 to 11 metabolic equivalents (MET).
      3) Should be reduced in cadence for individuals who are less fit (functional capacity, <8 MET).
   g. Organizations such as the ACSM, the American Council on Exercise (ACE), and the Aerobics and Fitness Association of America (AFAA) are excellent resources for more detailed information and continuing education.
   h. **Water Exercise**
      1) Allows the buoyancy properties of water to reduce the weight-bearing load, decreasing the incidence of musculoskeletal injury.
      2) May allow those with injuries to exercise during rehabilitation.
      3) May be altered in intensity by changing the speed of movement or the depth of the water or by using resistive devices (e.g., fins, hand paddles).
      4) Involves walking, jogging, and dance activity.
      5) Typically combines the benefits of the buoyancy and resistive properties of water, providing an aerobic stimulus as well as enhancing muscular strength and endurance.
      6) May benefit special population groups:
         a) Obese.
         b) Pregnant.
         c) Arthritic.
         d) Elderly.
   i. **Cycling**
      1) A nonweight-bearing activity a with low incidence of musculoskeletal injury.
      2) An ergometer is recommended for accurate exercise testing and training so that workload can be quantified.
      3) The major limiting factor to cycling is local muscle fatigue of the upper leg.

E.   INTENSITY

Intensity is the relative (physiological) difficulty of the exercise.

1.   Intensity and duration interact and are inversely related.

   a.   Improvements in aerobic fitness from low-intensity, longer duration exercise are similar to those with higher intensity, short-duration exercise.

   b.   This becomes a consideration when developing an exercise prescription for individuals who do not enjoy high-intensity physical activity.

2.   Risk of orthopedic and other complications increases with higher intensity activity.

3.   Factors to consider when determining intensity for a particular client include:

   a.   Level of fitness.

   b.   Medical conditions.

   c.   Medications that may influence exercise performance.

   d.   Risk of cardiovascular or orthopedic injury.

   e.   Individual preference.

   f.   Program objectives.

4.   The ACSM recommends that exercise intensity be prescribed within a range of 64% to 94% of maximum HR, 50% to 85% of oxygen uptake reserve ($\dot{V}O_2R$) or HR reserve (HRR) (*Figure 8-1*).

   a.   Lower intensities (30–50% of $\dot{V}O_2R$) elicit a favorable response in individuals with low fitness levels.

   b.   An intensity of 60% to 80% of HRR or $\dot{V}O_2R$ is reasonable for improvement of cardiovascular endurance fitness.

   c.   Use of the actual maximal HR from a graded exercise test is preferable to estimating the maximal HR based on age.

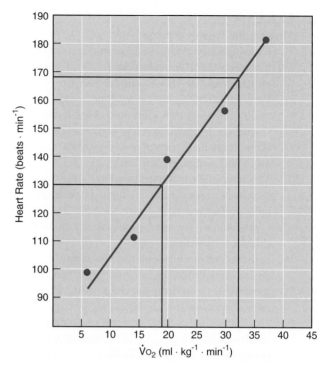

FIGURE 8-2. A line of best fit has been drawn through the data points on this plot of heart rate and oxygen consumption data observed during a hypothetical maximal exercise test in which maximal oxygen consumption ($\dot{V}O_2$max) was observed to be 38 mL·kg^{-1} min^{-1} and maximal heart rate was 184 bpm. A target heart rate range was determined by finding the heart rates that correspond to 50% and 85% of $\dot{V}O_2$max. For this individual, 50% of $\dot{V}O_2$max was approximately 19 mL·kg^{-1}·min^{-1}, and 85% of $\dot{V}O_2$max was approximately 32 mL·kg^{-1}·min^{-1}. The corresponding target heart rates are approximately 130 and 168 bpm, respectively. (From *ACSM's Guidelines for Exercise Testing and Prescription*. 6th Ed. Baltimore, Lippincott Williams & Wilkins, 2000, p. 148.)

	220	220
Age	-25	-25
Max Heart Rate	195	195
Resting Heart Rate	-75	-75
Heart Rate Reserve	120	120
50-85%	x .6	x .8
	72	96
Resting Heart Rate	+75	+75
Target Heart Rate	60% HRR=147 147	80% HRR=171 171

FIGURE 8-1. Calculation of 50% to 85% of the heart rate reserve (HRR) based on a 25-year-old individual with a resting heart rate of 75 bpm. (From Karvonen M, Kentala K, Mustala O: The effects of training on heart rate: A longitudinal study. *Annales Medicinae Experimentalis et Biological Fennial* 35:307–315, 1957.)

5.   The RPE may be used as an adjunct to the HR for regulating intensity.

   a.   The ACSM recommends an intensity that will elicit an RPE within a range of 12 to 16 on the original 6 to 20 (Borg) scale.

   b.   The RPE is considered to be a reliable indicator of exercise intensity; some learning is required on the part of the participant.

   c.   The RPE is particularly useful when a participant is unable to monitor his or her pulse accurately or when the HR response to exercise is altered by medications.

   d.   **The RPE should be individually determined on different exercise modalities.**

6.   The HR-$\dot{V}O_2$ relationship can be plotted to determine the exercise intensity (*Figure 8-2*).

7. An abnormal response to a graded exercise test or individual exercise limitations must be considered when prescribing intensity.
    a. The ACSM recommends that exercise at intensities eliciting the following signs/symptoms should be avoided:
        1) Exercise-induced angina.
        2) Inappropriate BP changes.
        3) Musculoskeletal discomfort.
        4) Leg pain.
        5) Any sign or symptom that causes premature termination of the exercise test.
    b. The training HR is set at 10 bpm lower than the HR when signs or symptoms of intolerance are present (see above).

F. DURATION

Duration is the time or length of an individual exercise session.

1. The ACSM recommends 20 to 60 minutes of continuous or intermittent aerobic activity.
2. Caloric expenditure and cardiovascular endurance conditioning goals may be achieved with exercise sessions of moderate duration (20–30 min).
3. High-intensity/short-duration exercise programs are associated with increased potential for injury.
4. Excessive duration is associated with decreased compliance.
5. Increases in exercise duration should be instituted as adaptation occurs without signs of intolerance.
6. Deconditioned individuals may benefit from multiple, short-duration exercise sessions (5–10 min) with frequent rest periods.
7. An inverse relationship exists between the intensity and duration of training.
8. Greater musculoskeletal and cardiovascular risk may occur with short-duration, high-intensity exercise compared to lower intensity, longer duration exercise.
9. Interval training programs using bouts of lower intensity exercise can be effective for improving cardiovascular endurance fitness.
    a. Intermittent exercise may allow for increased caloric expenditure and enhanced interest compared with continuous aerobic activity.
    b. Intermittent exercise may be particularly useful for beginning or deconditioned exercisers.
    c. Intermittent exercise programmed for health/fitness purposes should be aerobic in nature and not exceed an intensity of 85% of HRR.

G. FREQUENCY

Frequency is the number of exercise sessions per day and per week.

1. The ACSM recommends physical activity on most (preferably all) days of the week.
2. Frequency interacts with both intensity and duration.
3. Individual goals, preferences, limitations, and time constraints may affect frequency.
4. Frequency also is influenced by lifestyle and convenience.
5. Deconditioned people may benefit from lower intensity, shorter duration exercise performed at higher frequencies per day and/or per week.
6. An exercise frequency of greater than 5 days per week generally is used athletic performance enhancement or weight loss.

H. PROGRESSION

Progression is the periodic changes in exercise prescription (e.g., intensity, duration, frequency) necessary to increase fitness.

1. The rate of progression depends on health/fitness status, age, goals, and compliance.
2. Improvement depends on systematic progression of frequency, intensity, and/or duration.
3. Increasing the frequency and duration of an activity before increasing the intensity is preferred.
4. **Adaptation**
    a. Occurs when an individual can adequately respond to the demands of a particular exercise stressor.
    b. Depends on health/fitness status and the relative mix of frequency, intensity, duration, and mode of exercise.
5. Most participants adapt more easily and comfortably to smaller increases in the intensity, duration, and frequency of exercise.
6. Few objective markers are available for short-term adaptation (1–3 weeks). Some indicators may be:
    a. Improvements in motor patterns.
    b. Lower RPE or exercising HR at the same workload.
    c. Subjective evaluation through communication between the exercise professional and the individual.
7. The rate of adaptation is affected by compliance with the exercise program.
8. Increase the duration by 10% to 20% per week until the relevant goal is attained.
9. Once the duration goal is attained, increase the intensity by 5% to 10% every sixth training session.

I. STAGES OF CONDITIONING

1. Initial

a. Warm-up: 10–15 minutes.

b. Moderate intensity: 40–60% of HRR.

c. Interval: 15 minutes, progressing to 30 minutes.

d. Frequency: 3–4 days per week.

2. Improvement

a. 50% to 85% of HRR.

b. Progress duration by 10% to 20% per week or as tolerated if longer.

c. Progress intensity by 5% to 10% every 2 weeks until the relevant goal is attained.

d. Lasts approximately 4 to 8 months.

3. Maintenance

a. Goals have been attained.

b. Attainment of average fitness (50th percentile in all heath-related fitness parameters) is a reasonable goal.

c. Maintain fitness with a variety of activities.

J. WARM-UP

Warm-up involves low-intensity, large-muscle-group activity specific to the exercise to be performed.

1. Physiological changes induced by appropriate warm-up exercises include:

a. Increased muscle temperature.

b. Increased muscle blood flow.

c. Increased ease of dissociation of oxygen from hemoglobin.

d. Increased muscle enzyme activity.

e. Increased elasticity of muscle and connective tissue.

f. Decreased muscle viscosity.

2. Benefits of specific warm-up routines include enhanced performance and, perhaps (inconsistently demonstrated in the literature), prevention of musculoskeletal and cardiovascular complications.

3. Five to 10 minutes should be allowed for the warm-up.

4. Stretching may be included after the large muscle activity.

K. COOL-DOWN

Cool-down is low- to moderate-intensity, large-muscle-group activity performed for approximately 5 to 10 minutes. Physiological changes induced by appropriate cool-down exercises include:

1. Enhanced venous return.

2. Enhanced transport of metabolic byproducts away from skeletal muscle.

3. Gradual return of HR and BP to preexercise levels.

4. Skeletal muscle and connective tissue may be less viscous and more pliable after the exercise stimulus; therefore, the cool-down period may be an appropriate time to enhance flexibility through stretching.

L. SPECIFICITY

1. Training effects resulting from an exercise program are specific to the exercise performed and to the muscles involved. For example, running has little carry-over to swimming.

2. Cross-training with a variety of exercises may provide better transfer effects to daily work and leisure-time pursuits.

M. CONTRAINDICATIONS TO EXERCISE

The ACSM specifies medical conditions that preclude safe participation in exercise testing and exercise programs. See *Table 6-1* for a complete listing of these conditions.

N. TERMINATION OF AN EXERCISE SESSION

The ACSM specifies the conditions that require termination of a test or an exercise session. See *Table 6-12* for a complete listing of these conditions.

IV. Flexibility

A. Refers to the range of motion (ROM) or mobility of a joint.

B. Is necessary for optimal musculoskeletal health and physical activity.

C. Optimal musculoskeletal function requires that an adequate ROM be maintained in all joints.

D. Activities that enhance or maintain musculoskeletal flexibility should be included in comprehensive preventive or rehabilitative exercise programs.

E. Although flexibility can improve acutely, scientific evidence regarding how long the effect may last is lacking. Ballistic (bouncing) stretching and proprioceptive neuromuscular facilitation are not recommended inclusions for most general exercise programs.

F. STATIC STRETCHING

1. Involves slow stretching to the point of discomfort, then holding that position for 15 to 30 seconds.

2. Perform two to four repetitions of static stretches 2 to 7 days per week.
3. Incidence of musculoskeletal injury is small with proper mechanics and form.

G. RISKS OF STRETCHING

1. Correct body alignment and joint position are critical for effectiveness and to minimize the risk of musculoskeletal injury.
2. Some common stretching exercises may be potentially harmful to the musculoskeletal system and, in the general population, should be avoided or modified (*Figure 8-3*)

V. Muscular Strength and Endurance

Muscular strength is the amount of resistance that a muscle or a group of muscles can move. **Muscular endurance** is the ability of a muscle or a group of muscles to continue moving a resistance.

A. INTRODUCTION

1. Maintenance or Improvement of Muscular Strength and Endurance
   a. Muscular strength and endurance are critical to the performance of activities of daily living.
   b. Increased strength enables performance of normal physical activity with less physiological strain and at reduced risk for musculoskeletal injury.
   c. Improvements in muscular strength and endurance generally result from enhanced neuromuscular and metabolic function and, perhaps, increased size of individual muscle fibers.
   d. The ability to realize substantial increases in muscle size is hormonally mediated and, probably, genetically limited.
   e. **Resistance training should be included as an integral part of comprehensive preventive and rehabilitative exercise programs.**
   f. Little scientific evidence indicates a difference in the training stimulus required to improve muscular strength and endurance for trained versus healthy, untrained populations.
2. Health benefits of resistance training include:
   a. Improved performance of activities of daily living with less physiological stress.
   b. Maintenance of functional independence.
   c. Decreased risk of bone mineral loss.
   d. Maintenance of lean body mass.
   e. Decreased risk of low back pain.

3. **Intensity** usually is prescribed as the percentage of the maximal voluntary contraction.
   a. Volitional fatigue is the inability to move a resistance through an ROM with proper biomechanical form.
   b. The number of repetitions to volitional fatigue varies inversely with resistance.
   c. Exercise to volitional fatigue is safe provided that good technique is maintained.
   d. Adaptation of the resistance training exercise prescription often is necessary in individuals with cardiovascular disease, hypertension, or those with complications associated with diabetes as well as other chronic disease conditions.
   e. A particular set of resistance training exercises should be terminated when the resistance cannot be moved through the full ROM during successive repetitions with good technique, including proper breathing.
   f. Relative exercise intensity should be similar for men and women.
   g. Resistance may be increased (by 2.5–5 pounds) when the desired number of repetitions can be completed with good technique.
   h. One exercise session per week has been shown to maintain strength for up to 3 months provided that intensity remains constant.
   i. The increase of intensity of resistance training can be achieved by altering any one of the following variables while keeping the others constant.
      1) Number of repetitions.
      2) Decreasing speed of movement.
      3) Avoiding "locking out" a joint during multijoint exercises (e.g., bench press, leg press).
   j. Intensity should be reduced for people with cardiovascular or other chronic disease.
   k. The HR is not a valid indicator of resistance exercise intensity.

B. MODES OF EXERCISE FOR RESISTANCE TRAINING

1. Free weights require some skill to perform exercises properly and safely, and they often require a partner for safety.
2. Machines (e.g., Nautilus, Universal, Keiser) may be safer than free-weight exercise, particularly for novice participants.
3. Springs, surgical tubing, and electronic devices also may be used for resistance training.
4. Choice of modality should be based on safety and individual preference.

CONTRAINDICTATED/HIGH-RISK EXERCISE	ALTERNATIVE EXERCISE
Straight Leg Full Sit-ups 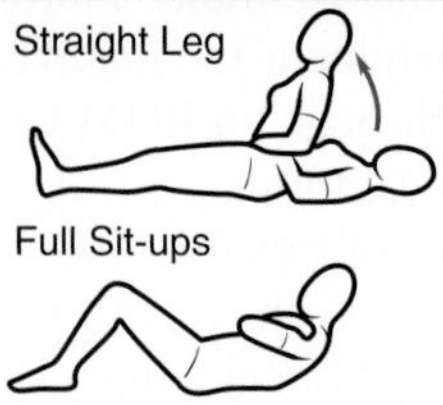 Risk: Stress on lower back due to utilization of hip flexors with origin in the lumbar spine; exercise primarily targets hip flexors	Crunches 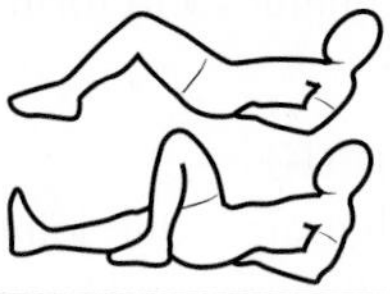
Double Leg Raises 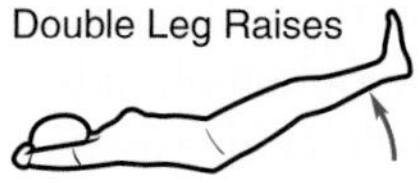 Risk: Hyperextends low back due to utilization of hip flexors with origin in the lumbar spine	Single Leg Raises-Opposite Knee Flexed 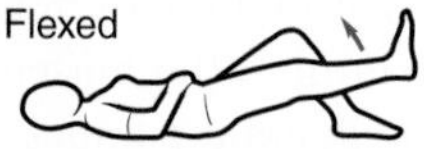
Full Squats 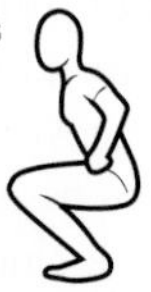 Risk: Patellar tendon forces during deep knee bending are 7.6 times body weight (7), increasing the risk of chondromalacia meniscal tears; individuals with previous injury to ligamental structures and menisci are at increased risk for injury	Squats to 90 Degrees of Knee Flexion-Knee Over Ankle 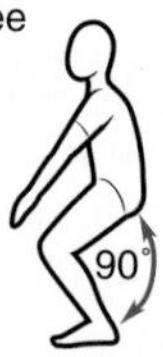 90
Hurdler's Stretch 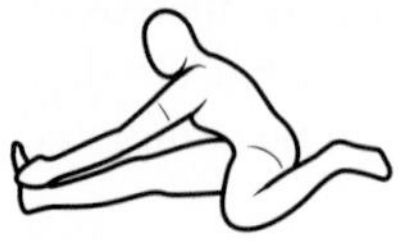 Risk: Knee flexion at end range of motion with rotational forces on hinge joint may stress the medial collateral ligament and menisci	Seated Hamstring Stretch 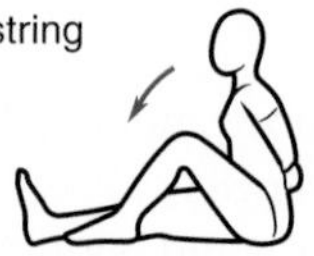
Plough 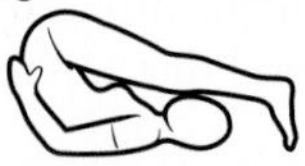 Risk: Loaded neck flexion can sprain cervical ligaments and increase pressure in cervical disks	Double Knee to Chest 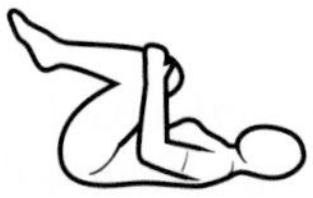
Back Hyperextension 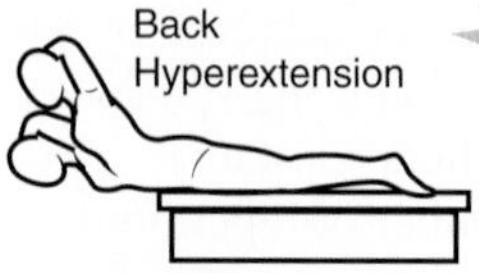 Risk: Hyperextension of the back	Back Extension to Normal Standing Lumbar Lordosis 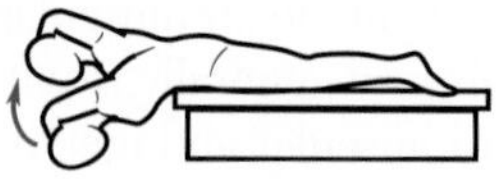
Full neck rolls 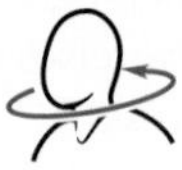 Risk: Stretches cervical ligaments, increases cervical disc pressure and may impinge arterial flow, resulting in dizziness	Lateral Neck Stretches 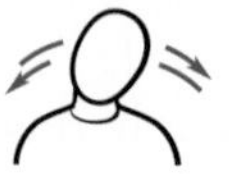
Flexion with rotation 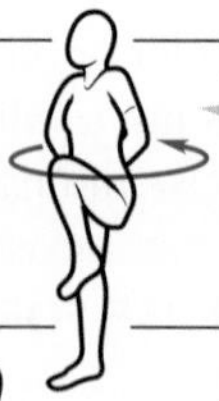 Risk: Flexion with rotation increases pressure on spinal disks	Supine Curl-ups with Flexion followed by Rotation 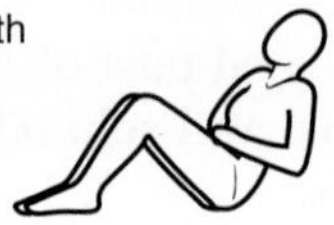
Standing toe touch 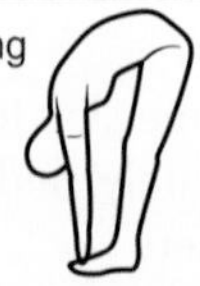 Risk: Increases pressure in lumbar disks and overstretches lumbar ligament	Standing Hamstring Stretch, Back Flat 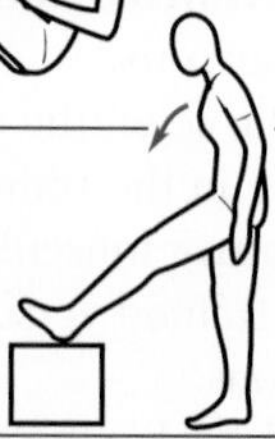

FIGURE 8-3. Common high-risk exercises and recommendations for alternative exercises. (Adapted from *ACSM's Resource Manual for Guidelines for Exercise Testing and Prescription.* 3rd Ed. Baltimore, Williams & Wilkins, 1998, p 644.)

C. EXERCISE PRESCRIPTION

1. Select a mode of exercise that is comfortable and provides full ROM.
2. Include 8 to 10 major muscle group exercises.
3. Program activity with attention to time efficiency, because exercise training programs lasting longer than 1 hour usually are associated with lower compliance.
4. The order of the exercises may be left to individual preference; however, arms should be exercised after the torso, if possible. Fatigue of the smaller arm muscles may limit the ability to adequately stress the larger torso muscles (triceps fatigue may limit bench press activity).
5. ACSM Recommendations
   a. Healthy individuals should perform **one set** of each exercise **to volitional fatigue**.
   b. Choose a (limited) range of repetitions between 3 and 20 (e.g., 3–6, 8–12, 6–10).
   c. These exercises should be performed on two or three nonconsecutive days per week. Training one day per week will maintain strength for several weeks.
   d. Different exercises for a given muscle group may be performed every two or three training sessions.
   e. **Proper breathing** instruction for individuals who are unfamiliar with resistive training is necessary.
      1) Exhaling with the concentric phase of the exercise and inhaling with the eccentric phase of each repetition is recommended.
      2) **The Valsalva maneuver** (a forced expiration against a closed airway) **should be discouraged** during resistance exercise, because it may be accompanied by a significant increase in arterial BP.
   f. Perform both the lifting and lowering phases of the exercise in a **controlled** manner at moderate to slow speeds (3-second concentric, 3-second eccentric) over the full ROM.
   g. Maintain proper mechanics.
      1) Heavy resistance should not be performed with improper technique.
      2) If correct biomechanical form cannot be maintained, the resistance should be decreased.
   h. Allow enough time for rest between exercises to perform the next exercise properly.
   i. Training with a partner may be beneficial for safety and motivation.

VI. Conditions Requiring Modification of Exercise Programs

A. OSTEOPOROSIS

1. Increased risk of fractures of the wrists, hips, and lumbosacral regions.
2. Reductions in bone mass are most prevalent in sedentary individuals and progress at a more rapid rate following menopause.
3. Weight bearing exercise is most effective in maintaining or increasing bone density, but such exercise may be harmful in advanced osteoporosis.
4. Resistance Training
   a. Include exercises that direct the load over the long axis of the bone (e.g., leg press, shoulder press).
   b. Frequency: two or three times per week.
   c. Repetitions: 8–10.
   d. Intensity: RPE of 13–15.
   e. Include functional exercises (e.g., balance).
   f. Include flexibility exercises 5 to 7 days per week.
   g. Spinal flexion may be contraindicated.
5. Aerobic Activity
   a. Mode: aquatic, walking, cycling.
   b. Frequency: 3–5 days per week.
   c. Duration: 20–60 minutes, continuous or intermittent.
   d. Intensity: 40–70% of HRR.
6. Special Considerations
   a. Pain is a contraindication to exercise.
   b. Avoid high-impact or ballistic activity.
   c. Excessive trunk flexion and twisting activities increase compressive forces and may increase the risk of vertebral fracture.

B. HYPERTENSION

1. **Hypertension** is defined as a resting systolic BP $\geq$140 mm Hg and/or a resting diastolic BP $\geq$90 mm Hg.
2. The majority of hypertensive cases may be classified as primary (of unknown origin) and typically warrant multifactorial therapy, including some or all of the following:
   a. Pharmacological management.
   b. Dietary management.
   c. Weight loss.
   d. Relaxation therapies.
3. Exercise is an effective tool in managing hypertension, with a reduction of 5 to 8 mm in both systolic and diastolic BP after daily exercise training.
4. If resting BP is 160/100 mm Hg or greater, drug therapy is indicated either before or coincident with initiation of an exercise program.

5. Aerobic Exercise
    a. Cardiovascular endurance activities (e.g., walking, cycling, swimming) are appropriate.
    b. Frequency: 3–7 days per week.
    c. Duration: 30–60 minutes.
    d. Intensity: 40–70% of HRR.
    e. Multiple bouts of short-duration (10–15 min), low-intensity activity (e.g., walking) throughout the day may provide a viable option for control of BP.
6. Resistance Exercise
    a. Resistance exercise should be included for those with hypertension, but not as the primary form of activity.
    b. Isometric exercise, Valsalva maneuvers, and maximal effort should be specifically avoided.
    c. Terminate a set when the RPE is between 13 and 15.
    d. High-repetition, low-intensity (e.g., resistance) programs are usually recommended.
7. Special Considerations
    a. Exercise is contraindicated if preexercise systolic BP is greater than 200 mm Hg or diastolic BP is greater than 110 mm Hg.
    b. Terminate an exercise session if exercise systolic BP is greater than 220 mm Hg or diastolic BP is greater than 105.
    c. For those on vasodilator medications, prolong cool-down and avoid abrupt postural change.
    d. β-Blockers attenuate the HR and necessitate use of the RPE.

C. DIABETES MELLITUS
1. A metabolic disorder characterized by hyperglycemia (fasting plasma glucose, >126 mg/dL).
2. Blood glucose levels that define diabetes according to the American Diabetes Association (ADA) in the 2004 Clinical Practice Guidelines are as follows:
    a. A fasting plasma glucose of less than 100 mg/dL (5.6 mmol/L) is normal.
    b. A fasting plasma glucose of 100 to 125 mg/dL (5.6–6.9 mmol/L) is impaired.
    c. A fasting plasma glucose of 126 mg/dL (7.0 mmol/L) or greater indicates a provisional diagnosis of diabetes.
3. This condition is associated with increased risk for cardiovascular disease, renal failure, neuropathic disorders, and ophthalmic dysfunction, including blindness.

4. Benefits of exercise include:
    a. Improved insulin sensitivity.
    b. Increased glucose control.
    c. Decreased body fat (for type 2 diabetes).
    d. Improved lipid profile.
5. Classification
   There are two major classifications of diabetes mellitus.
    a. Type 1 is caused by insulin deficiency and usually is an immune-mediated diabetes mellitus.
    b. Type 2 is caused by insulin resistance and generally is associated with obesity. Most cases of diabetes involve type 2.
    c. **The treatment goal for diabetes is glucose control,** which is accomplished through diet, medications. and exercise.
6. Complications
    a. Can include autonomic neuropathy, peripheral neuropathy, claudication, hypertension, retinopathy, and nephropathy.
    b. Often necessitate modification of the exercise program.
7. Aerobic Exercise
   Exercise has an "insulin-like" effect on blood glucose through enhanced insulin-receptor sensitivity. Therefore, avoidance of hypoglycemia during or after exercise is important.
    a. Frequency: 3–7 days per week.
        1) Those with type 2 diabetes should strive to expend at least 1,000 kcal per week.
        2) Daily exercise may provide for better glycemic control.
    b. Intensity: 50–80% of HRR.
    c. Duration: 20–60 minutes.
8. Resistance Training
    a. Lower intensity.
    b. Consider complications.
9. Special Considerations
    a. Monitor glucose pre- and postexercise, especially during the initial stages of an exercise program.
    b. Exercise is contraindicated if the fasting glucose level is greater than 250 mg/dL with ketones or greater than 300 mg/dL without ketones.
    c. Carbohydrate intake and insulin dosage should be adjusted before exercise (e.g., decrease insulin, increase carbohydrate intake).
    d. Avoid injecting insulin into exercising muscle; abdominal injection is recommended.
    e. Consume carbohydrates following late-evening exercise to avoid nocturnal hypoglycemia.

f. Maintain adequate hydration.

g. Clothing should allow proper thermoregulation so that any signs of hypoglycemia are not masked.

D. OBESITY

Obesity is an excess accumulation of body fat, particularly intra-abdominal fat, that is associated with increased health risks (e.g., hypertension, coronary artery disease, type 2 diabetes).

1. Currently, approximately 65% of Americans are estimated to be overweight (BMI, >25 kg/m^2), and more than 30% estimated to be obese (BMI, >30.0 kg/m^2).

2. Fat loss is best attained through a combination of diet and aerobic exercise.

3. Even modest weight loss (5–10%) is associated with clinically significant health improvements.

4. Prevention of further weight gain should be a priority.

5. The objective of exercise programs for the treatment of obesity should be to maximize caloric expenditure safely.

6. The rate of weight loss should be gradual and generally, not exceeding 2 pounds (7,000 kcal) per week.

7. Objective Evidence of Obesity

    a. BMI: greater than 30 kg/m2.

    b. Waist Circumference

        1) Males: greater than 102 cm.

        2) Females: greater than 88 cm.

    c. Body Fat

        1) Men: greater than 25%.

        2) Women: greater than 32%.

        3) Variability in measurement often makes this value difficult to interpret and apply.

        4) Use this measure in conjunction with BMI and waist circumference.

8. Aerobic Exercise

    a. Mode

        1) Walking is a generally accessible activity and should be within the tolerance limits of most obese clients.

        2) Cross-training with combinations of weight-bearing and nonweight-bearing activities may be effective.

        3) Nonweight-bearing activities (e.g., cycling, water exercises) should be included for client with lower extremity orthopedic problems.

    b. Frequency: 5–7 days per week.

    c. Intensity: 40–60% of HRR, progressing to 50–75%.

    d. Duration: 45–60 minutes.

        1) Initial weekly training volume should be approximately 150 minutes per week, progressing to 200 to 300 minutes.

9. Resistance training is recommended as an adjunct to an aerobic exercise program, but it is not the primary means for caloric expenditure.

10. Special Considerations

    a. Adequate thermoregulation often is a problem.

    b. Equipment modification may be necessary (e.g., wider seats on cycles and rowers).

    c. Behavior modification strategies should be included in the management of obesity.

E. PREGNANCY

1. Exercise generally is considered to be safe both during and after pregnancy if hyperthermia is avoided and adequate fuel is available for the mother and the fetus.

2. The American College of Obstetricians and Gynecologists (ACOG) have established contraindications to exercise during pregnancy (see http://www.acog.org).

3. Aerobic Exercise

    a. Frequency: 3–7 days per week.

    b. Intensity: RPE of 11–13.

    c. Duration: 30–40 minutes.

4. Resistance Training

    a. Decreased intensity.

    b. Avoid Valsalva maneuvers.

5. Special Considerations

    a. Avoid exercise in the supine posture after the first trimester.

    b. Pregnancy requires an additional 300 kcal per day, so additional calories must be consumed to meet the needs of exercise and pregnancy.

    c. Avoid motionless standing during and in the short term after exercise, because it may exacerbate venous blood pooling.

    d. Avoid all risk of abdominal trauma.

    e. Facilitate thermoregulation.

        1) Consider temperature and humidity when planning and performing exercise.

        2) Wear proper clothing.

        3) Maintain adequate hydration.

        4) Avoid extreme intensity and duration of exercise.

    f. Consume between 30 and 50 g of carbohydrate before exercise.

Review Test

DIRECTIONS: Carefully read all questions, and select the BEST single answer.

1. Which of the following is NOT an appropriate treatment activity for inpatient rehabilitation of a client on the second day after coronary artery bypass graft (CABG) surgery?
   A) Limit activities as tolerated to the development of self-care activities, ROM for extremities, and low-resistance activities.
   B) Limit upper body activities to biceps curls, horizontal arm adduction, and overhead press using 5-pound weights while sitting on the side of the bed.
   C) Progress all activities performed from supine to sitting to standing.
   D) Measure vital signs, symptoms, RPE, fatigue, and skin color and perform electrocardiography before, during, and after treatments to assess activity tolerance.

2. Which of the following situations indicates progression to independent and unsupervised exercise for a client after CABG surgery in an outpatient program?
   A) The client exhibits mild cardiac symptoms of angina, occurring intermittently during exercise and sometimes at home while reading.
   B) The client has a functional capacity of greater than 8 MET with hemodynamic responses appropriate to this level of exercise.
   C) The client is noncompliant with smoking cessation and weight loss intervention programs.
   D) The client is unable to palpate HR, deliver RPEs, or maintain steady workload intensity during activity.

3. Which of the following issues would you include in discharge education instructions for a client with congestive heart failure to avoid potential emergency situations related to this condition at home?
   A) Record body weight daily, and report weight gains to a physician.
   B) Note signs and symptoms(e.g., dyspnea, intolerance to activities of daily living), and report them to a physician.
   C) Do not palpate the pulse during daily activities or periods of light-headedness, because an irregular pulse is normal and occurs at various times during the day.
   D) Both A and B.

4. Initial training sessions for a person with severe chronic obstructive pulmonary disease most likely would NOT include
   A) Continuous cycling activity at 70% of $\dot{V}O_2max$ for 30 minutes.
   B) Use of dyspnea scales, RPE scales, and pursed-lip breathing instruction.
   C) Intermittent bouts of activity on a variety of modalities (exercise followed by short rest).
   D) Encouraging the client to achieve an intensity either at or above the anaerobic threshold.

5. Symptoms of claudication include
   A) Cramping, burning, and tightness in the calf muscle, usually triggered by activity and relieved with rest.
   B) Acute, sharp pain in the foot on palpation at rest.
   C) Crepitus in the knee during cycling.
   D) Pitting ankle edema at a rating of 3+.

6. Treatment for claudication during exercise includes all of the following EXCEPT
   A) Daily exercise sessions.
   B) Intensity of activity to maximal tolerable pain, with intermittent rest periods.
   C) Cardiorespiratory building activities that are nonweight bearing if the plan is to work on longer duration and higher intensity to elicit a cardiorespiratory training effect.
   D) Stopping activity at the onset of claudication discomfort to avoid further vascular damage from ischemia.

7. A client with angina exhibits symptoms and a 1-mm, down-sloping ST-segment depression at a HR of 129 bpm on his exercise test. His peak exercise target HR should be set at
   A) 128 bpm.
   B) 109 to 119 bpm.
   C) 129 bpm.
   D) 125 to 128 bpm.

8. Special precautions for clients with hypertension include all of the following EXCEPT
   A) Avoiding muscle strengthening exercises that involve low resistance.
   B) Avoiding activities that involve the Valsalva maneuver.
   C) Monitoring a client who is taking diuretics for arrhythmias.
   D) Avoiding exercise if resting systolic BP is greater than 200 mm Hg or diastolic BP is greater than 115 mm Hg.

9. According to the most recent National Institutes of Health's *Clinical Guidelines for the Identification, Evaluation, and Treatment of Overweight and Obesity in Adults,* recommendations for practical clinical assessment include
    A) Determining total body fat through the BMI to assess obesity.
    B) Determining the degree of abdominal fat and health risk through waist circumference.
    C) Using the waist-to-hip ratio as the only definition of obesity and lean muscle mass.
    D) Both A and B.

10. A client with type 1 diabetes mellitus checks her fasting morning glucose level on her whole-blood glucose meter (fingerstick method), and the result of 253 mg/dL (14 mmol/L). A urine test is positive for ketones before her exercise session. What action should you take?
    A) Allow her to exercise as long as her glucose is not greater than 300 mg/dL (17 mmol/L).
    B) Not allow her to exercise this session, and notify her physician of the findings.
    C) Give her an extra carbohydrate snack, and wait 5 minutes before beginning exercise.
    D) Readjust her insulin regimen for the remainder of the day to compensate for the high morning glucose level.

11. A 62-year-old, obese factory worker complains of pain in his right shoulder on arm abduction; on evaluation, decreased ROM and strength are noted. You also notice that he is beginning to use accessory muscles to substitute movements and to compensate. These symptoms may indicate
    A) A referred pain from a herniated lumbar disk.
    B) Rotator cuff strain or impingement.
    C) angina.
    D) Advanced stages of multiple sclerosis.

12. All of the following are special considerations in prescribing exercise for the client with arthritis EXCEPT
    A) The possible need to splint painful joints for protection.
    B) Periods of acute inflammation result in decreased pain and joint stiffness.
    C) The possibility of gait abnormalities as compensation for pain or stiffness.
    D) The need to avoid exercise of warm, swollen joints.

13. What common medication taken by clients with end-stage renal disease requires careful management for those undergoing hemodialysis?
    A) Antihypertensive medication.
    B) Lithium.

C) Cholestyramine.
D) Cromolyn sodium.

14. Which of the following is an appropriate exercise for clients with diabetes and loss of protective sensation in the extremities?
    A) Prolonged walking.
    B) Jogging.
    C) Step-class exercise.
    D) Swimming.

15. A client taking a calcium-channel blocker most likely will exhibit which of the following responses during exercise?
    A) Hypertensive response.
    B) Increased ischemia.
    C) Improved anginal thresholds.
    D) Severe hypotension.

16. During the cool-down phase of an exercise session, clients should be encouraged to
    A) Rehydrate.
    B) Decrease the intensity of activity quickly to decrease cardiac afterload.
    C) Limit the cool-down period to 5 minutes.
    D) Increase the number of isometric activities.

17. Muscular endurance training is best accomplished by
    A) Performing four to six repetitions per set.
    B) Using high resistance.
    C) Incorporating high repetitions.
    D) Performing isometric exercises only.

18. Transitional care exercise and rehabilitation programs are NOT appropriate for
    A) Clients with functionally limiting chronic disease.
    B) Clients with comorbid disease states.
    C) Asymptomatic clients with a functional capacity of 10 MET.
    D) Clients at 1 week after CABG surgery.

19. Many clients have VVI-mode programmed pacemakers. Which of the following is TRUE regarding exercise programming with VVI pacemakers?
    A) Persons with VVI pacemakers may be chronotropically (HR) competent with exercise but require longer warm-up and gradual increase in intensity during the initial exercise portion of their session.
    B) Persons who are chronotropically competent are tachycardic at rest and should not exercise at low intensities.
    C) BP response is not a good marker of intensity effort in those with VVI pacemakers and need not be evaluated during an exercise session.

D) Persons with VVI pacemakers must avoid exercise on the bicycle ergometer because of the location of the ventricular lead wire and potential for displacement.

20. Controlling pool water temperature (83–88°F), avoiding jarring and weight-bearing activities, and avoiding movement in swollen, inflamed joints are special considerations for exercise in
A) Clients after atherectomy.
B) Clients with angina.
C) Clients with osteoporosis.
D) Clients with arthritis.

21. Which of the following is a resistive lung disease?
A) Asthma.
B) Tuberculosis.
C) Cystic fibrosis.
D) Emphysema.

22. A specific benefit of regular exercise for patients with angina is
A) Improved ischemic threshold at which angina symptoms occur.
B) Increased myocardial oxygen demand at the same submaximal levels.
C) Eradication of all symptoms.
D) Elevation of BP.

23. Which of the following is NOT a benefit of increased flexibility?
A) Increased muscle viscosity, allowing easier and smoother contractions.
B) Reduced muscle tension and increased relaxation.
C) Improved coordination by allowing greater ease of movement.
D) Increased ROM.

24. Which of the following statements regarding warm-up is FALSE?
A) Muscle blood flow is increased as a result of warm-up.
B) Peripheral vasodilation occurs as a result of warm-up.
C) Peripheral vasoconstriction occurs as a result of warm-up.
D) Between 5 and 10 minutes should be allotted for a warm-up period.

25. Which of the following statements regarding cool-down is FALSE?
A) The emphasis should be large muscle activity performed at a low to moderate intensity.
B) Increasing venous return should be a priority during cool-down.
C) The potential for improving flexibility may be improved during cool-down as compared with warm-up.

D) Between 1 and 2 minutes are recommended for an adequate cool-down.

26. All of the following are examples of aerobic exercise modalities EXCEPT
A) Weight training.
B) Walking.
C) Bicycling.
D) Stair climbing.

27. A target HR equivalent to 85% of HRR for a 25-year-old male with a resting HR of 75 bpm would be equal to
A) 195 bpm.
B) 166 bpm.
C) 177 bpm.
D) 102 bpm.

28. The appropriate exercise HR for an individual on β-blocking medication would generally be
A) 75% of HRR.
B) 30 bpm above the standing resting HR.
C) 40% of HRR.
D) $(220 - age) \times 0.85$.

29. The recommended cardiorespiratory exercise training goal for apparently healthy individuals should be
A) 15 minutes, six times per week, at 90% of HRR.
B) 30 minutes, three times per week, at 85% of HRR.
C) 60 minutes, three times per week, at 85% of HRR.
D) 30 minutes of weight training, three times per week, at 60% of HRR.

30. In an effort to improve flexibility, the ACSM recommends
A) Proprioceptive neuromuscular facilitation.
B) Ballistic stretching.
C) The plough and hurdler's stretches.
D) Static stretches held for 10 to 30 seconds per repetition.

31. An appropriate exercise for improving the strength of the low back muscles are
A) Straight leg lifts.
B) Parallel squats.
C) Spinal extension exercises.
D) Sit-ups with feet anchored.

32. Which of the following statements true regarding exercise leadership is FALSE?
A) The exercise leader should be fit enough to exercise with any of his or her participants.
B) Most people are not bored by exercise and can easily find time to participate in an exercise program.

C) The exercise leader should adjust the exercise intensity based on individual differences in fitness.

D) Periodic fitness assessment may provide evidence of improvement in fitness for some participants.

33. Which of the following statements regarding exercise for the elderly is FALSE?
A) A decrease in maximal HR is responsible for reductions in the maximal oxygen consumption as we age.
B) A loss of fat-free mass is responsible for the decrease in muscular strength as we age.
C) The ACSM recommends a cardiorespiratory training intensity of 50% to 70% of HRR for older adults.
D) Resistance exercise training is not recommended for older adults.

34. Which of the following medications have been shown to be most effective in preventing or reversing exercise-induced asthma?
A) β_2-Agonists.
B) β-Blockers.
C) Diuretics.
D) Aspirin.

35. The exercise leader or health/fitness instructor should modify exercise sessions for participants with hypertension by
A) Shortening the cool-down to less than 5 minutes.
B) Eliminating resistance training completely.
C) Prolonging the cool-down.
D) Implementing high-intensity (>85% of HRR), short-duration intervals.

36. Normal values for fasting blood sugar are
A) Greater than 140 mg/dL.
B) Between 60 and 140 mg/dL.
C) Less than 60 mg/dL.
D) Between 200 and 400 mg/dL.

37. The goal for the obese exercise participant should be to
A) Sweat as much as possible.
B) Exercise at 85% of HRR.
C) Perform resistance exercise three to five times per week.
D) Expend 300 to 500 calories per exercise session.

38. Which of the following statements regarding exercise for persons with controlled cardiovascular disease is TRUE?
A) Resistance exercise training is dangerous and should be avoided.

B) A physician-supervised exercise test is not necessary to establish exercise intensity.
C) Anginal pain is normal during exercise, and participants should be pushed through the pain.
D) Exercise intensity should be set at an HR of 10 bpm less than the level at which signs/symptoms were evidenced during an exercise test.

39. All of the following factors are important to consider when determining exercise intensity EXCEPT
A) An individual's level of fitness.
B) The risk of cardiovascular or orthopedic injury.
C) Any previous history participating in organized sports.
D) Individual preference and exercise objectives.

40. When determining the intensity level, the RPE is a better indicator than percentage of maximal HR for all of the following groups EXCEPT
A) Individuals on β-blockers.
B) Aerobic classes that involve excessive arm movement.
C) Individuals older than 65 years.
D) Individuals involved in high-intensity exercise.

41. Using the original Borg scale, it is recommended that the exercise intensity elicit an RPE within the range of
A) 8 to 12.
B) 12 to 16.
C) 14 to 18.
D) 6 to 10.

42. The MINIMAL duration of exercise necessary to achieve improvements in health for deconditioned individuals is
A) 20 minutes continuously.
B) 30 minutes continuously.
C) Multiple sessions of more than 10 minutes in duration throughout the day.
D) Two sessions of 20 minutes throughout the day.

43. Which of the following is a method of strength and power training that involves an eccentric loading of muscles and tendons followed immediately by an explosive concentric contraction?
A) Super sets.
B) Split routines.
C) Plyometrics.
D) Periodization.

44. The safety of resistance exercise is dependent on all of the following EXCEPT

A)   Having a personal trainer.
B)   Proper breathing.
C)   Speed of movement.
D)   Body mechanics.

45.   The recommended muscular strength and endurance training program for apparently healthy individuals should be
A)   One set of 8 to 12 reps, 8 to 10 separate exercises, 2 days per week.
B)   Two sets of six to eight reps, 8 to 10 separate exercises, 2 days per week.
C)   One set of 8 to 12 reps, 8 to 10 separate exercises, 4 to 5 days per week.
D)   Two sets of six to eight reps, 8 to 10 separate exercises, 4 days per week, and alternating days for legs and upper body.

46.   Which the following statements regarding intensity of resistance training is FALSE?
A)   The number of repetitions to volitional fatigue will vary inversely with resistance.
B)   It is necessary to determine the 1-RM to establish training intensity.

C)   Exercise to volitional fatigue is not dangerous from a musculoskeletal standpoint provided that good exercise form is maintained.
D)   Exercise intensity should be similar for males and females.

47.   The recommended cardiorespiratory endurance exercise training program for older individuals should be
A)   40% to 60% of maximum HR, 20 to 30 minutes continuously, 3 days per week.
B)   50% to 70% of HRR, 20 to 30 minutes (multiple sessions of 5–10 min), 3 days per week.
C)   40% to 60% of maximum HR, 20 to 30 minutes (multiple sessions of 5–10 min), 3 days per week.
D)   50% to 70% of HRR, 20 to 30 minutes continuously, 3 days per week.

48.   Osteoporosis is more prevalent in
A)   Women who have never been pregnant.
B)   African-American women.
C)   Women who are involved in activities that place stress on the wrists, hips, or lumbosacral region.
D)   Postmenopausal women.

ANSWERS AND EXPLANATIONS

1–B.   Strenuous and resistive upper body exercises and activity may cause injury to the sternum immediately after CABG surgery. Such exercises should be avoided until the sternum and chest incisions have healed.

2–B.   Progression to more independent self-managed programs is encouraged for those who have a good functional capacity, exhibit appropriate hemodynamic and electrocardiographic responses to exercise and recovery, are asymptomatic, have stable resting HR and BP, manage risk factor intervention strategies safely and effectively, demonstrate knowledge of the disease process, and are compliant with their program.

3–D.   Symptoms of worsening heart failure (e.g., leg edema, activity intolerance, dyspnea, orthopnea, paroxysmal dyspnea) must be explained to clients. A weight gain of 3 to 5 pounds since the last appointment should be reported. During symptoms of light-headedness or chest discomfort, palpating the pulse provides helpful information if the heartbeat suddenly becomes irregular during these episodes. Development of an arrhythmia should be reported to the physician.

4–A.   A client with severe chronic obstructive pulmonary disease who is just beginning an exercise program would not be able to tolerate vigorously intense exercise for prolonged periods because of limitations such as dyspnea, muscle weakness, and cardiovascular deconditioning as a result of previous inactivity.

5–A.   Sharp, palpable pain over an area typically indicates fasciitis or tendonitis. Crepitus in the knee indicates inflammation, arthritis, and other joint structural problems. Ankle edema indicates of poor venous return in conditions such as right heart failure and is not an indication of an atherosclerotic artery.

6–D.   Clients with claudication are encouraged to exercise at an intensity that causes intense pain (grade III) or unbearable pain (grade IV). This is followed by a full-recovery rest period.

7–B.   Peak exercise HR is set at 10 to 20 bpm below the ischemic level (which was symptomatic, downsloping ST-segment depression at 129 bpm).

8–A.   Low-resistance muscle-strengthening exercises can be performed by those diagnosed with hypertension if they follow appropriate lifting techniques and avoid the Valsalva maneuver. In addition, hemodynamic parameters (HR and BP) and medications should be controlled.

9–D. The BMI can be used to classify overweight and obesity levels. In addition, waist circumference has been found to be a better marker of abdominal fat content than the waist-to-hip ratio.

10–B. Whole-blood glucose values generally are 10% to 15% lower than plasma glucose levels. Those with type 1 diabetes should avoid exercise when ketones are present at a glucose level of greater than 240 mg/dL (14 mmol/L) or if glucose levels exceed 300 mg/dL (17 mmol/L) regardless of whether ketosis is present. Carbohydrate snacks are taken only when glucose levels are too low to help maintain proper glycemic control during exercise. Only a physician can prescribe changes in medication regimen.

11–B. The subdeltoid bursa, supraspinatus muscle, and nerves become impinged between the coracoid and acromion process with shoulder abduction. The resulting pain leads to decreased ROM, disuse, and muscle atrophy. Such impingement of the rotator cuff is common in assembly line workers who perform repetitive overhead tasks.

12–B. During periods of acute arthritic inflammation, affected joints will be painful, stiff, hot, and swollen. These joints should not be exercised and may need to be protected to allow the client to perform other motor tasks.

13–A. The process of hemodialysis interacts with antihypertensive medications and lowers the drug level, causing a potentially severe hypertensive response. To avoid such a reaction, clients may skip their hypertension medication on dialysis days.

14–D. Prolonged walking, jogging, and step classes are high-impact or weight-bearing activities that can lead to sores, ulcers, or fractures in those with loss of sensation in the feet (peripheral neuropathy).

15–C. Clients with angina who are taking calcium-channel blockers will improve their exercise capacity response to exercise regimens.

16–A. A longer cool-down period of 10 to 15 minutes (or longer for certain disease states) and a gradual decrease in intensity will provide a smoother recovery period and avoid sudden adverse hemodynamic responses and associated symptoms.

17–C. Muscular endurance (the ability to sustain prolonged muscular contractions) is best accomplished by using lighter weights and performing more repetitions per set.

18–C. Transitional or home care rehabilitation can be provided through nursing homes, rehabilitation hospitals, or clinics to those needing supervised care for exercise or activities of daily living.

19–A. Chronotropically competent VVI clients often are bradycardic at rest but have good atrioventricular conduction. Gradual increases in activity are recommended to allow the sinus node time to respond. The BP should be monitored during exercise to help assess intensity levels.

20–D. Clients with arthritis should avoid exercising joints that are acutely inflamed and will benefit from nonweight-bearing pool exercises in warm water. Clients with cardiac diagnoses are not limited to nonweight-bearing activities and do not have inflamed joints as a result of their disease. Clients with osteoporosis benefit from exercise that decreases the rate of bone loss.

21–B. Obstructive lung diseases are "flow" obstructions, including asthma, cystic fibrosis, interstitial lung disease, chronic bronchitis, and emphysema. Restrictive lung diseases are those involving restricted lung capacity because of disease or damage of the lungs, including lupus, pulmonary edema, tuberculosis, and lung cancer.

22–A. The ischemic threshold is predictable in stable angina patients. A benefit of regular exercise for patients with angina is an improved ischemic threshold at which angina symptoms occur. In addition, myocardial oxygen demand decreases, as do the BP and HR response to submaximal exercise.

23–A. Increased flexibility provides numerous benefits, including reduced muscle tension, increased relaxation, increased ease of movement, improved coordination, increased ROM, improved body awareness, improved capability for circulation and air exchange, decreased muscle viscosity (causing contractions to be easier and smoother), and decreased soreness associated with other exercise activities.

24–C. Peripheral vasoconstriction would be a negative consequence of warm-up if it occurred. Appropriate warm-up activities promote increased muscle blood flow and increased oxygen delivery. This is accomplished through peripheral vasodilation. Typically, a 5- to 10-minute time frame will allow for a gradual increase in HR, an increase in body temperature, and a slight reduction in pH. These changes will facilitate increased oxygen consumption. Although more research is needed to determine the effects of warm-up on musculoskeletal injury rates, it seems that even from a psychological perspective, warm-up may prevent injury during exercise.

25–D. The primary purpose of cool-down is to increase venous return, and this is accomplished by low-intensity, large-muscle activity. This type of activity also aids the removal of lactic acid. Evidence of an effective cool-down is an HR of less than 100 bpm and a systolic BP within 10 mm Hg of preexercise levels. Between 5 and 10 minutes will allow these changes to occur and provide time for some attention to flexibility exercises. The potential for improving flexibility is increased when the body is warm and the muscles and connective tissue are more pliable, as is the case after (versus before) exercise.

26–A. Weight training is not considered to be an aerobic exercise. Although some increases in maximal oxygen consumption have been shown from circuit weight training, this is not considered to be the most effective means for improving cardiorespiratory fitness. Large-muscle group activity, performed in rhythmic fashion for a prolonged period, is the most efficient means of taxing the aerobic energy system.

27–C. Using 220 minus age (25) yields 195. Subtract 75 (resting HR) to yield the HRR (120). Multiply 120 by 0.85 (85%) to yield 102, and then add the resting HR (75) back in to yield 177 as the target HR.

28–A. β-Blocking medications blunt the HR response at rest and during exercise, but the linear relationship between HR and oxygen consumption remains consistent with β-blocking medication. It is appropriate to program exercise at a percentage of HRR (75% is well within the correct range, but 40% HRR is not within guideline standards).

29–B. Although additional improvements in maximal oxygen consumption may be seen when exercise is performed at greater than 85% of HRR or when duration exceeds 30 minutes and at frequencies greater than three times per week, these improvements are minimal and accompanied by increased risk of musculoskeletal injury.

30–D. The proprioceptive neuromuscular facilitation is impractical, because it requires a partner and potential for injury exists if the stretch is applied too vigorously. Ballistic stretching may induce soreness and actually impede the ability to stretch. The plough and hurdler's stretches are potentially harmful exercises that compromise the neck and knee, respectively. Isometric activity involves exerting force against an immovable

object and is considered to be an inefficient form of muscle strengthening exercise. Static stretches held for 10 to 30 seconds per repetition are effective and carry a low risk of injury.

31–C. Straight leg lifts are potentially harmful to the low back and actually tax the hip flexors and the abdominals. Squats primarily involve the gluteals and the quadriceps. The erector spinae are the prime movers for spinal extension. Spinal flexion requires the abdominals to contract while placing the low back muscles on a slight stretch. Sit-ups exercise the abdominal musculature and, if performed with the feet anchored or to a full ROM, will involve the hip flexors.

32–B. Unless creative program strategies are employed, most people become bored with exercise. The exercise leader may be able to increase exercise program compliance by offering variety in programming, providing adequate instruction and encouragement, keeping participants free of injury, and demonstrating progress through exercise testing. A comprehensive exercise program that can be completed in no more than 1 hour, three times per week, should be developed for all participants who are interested in health/fitness. The idea is to minimize the time commitment while providing for maximal response.

33–D. Resistance exercise training for older adults is highly recommended to slow the typical age-related loss of lean tissue. Additional benefits include increases in bone density and improved functional capacity. Attention should be given to the overall health status of the individual, and appropriate modifications should be made if cardiovascular, metabolic, or musculoskeletal problems are present.

34–A. β₂-Agonists provide effective bronchodilation with relatively minimal side effect. β-Blockers are prescribed for cardiovascular concerns, including hypertension. Diuretics also are used to treat hypertension and congestive heart failure. Aspirin is used to reduce pain and fever, but it provides no pulmonary effect. Theophylline has a slow onset of action and many associated side effects.

35–C. A prolonged cool-down of 5 to 10 minutes will enhance venous return and the hypotensive effects that are associated with many antihypertensive medications.

36–B. Blood sugar levels of 60 mg/dL or less are considered to be hypoglycemic, whereas levels of 140 mg/dL or greater are indicative of hyperglycemia.

37–D. The goal for weight loss would be to expend 300 to 500 kcal per exercise session in combination with a reduced caloric intake that would yield a total caloric deficit of no more than 1,000 kcal per day or 7,000 kcal per week. The recommended rate of weight loss should not exceed 1 or 2 pounds per week to ensure adequate nutrition and health. The emphasis in weight-loss exercise programs should be large-muscle-group, aerobic-type exercise at a level of intensity that will allow the greatest caloric expenditure for the time spent exercising, with attention also being given to musculoskeletal and cardiovascular safety.

38–D. According to the ACSM, individuals with known disease should have a clinical exercise test before exercise participation to determine safe levels of exercise for the participant. Exercise intensity should be set at 1 MET below the level where signs/symptoms are evidenced. An HR of 10 bpm less than the HR where signs/symptoms are evidenced also may be used. Whenever anginal pain is evidenced during exercise, the exercise should be terminated and appropriate medical attention sought.

39–C. The risk of orthopedic and, perhaps, cardiovascular complications may be increased with high-intensity activity. Factors to consider when determining the appropriate intensity include the individual's level of fitness, use of medications that may influence exercise performance, risk of cardiovascular or orthopedic injury, individual preference regarding exercise, and individual program objectives.

40–D. The RPE is particularly useful when participants are incapable of monitoring their pulse or when medications such as β-blockers alter the HR response to exercise. Excessive arm movements (e.g., in high-intensity exercise) make it difficult to feel and accurately count the pulse rate.

41–B. The RPE is particularly useful when participants are incapable of monitoring their pulse or when medications such as β-blockers alter the HR response to exercise. The ACSM recommends an exercise intensity that will elicit an RPE within a range of 12 to 16 on the original Borg scale.

42–C. The ACSM recommends 20 to 60 minutes of continuous aerobic activity. Typically, adequate caloric expenditure and cardiorespiratory conditioning goals may be met with exercise sessions of moderate duration (20–30 min). Individuals who are very deconditioned may benefit from multiple exercise sessions of short (≤10 min) duration. Increases in duration may be instituted as evidence of adaptation without undue fatigue or injury occurs.

43–C. Plyometrics is a method of strength and power training that involves an eccentric loading of muscles and tendons followed immediately by an explosive concentric contraction. This stretch-shortening cycle may allow enhanced force generation during the concentric (shortening) phase.

44–A. The safety of resistance exercise is dependent on the proper execution of a given exercise. Spotting, proper breathing, speed of movement, and body mechanics are all central to safe exercise performance.

45–A. The ACSM recommends that one set of 8 to 12 repetitions of exercise should be performed to volitional fatigue at least 2 days each week.

46–B. Intensity is defined as a percentage of one's momentary ability to perform an activity (e.g., how difficult the exercise is, amount of effort during the exercise). It is the percentage of the maximal voluntary contraction in resistance exercise. It is not the percentage of 1-RM unless all other variables (e.g., individual exercise, speed of movement, number of repetitions) are kept constant.

47–B. The health status of the individual should be carefully considered when establishing intensity. Generally, a conservative approach should initially be taken. The ACSM recommends an intensity of 50% to 70% of HRR for older adults.

48–D. Osteoporosis is reduction in bone mass per unit volume. Reduced bone mass is more prevalent in sedentary individuals and progresses at a more rapid rate in women following menopause. This condition increases the risk for fractures of the wrists, hips, and lumbosacral regions and is considered to be a significant source of debilitation in older adults.

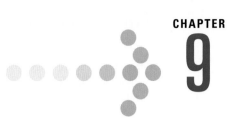

Nutrition and Weight Management

JANET R. WOJCIK AND BRENDA M. DAVY

I. Weight-Related Terms

A. OVERWEIGHT
As defined by the Centers for Disease Control and Prevention (CDC), **overweight** refers to increased body weight in relation to height when compared to some standard of acceptable or desirable weight.

B. OBESITY
As defined by the CDC, **obesity** refers to an excessively high amount of body fat or adipose tissue in relation to lean body mass based on any of the following methods of assessment:
1. **Body Composition Assessment**
   a. Assessment of body composition by comparing fat to nonfat (lean) components.
   b. Established norms for age and gender.
   c. Typically assessed by:
      1) **Skinfold** calipers.
      2) **Bioelectrical impedance.**
         a) Handheld devices.
         b) Specially-designed bathroom-style scales.
      3) **Hydrostatic (underwater) weighing.**
      4) **Dual x-ray absorptiometry.**
      5) **Air displacement plethysmography.**
   d. Error typically varies from 1–3% but can be higher.
   e. Field methods (e.g., skinfold, bioelectrical impedance) have the highest error compared to laboratory methods but are most commonly used in health/fitness settings.
2. **Body Mass Index (BMI)**
   a. Weight in kilograms/height in square meters ($kg \cdot m^{-2}$).
      1) To convert weight in pounds to weight in kilograms, divide by 2.2.
      2) To convert height in inches to height in meters, multiply by 0.0254 and then square the resulting number.
   b. Classification of disease risk:
      Overweight: $25.0–29.9\ kg \cdot m^{-2}$.
      Class I obesity: $30.0–34.9\ kg \cdot m^{-2}$.
      Class II obesity: $35.0–39.9\ kg \cdot m^{-2}$.
      Class III obesity: $\geq 40.0\ kg \cdot m^{-2}$.
   c. Does not designate body composition, so it may not be appropriate in athletic populations.
   d. Useful for comparing large numbers of people in research studies or historical data.

C. PERCENTAGE BODY FAT (% FAT)
1. Percentage of overall body weight that is fat mass.
2. To estimate total fat mass, multiply the total body weight by the percentage body fat.

D. LEAN BODY MASS (LBM)
1. Percentage of overall body weight that is nonfat (e.g., muscle, bone, blood, fluids, organs).
2. Related to resting metabolic rate (**RMR**).
3. To estimating lean body mass, subtract the fat weight from the total body weight.

E. ANOREXIA NERVOSA
1. A clinically diagnosed eating disorder.
2. Extremely thin appearance.
   a. Body weight is 15% below the lowest range from height/weight charts.
   b. BMI: $\leq 17.5\ kg \cdot m^{-2}$.
3. Refusal to consume food/self-starvation.
4. Preoccupation with food.
5. Distortion of body image (appearance is very thin, but self-perception is overweight).
6. Intense fear of weight gain.
7. More common in females, but males can be affected.
8. More common in caucasians.
9. Medical treatment required.

F. BULIMIA
1. A clinically diagnosed eating disorder.
2. Body weight may be of normal range, overweight, or underweight.

3. Binge behavior (eating large quantities of food) at least twice a week for several months.
4. Purge behavior:
   a. Vomiting.
   b. Laxative abuse.
   c. Excessive exercise.
   d. Sauna suits.
   e. Use of diuretics.
5. More common in females, but males may be at risk, especially if they participate in sports where body weight is a concern.
6. More common in caucasians, but incidence is increasing in other racial/ethnic groups.
7. Medical treatment required.

II. Relationship of Body Composition to Health

A. HIGH BODY FAT
High body fat, especially abdominal fat, is associated with risk of obesity-related diseases.
1. Diabetes.
2. Coronary artery disease.
3. Heart failure.
4. Stroke.
5. Certain cancers (e.g., pancreatic, colon, possibly breast and prostate).
6. Sleep apnea.
7. Arthritis.
8. Hypertension (high blood pressure).

B. LOW BODY FAT
Low body fat may be desirable for aesthetics or athletic performance, but it also may be indicative of disease processes, especially if weight loss is sudden. Association with the following should be considered:
1. Eating disorders (e.g., anorexia, bulimia).
2. Digestive and other diseases involving malabsorption of nutrients.
3. Certain cancers.

III. Health Implications of Body Fat Distribution Pattern

A. SIMPLE METHODS TO ASSESS BODY FAT DISTRIBUTION
1. **Waist-to-Hip Ratio (WHR)**
   a. Determined by dividing the circumference of the waist by the circumference of the hips.
   b. Levels indicating increased risk of type II diabetes, coronary heart disease (CHD), and hypertension:
      1) Men: >0.95.
      2) Women: >0.86.

2. **Waist Circumference**
   a. May be superior to WHR in determining disease risk.
   b. Levels indicating abdominal obesity:
      1) Men: >40 inches (102 cm).
      2) Women: >35 inches (88 cm).

B. BODY FAT DISTRIBUTION PATTERNS
1. **Central or Android Pattern ("Apple" Shaped)**
   a. Body fat accumulation in the abdominal area.
   b. More common in men.
   c. Also termed abdominal obesity.
2. **Peripheral or Gynoid Pattern ("Pear" Shaped)**
   a. Body fat accumulation in the hips and thighs.
   b. More common in women, at least before menopause.

C. HEALTH RISKS ASSOCIATED WITH ANDROID OBESITY (ABDOMINAL FAT)
1. Abdominal fat is more highly correlated with metabolic risk factors (e.g., insulin resistance, high blood pressure, elevated fasting blood glucose level, elevated blood lipid and lipoprotein levels) than with BMI.
2. Android obesity is the central feature of the **Metabolic Syndrome**, a condition in which several CHD risk factors are clustered (e.g., insulin resistance, dyslipidemia, elevated blood pressure).
3. Risk factors associated with this syndrome act synergistically to increase cardiovascular disease morbidity and mortality.

IV. Modifying Body Composition
One pound of body fat contains stored energy in the amount of 3,500 kilocalories (kcal). An energy deficit of 3,500 kcal generally is considered to be necessary to lose one pound. Genetic differences may be associated with variability of this value.

A. DIET ALONE
1. Losing more than 1 to 2 pounds of fat mass (≈0.5–1 kg) per week is not recommended, as it may lead to decreased lean body mass and lower resting metabolic rate.
2. Greater weight loss during the first several weeks of a diet program is common, but this loss likely due to water loss associated with glycogen depletion.

B. EXERCISE ALONE
1. To create a sufficient energy deficit, longer duration aerobic activities are usually emphasized.

2. The energy expenditure of different activities varies; therefore, it is difficult to prescribe a specific duration of exercise.
   a. It is necessary to approach a weekly caloric expenditure of 2,000 kcal or more for significant weight loss to occur and be maintained.
   b. This level is associated with 4 to 6 hours per week of aerobic, weight-bearing exercise.
3. The RMR remains elevated in the postexercise period, particularly after high intensity exercise. Whether this additional energy expenditure contributes significantly to weight loss is not known.
4. Classic resistance training exercise does not contribute significantly to exercise caloric expenditure; however, it does help to maintain or increase lean body mass.
5. Maintenance of lean body mass preserves RMR and may be important for weight management.

C. DIET PLUS EXERCISE
1. Reasonable energy deficits using a combination of diet and exercise may lead to a weight loss of 1 pound (0.5 kg) per week. For example, decreasing caloric intake by 250 kcal/day and increasing caloric expenditure by 250 kcal/day results in a total weekly deficit of 3,500 kcal.
2. Through exercise, lean body mass can be maintained or increased, especially with resistance training exercise.
3. Maintenance of healthy eating habits combined with exercise leads to better outcomes for long-term weight management.

V. Inappropriate Methods of Weight Loss

There is no "quick fix" for weight loss. Decreasing caloric consumption and increasing caloric expenditure through exercise remains the most effective method for long-term weight loss and maintenance. Myths of weight loss include the following:

A. SPOT REDUCTION
1. Spot reduction is the idea of exercising specific body parts to reduce fat in that area.
2. In reality, fat loss is spread over most of the body and throughout most tissue, though certain areas may be resistant to fat loss irrespective of the area exercised.

B. SAUNAS
1. Rationales for use include:
   a. Lose weight quickly.

b. May be used by athletes who need to compete at a reduced body weight (e.g., wrestlers, boxers, bodybuilders).
2. Inappropriate for weight loss, because:
   a. Weight lost is water weight.
   b. Risk of dehydration and electrolyte loss.
   c. Risk of heat-related illnesses (e.g., heat exhaustion, heat stroke).
   d. Water weight is quickly regained with fluid replenishment.

C. VIBRATING BELTS
1. Rationales for use include:
   a. Mechanical manipulation of a certain body part will "break down" fat.
   b. No sweat involved by user.
2. Inappropriate for weight loss, because:
   a. Does not lead to actual breakdown of stored body fat.
   b. Little or no energy expenditure by client.
   c. It is not possible to spot reduce a body part by exercising that body part.

D. BODY WRAPS
1. Rationales for use include:
   a. Lose weight quickly.
   b. May be used by athletes who need to compete at a reduced body weight (e.g., wrestlers, boxers, bodybuilders).
   c. Use as a "toning" mechanism for specific body part areas.
2. Inappropriate for weight loss, because:
   a. Weight lost is water weight.
   b. Risk of dehydration and electrolyte loss.
   c. Spot reduction is not possible.
   d. Water weight is quickly regained with fluid replenishment.

E. ELECTRIC STIMULATORS
1. Rationales for use include:
   a. Increase muscle size by electrical stimulation.
   b. Effortless calorie expenditure
2. Inappropriate for weight loss, because:
   a. Spot reduction is not possible.
   b. No significant energy expenditure.

F. SWEAT SUITS
1. Rationales for use include:
   a. Lose weight quickly.
   b. May be used by athletes who need to compete at a reduced body weight (e.g., wrestlers, boxers, bodybuilders).

2. Inappropriate for weight loss, because:
   a. Weight lost is water weight.
   b. Risk of dehydration and electrolyte loss.
   c. Risk of heat-related illnesses (e.g., heat exhaustion, heat stroke).
   d. Water weight is quickly regained with fluid replenishment.

G. FAD DIETS

1. Rationales for use include:
   a. Possibility of rapid weight loss.
   b. Special food combinations.
   c. Elimination of certain foods.
2. Inappropriate for weight loss, because:
   a. Any diet will lead to weight loss if energy intake is reduced.
   b. Very low energy intake (also known as "very low calorie diets") may lower RMR and stimulate physiological processes that conserve energy expenditure, thus making weight loss even more difficult.
   c. Risk of nutritional deficiencies because of elimination of certain foods or food groups.
   d. Long-term safety and efficacy generally are not known.
3. Clearly, some individuals are successful with fad diets. Current scientific evidence, however, does not support widespread or long-term use of these diets.

VI. Role of Diet and Exercise in Weight Control

A. Increased physical activity, even in the absence of weight loss, can reduce the risk of chronic and, especially, cardiovascular disease. Similarly, weight loss through caloric restriction in the absence of increased physical activity also may result in reduced risk of chronic disease.

B. Regular physical activity is the best predictor of long-term weight maintenance.

C. The optimal weight control approach is to combine a diet low in total fat (e.g., <30% of total energy) and rich in fruits, vegetables, whole grains, and lean sources of protein with regular (daily) physical activity.

VII. Estimating Adequate Daily Energy Intake

A. Total Energy Expenditure
   1. **Resting Metabolic Rate**
      The amount of energy, usually expressed in Kcal, required for basic physiological function in a quiet, resting state.
   2. **Thermic Effect of Food**
      The energy required for digestion, absorption, and assimilation of nutrients.
   3. **Thermic Effect of Exercise**
      The energy required for physical activity or exercise.

B. Measurement by indirect calorimetry is the gold standard measure for RMR.
   1. Usually performed in a hospital or research setting.
   2. The individual may stay overnight at facility or arrive in the morning; measurements are performed after an 8- to 12-hour fast.
   3. Two assessment techniques:
      a. Sealed room/chamber.
      b. Portable metabolic cart.
   4. Oxygen consumed plus carbon dioxide produced is measured over time and converted to energy expenditure.

C. Other Estimations of Resting Energy Expenditure and Energy Requirements for Additional Physical Activity
   1. **Harris-Benedict Equation**
      a. Calculation of RMR in kilocalories per day.
      b. Males: RMR = 66 + 13.8 (weight in Kg) + 5 (height in cm) − 6.8 (age).
      c. Females: RMR = 655 + 9.6 (weight in Kg) + 1.8 (height in cm) − 4.7 (age).
      d. To estimate daily caloric requirements multiply by the factor that best represents the activity level of the person:
         1) Bed rest = 1.2
         2) Sedentary = 1.3
         3) Active = 1.4
         4) Very active = 1.5
   2. **Estimation of RMR Based on Fat-Free Mass**
      a. Fat-free mass may be obtained from body composition assessment.
      b. RMR = 370 + (21.6 × fat free mass in kg).
      c. The activity correction factors cited above can be used.

D. Regardless of the methods used, a client can be given appropriate energy intake and expenditure targets depending on whether body weight should be lost, gained, or maintained as well as to account for energy expenditure through exercise or athletic events. Many tables and charts exist for common energy expenditures of physical activities.

VIII. Dietary Guidelines for Management of Body Weight

A. RECOMMENDED ENERGY AND MACRONUTRIENT INTAKE FOR HEALTHY WEIGHT MANAGEMENT

1. Minimum energy intake to consume a nutritionally adequate diet is approximately 1,200 kcal/day. Dietary intake below this minimum level may be deficient in essential nutrients and, thus, may require supplementation.
2. Energy needs for weight maintenance may be estimated based on usual activity level as follows:
   a. Very light activity: 30–31 kcal/kg per day.
   b. Light activity: 33–38 kcal/kg per day.
   c. Moderate activity: 40–47 kcal/kg per day.
   d. High activity: 44–50 kcal/kg per day.
   e. Individuals with high-energy needs should consume additional energy in the form of nutrient-dense foods (e.g., fruits, vegetables, whole grains, lean sources of protein).
3. Carbohydrate intake should range from approximately **55% to 60%** of total energy for most individuals.
   a. Carbohydrates provide **4 kcal/g**.
   b. Athletes may need **7 to 10 g/kg** per day, or 65% to 70% of total energy from carbohydrates
   c. Fiber intake should be 20–35 g/day.
4. Protein intake should be **10% to 15%** of total energy, or 0.8g/kg for most individuals.
   a. Protein provides **4 kcal/g**.
   b. Athletes may need up to **1.7 g/kg**.
   c. No benefit is likely to be gained by exceeding a protein intake of 1.7g/kg.
5. Fat intake should be in the range of **25% to 35%** of total energy; a lower fat intake (<30% of total energy) may facilitate weight control.
   a. Fats provide **9 kcal/g**.
   b. Saturated fat intake should be less than 10% of total energy.
   c. Emphasis should be on mono- and polyunsaturated fats (e.g., olive oil, canola oil).
   d. A very low fat intake (<10% of total energy) can lead to deficiencies of fat-soluble vitamins and essential fatty acids.

B. WEIGHT REDUCTION

1. In general, women desiring weight loss should consume 1,200 to 1,500 kcal/day, and men should consume 1,800 to 2,000 kcal/day.
2. Optimal macronutrient composition for promoting weight reduction has not been determined.
3. Weight loss is best achieved with the combination of reduced total energy intake and reduced fat intake (<30% of total energy).

C. WEIGHT GAIN

1. For weight gain to occur, energy intake must exceed energy expenditure.
2. Those desiring weight gain should aim for an additional 400 to 500 kcal/day above their current energy intake.
3. To increase energy intake:
   a. Increase portion sizes at meals.
   b. Consume more nutrient-rich, energy-dense foods (e.g., nuts, trail mix, energy or sports bars, fig bars, dried fruit, granola, shakes, smoothies).
   c. Snack between meals.
   d. Eat one extra meal per day.

IX. Food Guide Pyramid

A. Developed by the U.S. Department of Agriculture (USDA) in 1992 to encourage Americans to develop and maintain healthy eating habits (*Figure 9-1*).
   1. Foods in the lower portion of the pyramid (carbohydrates from breads, cereals, rice, and pasta) should make up the majority of the diet. Consumption of complex carbohydrates and whole grains should be favored over consumption of simple and processed carbohydrates, such as white flour (including white flour pasta), white rice, and heavy use of sugar and other sweeteners.
   2. From the base of the pyramid to the peak, the recommended number of servings decreases.
   3. Foods at the top of the pyramid should be consumed less often.
   4. Serving sizes are based on USDA standard portions, which may not be typical of the serving sizes actually consumed by the general population, so people may eat far more than the recommended servings.
   5. Smaller persons may benefit from maintaining the lower range of serving recommendations.
   6. Larger or very active persons may need higher ranges of serving recommendations.

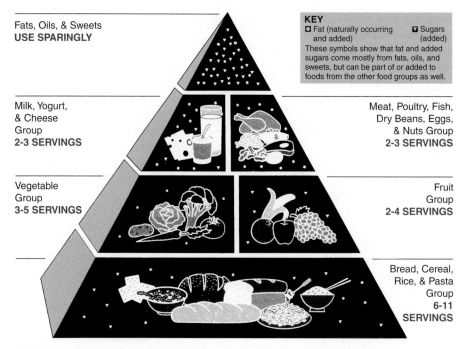

FIGURE 9-1. The U.S. Department of Agriculture Food Guide Pyramid. (U.S. Department of Agriculture/U.S. Department of Health and Human Services.)

B. The food pyramid has been somewhat controversial.
1. Certain dietary fats, such as omega-3 fatty acids found in "fatty" fish (e.g., salmon) and monosaturated fats (e.g., olive oil, canola oil) are considered to be "healthy fats" and should be emphasized in the diet.
2. Bread and cereal products made from whole grains should be encouraged over those made from white flour.
3. Lower-fat alternatives of meat and dairy are emphasized.

C. The Food Pyramid Guidelines are being revised to reflect the latest research and will account for age, gender, body weight, and physical activity.

X. Macronutrients and Kilocalories

A. Energy with respect to food consumption and physical activity is typically expressed in **Calories** or kilocalories. Other common units of energy include the joule (J), kilojoule (kJ), and watts (W).

B. CARBOHYDRATES
1. Composed of **carbon**, **hydrogen, and oxygen**.
2. Often abbreviated as **CHO**.
3. Contain energy in the amount of 4 kcal/g.
4. Generally recommended to make up between 55% and 60% of total energy intake for healthy adults.
5. Athletes preparing for an endurance event may

consume 70% of total energy intake as carbohydrates.
6. Carbohydrates are stored and metabolized in the body for energy.
   a. Blood glucose is an immediately available source of carbohydrate.
   b. Muscle glycogen is the largest, long-term storage form of carbohydrate.
   c. Liver glycogen is another long-term storage form of carbohydrate.

C. PROTEIN
1. Composed of **amino acids**.
   a. Contain an **amino group** (NH_2^+) plus carbon, oxygen, and hydrogen.
   b. Eight amino acids are considered to be essential, because they cannot be synthesized in the body and, therefore, must be consumed.
   c. Complete proteins are found in animal-based food products and contain all essential amino acids.
   d. Incomplete proteins are found in plant-based products and do not contain all essential amino acids. Consuming a variety of protein sources will ensure that an individual's protein and amino acid needs are met.
2. Contains energy in the amount of 4 kcal/g.
3. Body proteins are continuously broken down,

and those amino acids are recycled in combination with the amino acids that are consumed.

D. FAT

1. **Triglycerides** are composed of a **glycerol** molecule combined with three **fatty acids**.
2. Contains energy in the amount of 9 kcal/g (more energy per weight than carbohydrate or protein).
3. Triglycerides represent the largest potential energy store in the body and are found in:
   a. Subcutaneous fat.
   b. Intra-abdominal fat that surrounds internal organs.
   c. Intramuscular fat, another readily available energy source.

E. ALCOHOL

1. Is not a macronutrient and often is viewed as "empty calories" (e.g., does not contain substantial nutrients other than energy).
2. Contains energy in the amount of 7 kcal/g.
3. Metabolized by the liver.

XI. Vitamins

A. Organic compounds essential for life.

B. Must be consumed, because they are not manufactured in the body.

C. Used in physiological functions (e.g., blood coagulation, digestion, enzyme reactions).

D. Dietary Reference Intakes are new standards and include:

1. **Estimated Average Recommendations**
   a. Means and standard deviations.
   b. Recommendations by age and gender.
2. **Recommended Daily Allowances (RDAs)**
   a. Recommendations by age and gender.
   b. Goal for an intake that will meet the needs of 97% to 98% of individuals in a life stage and/or gender group.
3. **Adequate Intake (AI)**
   a. Recommendations by age and gender.
   b. Goal for an intake that is believed to cover the needs for all individuals in a group.
   c. Not as much supporting scientific evidence as for RDAs.
4. **Upper Limits (ULs)**
   a. Recommendations by age and gender.
   b. Possibility of toxicity above these levels.
   c. Represent intake from food, water, and supplements.

E. CLASSIFICATIONS OF VITAMINS

1. **Fat-Soluble Vitamins**
   a. **Vitamins A, D, E, and K.**
   b. Stored in body fat after absorption.
   c. Can build to toxic levels if oversupplemented (especially vitamin A).
2. **Water-Soluble Vitamins**
   a. **Vitamins C and B complex.**
   b. Excess amounts excreted; must be consumed on a regular basis.
   c. Oversupplementation can be dangerous for vitamin C, niacin, and vitamin B_6.

F. See *Table 9-1* for a description of vitamins, RDAs, food sources, and adverse effects of overconsumption.

G. Clients who may have deficiencies because of low energy consumption or other medical problems should consult a registered dietitian.

XII. Calcium and Iron in Health

A. CALCIUM

1. Mineral important for:
   a. Bone formation and maintenance.
   b. Tooth formation and maintenance.
   c. Muscle contraction.
   d. Nerve conduction.
   e. Blood clotting.
2. Deficiencies can occur in women because of:
   a. Lower overall energy consumption compared to men.
   b. Lower consumption of dairy products.
3. AI for Calcium
   a. Males and females aged 9–18 years: 1,300 mg/day.
   b. Males and females aged 19–50 years: 1,000 mg/day.
   c. Males and females aged 30–50 years: 1,000 mg/day.
   d. Males and females aged 50 years and older: 1,200 mg/day.
   e. Tolerable UL for all: 2,500 mg/day.
   f. Pregnant and lactating females: 18 years old and younger, 1,300 mg/day; older than 18 years, 1,000 mg/day.
4. Deficiencies can lead to bone loss quicker than replenishment (osteopenia) or bone loss that is not replaced (osteoporosis).
5. Food Sources of Calcium
   a. Dairy products (e.g., milk, cheese, yogurt).
   b. Canned fish that includes bones (e.g., salmon, sardines).

TABLE 9-1. Fat- and Water-Soluble Vitamins

Vitamin	Functions	RDA^a/AI^b*	Food Sources	Effects of Overconsumption
Fat Soluble				
Vitamin A	Vision, gene expression, immune function	Youths 9–13 years: 600 µg Males ≥14 years: 900 µg Females ≥14 years: 700 µg Pregnancy and lactation: 770–1,300 µg	Liver, dairy products, fish, sweet potatoes, carrots, cantaloupe	Liver toxicity
Vitamin D (calciferol)	Maintains blood calcium and phosphorus, B$_1$ metabolism	Youths 9–13 years: 5 µg* Males 14–50 years: 5 µg* Females 14–50 years: 5 µg* Males 50–70 years: 10 µg* Females 50–70 years: 10 µg Males ≥70 years: 15 µg* Females ≥70 years: 15 µg* Pregnancy and lactation: 5 µg*	Dairy products, fatty fish, fortified cereals, fortified milk products	Hypercalcemia (calcium imbalances can be life-threatening)
Vitamin E (α-tocopherol)	Antioxidant	Youths 9–13 years: 11 mg Males ≥14 years: 15mg Females ≥14 years: 15 mg Pregnancy and lactation: 15–19 mg	Nuts, fruits, vegetables, meats, vegetable oils	Possible hemorrhagic toxicity from over-supplementation
Vitamin K	Blood clotting, bone metabolism	Youths 9–13 years: 60 µg* Males 14–18 years: 75 µg* Males ≥19 years: 120 µg* Females 14–18 years: 75 µg* Females ≥19 years: 120 µg* Pregnancy and lactation: 75–90 µg*	Green leafy vegetables, broccoli, brussel sprouts, cabbage plant oils and margarine	None reported in healthy persons; persons taking anticoagulants must monitor intake
Water Soluble				
Vitamin C (ascorbic acid)	Antioxidant	Youths 9–13 years: 45 mg Males 14–18 years: 75 mg Males ≥19 years: 90 mg Females 14–18 years: 65 mg Females ≥19 years: 75 mg Smokers (all): 35 mg Pregnancy and lactation: 80–120 mg	Citrus fruits, tomatoes, tomato juice, potatoes cabbage, strawberries, cauliflower, broccoli, Brussels sprouts	Excess iron absorption, possible kidney stones, possible stomach upset
Vitamin B$_1$ (thiamin)	Coenzyme in carbohydrate metabolism	Youths 9–13 years: 0.9 mg Males 14–50 years: 1.2 mg Males ≥50 years: 1.2 mg Females 14–18 years: 1.0 mg Females 19–50 years: 1.1 mg Females ≥50 years: 1.1 mg Pregnancy and lactation: 1.4 mg	Whole-grain breads and cereals, fortified breads and cereals	None known
Vitamin B$_2$ (riboflavin)	Coenzyme in many metabolic pathways	Youths 9–13 years: 0.9 mg Males ≥14 years: 1.3 mg Females 14–18 years: 1.0 mg Females ≥19 years: 1.1 mg Pregnancy and lactation: 1.4–1.6 mg	Organ meats, milk, bread, fortified cereals	None known
Vitamin B$_6$) (pyridoxine	Coenzyme in amino acid metabolism	Youths 9–13 years: 1.0 mg Males 14–50 years: 1.2 mg Males ≥50 years: 1.7 mg Females 14–18 years: 1.2 mg Females 19–50 years: 1.3 mg Females ≥50 years: 1.5 mg Pregnancy and lactation: 1.4 mg	Organ meats, fortified cereals, fortified soy-based meat substitutes	Possible neuropathy from oversupplementation
Vitamin B$_{12}$ (cobalamin)	Coenzyme in nucleic acid metabolism, prevents megaloblastic anemia	Youths 9–13 years: 1.8 µg Males ≥14 years: 2.4 µg Females ≥14 years: 2.4 µg Pregnancy and lactation: 2.6–2.8 µg	Red meat, chicken, fish, fortified cereals	None known

TABLE 9-1. Fat- and Water-Soluble Vitamins *(continued)*

Vitamin	Functions	RDA^a/AI^b*	Food Sources	Effects of Overconsumption
Pantothenic acid	Coenzyme in fat metabolism	Youths 9–13 years: 4 mg* Males ≥14 years: 5 mg* Females ≥14 years: 5 mg* Pregnancy and lactation: 6–7 mg*	Beef, chicken, liver, egg yolks, potatoes, cereals, whole grains, tomato products, broccoli	None known
Biotin	Coenzyme in synthesis of fat, glycogen, and amino acids	Youths 9–13 years: 20 μg* Males 14–18 years: 25 μg* Males ≥19 years: 30 μg* Females 14–18 years: 25 μg* Females ≥19 years: 30 μg* Pregnancy and lactation: 30–35 μg*	Liver, meats, fruits	None known
Folate (folacin, folic acid)	Coenzyme in amino acid and nucleic acid metabolism, prevents megaloblastic anemia	Youths 9–13 years: 300 μg Males ≥14 years: 400 μg Females ≥14 years: 400 μg Pregnancy and lactation: 500–600 μg	Dark leafy green vegetables, whole grain breads, fortified cereals	Excessive intake may mask vitamin B_{12} deficiency
Niacin	Coenzyme in many metabolic reactions	Youths 9–13 years: 12 mg Males ≥14 years: 16 mg Females ≥14 years: 14 mg Pregnancy and lactation: 17–18 mg	Red meat, chicken, fish, whole grain products, fortified cereals	Stomach upset and skin flushing from oversupplementation
Choline	Precursor for acetylcholine and phospholipids	Youths 9–13 years: 375 mg* Males ≥14 years: 550 mg* Females 14–18 years: 400 mg* Females ≥19 years: 425 mg* Pregnancy and lactation: 450–550 mg*	Liver, milk, eggs, peanuts, low blood pressure	Liver toxicity, fishy body odor, sweating, excess salivation

^{a}Recommended Dietary Allowance: the goal for intake that will meet the needs of almost all (97–98%) individuals in a life stage and/or gender group.

^{b}Adequate Intake: the goal for intake that is believed to cover the needs of individuals in a group (insufficient scientific data to determine percentage of individuals covered).

Reprinted with permission from *Dietary Reference Intakes for Vitamin A, Vitamin K, Arsenic, Boron, Chromium, Copper, Iodine, Iron, Manganese, Molybdenum, Nickel, Silicon, Vanadium, and Zinc* (2002) by the National Academy of Sciences; courtesy of the National Academies Press, Washington, DC.

   c. Dark green vegetables (e.g., spinach, kale, other greens).
   d. Orange juice and some breads may be calcium fortified (check labels).

B. IRON
   1. Mineral important for:
      a. Maintenance of red blood cells (hemoglobin).
      b. Prevention of certain types of anemia.
      c. Cofactor in enzymatic reactions.
   2. Deficiencies can occur in women because of:
      a. Lower overall energy consumption compared to men.
      b. Lower consumption of meat.
      c. Menstrual blood loss.
   3. AI for Iron
      a. Males and females aged 9–13 years: 8 mg/day.
      b. Males aged 14–18 years: 11 mg/day.
      c. Females aged 14–18 years: 15 mg/day.
      d. Males aged 18 years and older: 8 mg/day.
      e. Females aged 19–50 years: 18 mg/day.
      f. Females aged 50 years and older: 8 mg/day.
      g. Tolerable UL for all: 40–45 mg/day.
   4. Deficiencies can lead to anemia, which can lead to fatigue and reduced exercise performance.
   5. Food Sources of Iron
      a. Meats (e.g., beef, pork, chicken).
      b. Legumes.
      c. Eggs.
      d. Grains, breads, and cereals often are iron-fortified (check labels).
      e. Dark green vegetables (e.g., spinach, kale, other greens).
   6. Vegetarians
      a. Need to ensure an AI of iron from nonmeat food sources.
      b. May have iron requirements double those of nonvegetarians.

C. Women who appear to be prone to calcium and/or iron deficiencies may wish to consult a registered dietitian for advice. Iron supplements should be used only at the recommendation of a physician, because iron overload can occur.

XIII. Maintaining Hydration

A. WATER
1. Is an essential nutrient necessary for life.
2. Accounts for approximately **60% to 70%** of total body weight.
3. Is necessary for bodily functions such as:
   a. Transport of nutrients and waste products.
   b. Solvent for chemical reactions.
   c. Lubrication for and between cells.
   d. Regulation of body temperature.
4. Risk of dehydration risk is increased in:
   a. Infants and young children, because of immature body temperature regulation.
   b. The elderly, because of insufficient fluid intake.
   c. Persons with chronic diseases, insufficient intake, and medications, which increase excretion or affect electrolytes, such as sodium (Na^+) or potassium (K^+).
      1) Physically active and athletic persons can experience insufficient intake and large volumes lost through sweat loss.
      2) Electrolyte imbalance can interfere with the ability to dissipate heat.
5. Recommendations for Water Consumption
   a. Healthy Adults
      The Institute of Medicine recommends the following daily intake of total water from all beverages and foots:
      1) Women: $\approx$2.7 L (91 ounces).
      2) Men: $\approx$3.7 L (125 ounces).
   b. Active Individuals
      1) For most persons, water is sufficient.
      2) Consume a healthy diet, and maintain hydration as recommended for healthy adults.
      3) Two hours before exercise, consume 400 to 600 mL (16–20 fluid ounces) of water to allow for excretion before exercise; during exercise, consume water every 15 to 20 minutes (150–350 mL per drink).
      4) Individuals will vary in terms of how much water consumption during exercise feels comfortable.
      5) Water temperatures of 15° to 21°C (59–72°F) is typically preferred.
      6) Slight flavoring or sweetening of water may encourage drinking or use of sports drinks.
      7) After exercise, consume water to replace lost water weight; consumption should be 450 to 675 mL (16–24 fluid ounces) for each pound of body weight lost.
      8) Additional hydration may be obtained by sports drinks for events lasting longer than 60 minutes.

B. SPORTS DRINKS
1. Contain carbohydrates, in the form glucose or glucose polymer, as well as electrolytes, such as sodium (Na^+) and potassium (K^+), for repletion of both, formulated in a concentration that is easily absorbed and usually not irritating to the stomach.
2. May be appropriate for intense activities with a duration of 60 minutes or longer (e.g., distance running, cycling, sports team practice).
3. Recommended for activities performed in higher heat and/or humidity.
4. Electrolyte depletion can be an issue in long-duration events (e.g., distance running, cycling, sports team practices); water alone may overdilute electrolytes and lead to hyponatremia (low blood sodium).

XIV. Common Nutritional Ergogenic Aids

A. Ergogenic aids are substances believed to improve muscle size, strength, endurance, or athletic performance.

B. CARBOHYDRATE SUPPLEMENTS
1. A pre-event meal with adequate carbohydrate is important for maintenance of blood glucose levels during exercise.
   a. Maintenance of blood glucose during exercise may be achieved by drinking an 8% carbohydrate or carbohydrate/electrolyte solution.
   b. Between 30 and 60 g of carbohydrate per hour of **continuous exercise** is recommended to maintain blood glucose levels.
   c. More than 17 g of carbohydrate per 8 ounces of fluid may lead to stomach irritation and cramps.
2. Replenishing muscle glycogen stores following exercise is best achieved by consuming 1.0 to 1.5 g/kg of carbohydrate within 30 to 60 minutes after exercise.
   a. This amount is difficult to consume within 30 minutes.
   b. Some recommend consumption within the first 2 hours after exercise.
3. Carbohydrate in excess of energy needs will be converted to body fat.
4. Glucose or glucose polymer solutions are recommended, because fructose may cause gastrointestinal distress.

5. Experimental research supports efficacy and safety.

C. PROTEIN/AMINO ACIDS

1. Purported to increase muscle mass.
2. No evidence supports any benefit from consuming more than 1.7 g/kg, even in strength/power athletes.
3. May lead to dehydration and excess protein in the urine, and may unduly stress the kidneys.
4. Adequate dietary protein can be easily obtained through food intake.
5. No evidence supports any benefit from supplementation with amino acids.

D. VITAMINS AND MINERALS

1. Purported to improve athletic performance by increasing energy availability, etc.
2. Toxic concentrations are a risk with megadosing.
3. Athletes with adequate nutrition rarely experience nutritional deficiencies.
4. Supplements do not substitute for inadequate nutrition; nutrient cofactors found only in whole foods are not present in supplements.
5. Supplementation of a single vitamin or mineral may affect the metabolism of other nutrients (e.g., some compete for absorption in the gut).

E. SODIUM BICARBONATE

1. Purported to enhance performance in short-term, high-intensity exercise by inducing alkalosis (raising blood pH) to buffer hydrogen ion (H^+) and lactic acid.
2. May result in abdominal cramps and diarrhea approximately 1 hour after ingestion.
3. Safety is unknown.
4. Research results are equivocal.
5. Use is not recommended.

F. BEE POLLEN

1. Purported to promote exercise endurance.
2. No evidence supports any ergogenic effect.
3. May result in serious allergic reaction in sensitive persons.
4. Use is not recommended.

G. CREATINE

1. Purported to increase the muscle-free creatine pool, thereby increasing creatine phosphate synthesis and increased ability to perform short-term, high-intensity exercise or bouts of short-term exercise.
2. Buffers hydrogen ions (H^+) to increase the amount of work performed during exercise.
3. Studies suggest a possible ergogenic benefit in short-term, high-intensity anaerobic exercise.
4. No known benefits in endurance exercise.
5. Long-term effects of creatine supplementation are unknown.

H. SALT TABLETS

1. Used to replace electrolytes lost from endurance exercise or exercise in the heat.
2. May irritate the stomach lining, cause nausea, and further increase the need for water.
3. Use is not recommended, because water is lost at a higher rate than electrolytes during exercise.

I. DIET PILLS

1. Include appetite suppressants and stimulants.
2. Used by athletes to suppress appetite or to increase alertness and improve exercise performance, because they mimic the actions of epinephrine and norepinephrine.
3. Side Effects
   a. Headaches.
   b. Dizziness.
   c. Agitation.
   d. Increased blood pressure.
   e. Increased heart rate.
   f. Increased cardiac output.
   g. Increased respiration.
4. May interfere with normal perception mechanisms for pain, fatigue, or heat stress.
5. Use is not recommended.

J. CHROMIUM PICOLINATE

1. Purported to improve glucose tolerance, decrease body fat, and increase lean body mass.
2. Some evidence for efficacy in chromium-deficient individuals.
3. Toxicity of chromium supplementation has been hypothesized.
4. Efficacy and safety are unknown.
5. Use is not recommended.

XV. The Female Athlete Triad

A. A set of medical conditions that can occur in physically active women. This potentially life-threatening syndrome is marked by:
1. Inadequate food (energy) intake (eating disorder).
2. Menstrual cycle abnormalities (amenorrhea).
3. Osteoporosis.

B. DISORDERED EATING

May range from restriction of food intake, occasional bingeing and purging, to bulimia and anorexia nervosa and triggers other components of the triad.

1. Bulimia

Food restriction or fasting, followed by overeating/bingeing and then purging.

2. Anorexia Nervosa

Extreme restrictive eating behavior in which individuals continue to starve and perceives themselves as overweight despite being 15% or more below their ideal body weight.

C. AMENORRHEA

Absence of menstruation, which can result from excessive exercise and decreased food intake.

D. OSTEOPOROSIS

Loss of bone mineral density, which can result from chronically low levels of ovarian hormones. The amount of bone loss is correlated with:

1. Severity and length of menstrual irregularity.
2. Nutritional status, particularly calcium and vitamin D intake.
3. Amount of skeletal loading during activity.

E. TREATMENT

1. Daily calcium intake of 1,500 mg.
2. Oral contraceptives or hormone replacement.
3. Increasing energy intake by 250 to 350 kcal/day and/or reducing exercise training by 10% to 20%.
4. Physicians may consider bone-building pharmaceutical therapy.

F. PREVENTION

Focuses on instruction and counseling to reinforce the following:

1. Health and well-being.
2. Positive self-image.
3. Realistic fitness goals.
4. Sensible body composition.

XVI. Major Position Stands: Obesity, Nutrition and Physical Performance, and Weight Management

A. National Institutes of Health (NIH)/National Heart, Lung and Blood Institute (NHLBI) Guidelines for the Identification, Evaluation, and Treatment of Overweight and Obesity in Adults

1. Assessment of Body Weight by BMI.
   a. Underweight: <18.5 kg/m^2.
   b. Normal weight: 18.5–24.9 kg/m^2.
   c. Overweight: 25–29.9 kg/m^2.
   d. Class I obesity: 30–34.9 kg/m^2.
   e. Class II obesity: 35–39.9 kg/m^2.
   f. Extreme (class III) obesity: >40 kg/m^2.

2. If assessment of body weight status indicates that weight loss is advisable, readiness to make lifestyle changes should be assessed. This assessment should include:
   a. Reasons and motivation for weight loss.
   b. Previous attempts at weight loss.
   c. Support system (e.g., friends, family).
   d. Understanding the risks and benefits.
   e. Attitudes toward physical activity.
   f. Time availability.
   g. Potential barriers, including financial limitations.

3. The recommended initial weight loss goal is 10% of initial body weight, achieved over a 6-month period (1–2 pounds/week). Further weight loss may be considered after a period of weight maintenance.

4. In some patients, prevention of further weight gain may be an appropriate goal.

5. Therapies should include diet modification, increased physical activity, and behavior therapy.

6. Pharmacotherapy may be beneficial in some high-risk patients:
   a. Those with BMI $\geq$30.
   b. Those with BMI >27 and obesity-related comorbidities).

7. Weight loss surgery (bariatric surgery) may be indicated for patients with:
   a. BMI >40 (extreme obesity).
   b. BMI >35 and obesity-related comorbid conditions.

B. Joint Position of the American Dietetic Association, Dietitians of Canada, and the American College of Sports Medicine: Nutrition and Athletic Performance

1. Optimal nutrition enhances physical activity, athletic performance, and recovery from exercise.

2. Athletes should consume enough energy during high-intensity training to maintain their weight, maximize training effects, and maintain health.

3. Low energy intakes can lead to loss of muscle mass, menstrual dysfunction, loss or failure to gain bone density, and increased risk of fatigue, injury, and illness.

4. Optimal body fat levels vary with age, gender, sport, and heredity of the athlete.

5. If weight loss is desired, it should be undertaken before the competitive season and involve a trained health/nutrition professional.

6. Carbohydrate intake should range from 6 to 10g/kg per day.
7. Fat intake should not be less than 15% of total energy.
8. Protein Requirements
   a. Endurance athletes: 1.2–1.4g/kg per day.
   b. Strength/resistance-trained athletes: 1.6–1.7 g/kg per day.
9. Dehydration impairs athletic performance. Adequate fluid should be consumed as follows:
   a. Two hours before exercise: 400–600 mL (14–22 ounces).
   b. During exercise: 150–350 mL (6–12 ounces) every 15–20 minutes.
   c. After exercise: 450–675 mL (16–24 ounces) for each pound of body weight lost.
10. Nutritional Recommendation for Athletic Events
    a. Before exercise, consume a meal/snack to provide fluid for hydration and carbohydrate to maximize maintenance of blood glucose. Limit the fat and fiber to avoid gastrointestinal distress.
    b. During exercise (particularly endurance events lasting longer than 1 hour), consume fluids to maintain hydration and provide carbohydrate (30–60 g/hr).
    c. Following exercise, consume a mixed meal (containing carbohydrates, protein, and fat) to facilitate recovery.
11. Vitamin/mineral supplementation should not be necessary if an athlete is consuming adequate energy and a nutritionally balanced diet. If an athlete is dieting, sick or recovering from an injury, or eliminating foods or food groups, a multivitamin/mineral supplement may be indicated.
12. Vegetarian athletes may be at risk for inadequate caloric consumption, protein, or vitamin/mineral intake.

C. ACSM Position Stand: Appropriate Intervention Strategies for Weight Loss and Prevention of Weight Regain for Adults
1. Weight reduction should be achieved through a combination of decreased energy intake and increased energy expenditure.
2. Total energy deficit of 500 to 1,000 kcal/day is recommended.
3. A dietary fat intake of less than 30% of total energy (kcal) may facilitate weight loss.
4. A minimum of 150 minutes per week (2.5 hr/week) of moderate intensity physical activity should be encouraged.
5. A progressive increase in activity to 200 to 300 minutes per week (>2,000 kcal/week or 3.3–3.5

hr/week) is recommended, because this may facilitate long-term weight control.
6. Resistance exercise may increase muscular strength and function, but it may not prevent loss of fat-free mass with weight loss.
7. Pharmacotherapy may be indicated and is most effectively combined with other lifestyle modifications (e.g., increased activity, reduced energy intake).

XVII. National Cholesterol Education Program (NCEP) Adult Treatment Panel III (ATPIII) Guidelines: Detection, Evaluation, and Treatment of High Blood Cholesterol

A. Elevated low-density lipoprotein cholesterol (LDL-C) is a major cause of CHD, and LDL-C-lowering therapy reduces the risk of CHD. Thus, elevated LDL-C is the primary target of cholesterol-lowering therapy.

B. **RISK ASSESSMENT**
1. A fasting blood lipid/lipoprotein profile (total cholesterol, LDL-C, high-density lipoprotein cholesterol [HDL-C] and triglycerides) should be obtained once every five years in individuals over age 20.
2. Classifications
   a. LDL-C
      1) Optimal: <100 mg/dL.
      2) Near or above optimal: 100–129 mg/dL.
      3) Borderline high: 130–159 mg/dL.
      4) High: 160–189 mg/dL.
      5) Very high: ≥190 mg/dL.
   b. Total Cholesterol
      1) Desirable: <200 mg/dL.
      2) Borderline high: 200–239 mg/dL.
      3) High: ≥240 mg/dL.
   c. HDL-C
      1) Low: <40 mg/dL.
      2) High: ≥60 mg/dL.
3. Major Risk Factors that Modify LDL-C Goals
   a. Smoking.
   b. Hypertension.
   c. Low HDL-C.
   d. Family history of premature CHD.
   e. Age.
      1) Men: >45 years.
      2) Women: >55 years.
   f. Diabetes.
4. In individuals with CHD or CHD risk equivalents (e.g., diabetes, peripheral arterial disease), the LDL-C goal is less then 100 mg/dL.

5. For individuals with two or more risk factors, the LDL-C goal is less than 130 mg/dL.
6. For individuals with zero or one risk factor, the LDL-C goal is less than 160 mg/dL.

C. PRIMARY PREVENTION OF CHD

Primary prevention of CHD should include the adoption of lifestyle changes, including:
1. Reduced intake of saturated fat and cholesterol.
2. Increased physical activity.
3. Weight control.

D. SECONDARY PREVENTION OF CDH

Secondary prevention involves those with established CHD.
1. The LDL-C goal is less than 100 mg/dL.
2. Pharmacotherapy may be indicated.

E. COMPONENTS OF LDL-C-LOWERING THERAPY

1. **Therapeutic Lifestyle Changes (TLC)**
    a. Low intake of saturated fats (<7% of total energy).
    b. Monounsaturated fat intake of up to 20% of total energy.
    c. Polyunsaturated fat intake of up to 10% of total energy.
    d. Total fat intake of between 25% and 35% of total energy.
    e. Carbohydrate intake of between 50% and 60% of total energy, with an emphasis on complex carbohydrates (e.g., whole grains, fruits, vegetables).
    f. Fiber intake of 20 to 30 g/day (10–25 g/day soluble).
    g. Protein intake of approximately 15% of total energy.
    h. Cholesterol intake of less than 200 mg/day.
    i. Maintain a desirable body weight/prevent weight gain; weight reduction, if indicated
    j. Include at least moderate physical activity of 30 minutes on most, if not all, days of the week (minimum energy expenditure of 200 kcal/day).
    k. Consider plant stanols/sterols (2 g/day) and soluble (viscous) fiber (10–25 g/day; sources: fruits, beans, oats).
2. **Drug Therapy (as Adjunctive Therapy to TLC)**
    a. Hydroxymethylglutaryl–Coenzyme A Reductase Inhibitors (Statins)
        1) Decrease LDL-C and triglycerides.
        2) Increase HDL-C.
    b. Bile Acid Sequestrants
        1) Decrease LDL-C.
        2) Increase HDL-C.
    c. Nicotinic Acid
        1) Decreases LDL-C and triglycerides.
        2) Increases HDL-C.
    d. Fibric Acids
        1) Decrease LDL-C and triglycerides.
        2) Increases HDL-C.

F. METABOLIC SYNDROME

Along with lowered LDL-C, abnormalities associated with this condition are additional targets of therapy (e.g., dyslipidemia, elevated blood pressure, glucose intolerance).
1. **Diagnosis**
    Metabolic syndrome is diagnosed when three or more of the following are present:
    a. Abdominal Obesity
        1) Waist circumference in men: >40 inches.
        2) Waist circumference in women: >35 inches.
    b. Triglycerides: ≥150 mg/dL.
    c. HDL-C
        1) Men: <40mg/dL.
        2) Women: <50 mg/dL.
    d. Blood pressure: ≥130/85 mm Hg.
    e. Fasting glucose: ≥110 mg/dL.
2. **Management**
    a. Address the underlying causes (e.g., obesity, physical inactivity).
    b. Treat lipid and nonlipid risk factors (e.g., hypertension, elevated triglycerides, low HDL-C).
    c. Initiate TLC approach, particularly weight control and increased physical activity.

Review Test

DIRECTIONS: Carefully read all questions, and select the BEST single answer.

1. The eating habits of an athlete involved in long-distance running should differ from those of a sedentary individual of the same body weight in what way?
   A) The athlete should reduce fat intake to 10% of total calories.
   B) The athlete should increase protein intake to threefold the RDA.
   C) The athlete should have a greater intake of grains, fruits, vegetables, and lean sources of protein.
   D) There should be no change in calories.

2. Fiber is a type of carbohydrate that is not digestible (e.g., it will pass through the digestive system without being absorbed). The NCEP ATPIII guidelines recommend that soluble (viscous) fiber be included in the diet for the prevention and treatment of elevated blood lipid concentrations. Sources of soluble (viscous) fibers include
   A) Fruits, beans, and oats.
   B) Meat and dairy foods.
   C) Wheat bran and whole wheat products.
   D) All of the above.

3. The BMI is calculated using which of the following formulas?
   A) Weight/hip circumference.
   B) Weight/height^2.
   C) Height/weight^2.
   D) Hip circumference/height.

4. A common measure to assist in the evaluation of body fat distribution is
   A) Height/weight charts.
   B) Total body weight.
   C) WHR.
   D) Total body water.

5. Carbohydrate, protein, and fat provide which of the following amounts of energy (kcal/g)?
   A) 2, 4, and 6, respectively.
   B) 4, 6, and 8, respectively.
   C) 6, 8, and 9, respectively.
   D) 4, 4, and 9, respectively.

6. If total daily caloric consumption is 2,400 kcal and the total fat in that diet is 30%, how many grams of fat per day would be consumed?
   A) 80.
   B) 70.
   C) 90.
   D) 75.

7. When the body consumes more calories than it uses, the condition is called
   A) Ketogenesis.
   B) Positive caloric balance.
   C) Positive electrolyte balance.
   D) Negative energy balance.

8. Diets high in saturated fat can lead to elevations in blood ___ concentration, which may increase risk of heart disease. Optimal concentrations of this blood lipoprotein are ___.
   A) Very LDL-C, <120 mg/dL.
   B) LDL-C, <125 mg/dL.
   C) HDL-C, >30 mg/dL.
   D) LDL-C, <100 mg/dL.

9. An ideal weight-loss program should set a goal of ___ pounds per week, with an energy intake of not less than ___ kcal/day.
   A) 10, 1,600.
   B) 3–5, 1,500.
   C) 1–2, 1,200.
   D) None of the above.

10. Athletes who exercise in the heat and humidity have a special need for fluid replacement. Current guidelines suggest that athletes should
    A) Consume 16 to 24 fluid ounces of water for every pound of weight lost.
    B) Drink nothing but alcoholic beverages after engaging in exercise.
    C) Avoid drinking water after exercise because of the danger of cramps.
    D) Eat salt tablets with every meal during the hot summer months.

11. When counseling a patient with metabolic syndrome, your emphasis should be on addressing underlying causes of the syndrome, such as
    A) Obesity and physical inactivity.
    B) Excessive carbohydrate intake.
    C) Elevated LDL-C concentration.
    D) Lack of muscular strength.

12. Which of the following medical conditions is NOT part of the female athlete triad?
    A) Disordered eating.
    B) Osteoporosis.
    C) Amenorrhea.
    D) Anemia.

13. Which of the following waist circumference measurements indicates abdominal obesity?
    A) 0.98.
    B) >29.9.

C)   43 inches

D)   All of the above.

14.   What is the optimal approach for long-term management of body weight?

A)   Hypocaloric diet.

B)   Daily aerobic exercise.

C)   Resistance training.

D)   A low-fat, high-fiber diet and daily physical activity.

15.   Which eating disorder is marked by an overwhelming fear of becoming fat, a distorted body image, and extreme restrictive eating?

A)   Bulimia.

B)   Anorexia nervosa.

C)   Chronic dieting.

D)   Yo-yo dieting.

16.   Which of the following is not a feature of the metabolic syndrome?

A)   Dyslipidemia (low HDL-C, elevated triglycerides).

B)   Osteoporosis.

C)   Insulin resistance.

D)   Elevated blood pressure.

17.   All of the following are helpful suggestions for an athlete trying to gain weight EXCEPT

A)   Increase portion sizes at meals.

B)   Eat more high-calorie foods (e.g., candy bars, soft drinks).

C)   Eat one extra meal per day.

D)   Snack on energy- and nutrient-dense foods (e.g., fig bars, nuts and dried fruit).

18.   Athletes may have protein needs greater than those of sedentary individuals. What level of protein intake is the recommended UL for athletes?

A)   0.8 g/kg.

B)   1.4 g/kg.

C)   2.2 g/kg.

D)   1.7 g/kg.

19.   What is an appropriate initial weight loss goal for an obese individual desiring weight reduction?

A)   10% of initial body weight in first 6 months.

B)   20 pounds in 2 months.

C)   5 pounds per week for the first 6 weeks, then weight maintenance.

D)   BMI of less than 18.5.

20.   Women are likely to be deficient in both calcium and iron, because

A)   They tend to consume less overall energy than men.

B)   they tend to consume less dairy products.

C)   They tend to consume less protein from meat sources.

D)   All of the above.

21.   Which of the following foods would be in the group recommended to comprise most of the daily energy intake according to the Food Guide Pyramid?

A)   Oranges.

B)   Yogurt.

C)   Pasta.

D)   Olive oil.

22.   Which of the following diseases is NOT typically associated with obesity?

A)   Diabetes.

B)   Skin cancer.

C)   Coronary artery disease.

D)   Colon cancer.

23.   To lose one pound ($\approx$0.5 kg) of body fat, how much of an energy deficit must be created by diet and/or physical activity?

A)   2,000 kcal.

B)   2,500 kcal.

C)   3,000 kcal.

D)   3,500 kcal.

24.   Which fat-soluble vitamin is important for bone formation?

A)   Vitamin A.

B)   Vitamin D.

C)   Vitamin E.

D)   Vitamin K.

25.   Which energy source represents the largest potential energy store in the body?

A)   Fat.

B)   Blood glucose.

C)   Muscle glycogen.

D)   Protein.

ANSWERS AND EXPLANATIONS

1–C.   Important to any physical activity program is a plan for healthy eating. The nutritional needs of physically active individuals do not differ significantly from those of healthy adults except for energy or calorie intake. The primary source of additional calories will be from carbohydrates (e.g., whole grains, fruits, vegetables) and lean sources of protein (e.g., lean meat, beans, low-fat dairy products).

2–A.   Soluble (viscous) fiber is found in fruits (especially apples, oranges, pears, peaches, and grapes), vegetables, oat bran, oatmeal, rye, barley, and dried beans. Sources of insoluble fiber, which improves laxation, include wheat bran, brown rice, whole-grain breads, bran cereals, and pasta.

3–B.   The BMI is used more frequently than other measures to assess body fat. It is calculated as (weight in kg)/(height in m)^2.

4–C.   The WHR may be used to assess the distribution of body fat. Men and women tend to have body fat distributed at different sites: Men tend to exhibit extra weight around the waist (android pattern), whereas women (before menopause) tend to have extra weight distributed around the hips and buttocks (gynoid pattern).

5–D.   Each gram of carbohydrate and protein provides approximately 4 kcal of energy. Fat provides more than twice this amount of energy (9 kcal/g). The degree of fat saturation (saturated, monounsaturated, and polyunsaturated) does not change the 9 kcal/g amount of energy. Alcohol provides 7 kcal/g.

6–A.   Using the percentage distribution of 4 kcal of energy from carbohydrates and proteins and 9 kcal of energy from fat, a diet consisting of 2,400 kcal with 30% fat would consist of 80 grams of fat (2,400 kcal $\times$ 30% = 720 fat calories $\div$ 9 kcal/g = 80 g).

7–B.   When the body consumes more calories than are used, it is in a state of positive caloric (or energy) balance. A negative balance occurs when the body used more energy than it consumes. Ketogenesis is a condition in which the body metabolizes ketone bodies for energy, typically during severe carbohydrate restriction.

8–D.   Diets high in saturated fat can elevate blood LDL-C concentrations and increase the risk of heart disease. Elevated blood LDL-C level is one of the major risk factors for CHD. Optimal concentration of blood LDL-C is less than 100 mg/dL.

9–C.   Healthy weight loss programs should set a goal of 1 to 2 pounds per week. Energy intake should not fall below 1,200 kcal/day; otherwise, the diet may not include recommended amounts of essential nutrients. The most effective method for achieving and maintaining weight loss is a combined program of caloric management and regular physical activity.

10–A.   Athletes should drink plenty of cool, plain water before, during, and after activity—even if they do not feel thirsty. Athletes should consume at least 14 to 22 ounces of fluid in the 2 hours before exercise and 6 to 12 ounces every 15 to 20 minutes during the activity. After exercise, drink more than the amount needed to quench thirst. Every pound lost during activity should be replaced with at least 16 to 24 ounces of fluid (1 cup = 8 fl oz).

11–A.   For a patient with metabolic syndrome, treatment should be directed toward reducing the underlying causes of the syndrome (e.g., obesity, physical inactivity). Risk factors associated with the syndrome (e.g., hypertension, dyslipidemia) are effectively modified by weight reduction and increased physical activity.

12–D.   Disordered eating is the component of the female athlete triad that may lead to absence of menstruation (amenorrhea) and premature bone loss (osteoporosis). Anemia (low iron) is not considered to be part of the triad.

13–C.   A waist circumference of greater than 40 inches in men and 35 inches in women is associated with abdominal obesity.

14–D.   Modifying both diet and physical activity is the optimal approach for long-term weight control. Exercise may not produce significant weight loss by itself, but it is the best predictor of long-term success with weight control.

15–B.   Anorexia nervosa is an eating disorder marked by an overwhelming fear of becoming fat, a distorted body image, and the inability to eat. Bulimics binge on food, then purge by inducing vomiting or taking laxatives and diuretics. Chronic dieting (yo-yo dieting) is a continuous cycle of weight loss and weight gain.

16–B.   Metabolic syndrome is characterized by the coexistence of several risk factors for cardiovascular disease: dyslipidemia, insulin resistance, and elevated blood pressure. Abdominal obesity is thought to be the central feature of this syndrome.

17–B.   Individuals trying to gain weight should be encouraged to eat more energy- and nutrient-dense foods, to increase their portion sizes at meals, and to eat extra meal/snacks each day. Consuming foods with a high nutrient density allows individuals to meet their nutrient needs, whereas high-calorie foods devoid of nutrients (e.g., candy bars, chips, soft drinks) provide calories but not vitamins or minerals.

18–D.   Athletes may have increased protein requirements because of greater utilization of protein as an energy source and increased protein turnover. Up to 1.7 g/kg per day is recommended for an athlete, compared with 0.8 g/kg per day for a sedentary individual. Good sources of protein include lean meats, dried beans, and low-fat dairy foods.

19–A. The NIH/NHLBI Guidelines for the Identification, Evaluation, and Treatment of Overweight and Obesity in Adults advise an initial weight loss goal of 10% of initial body weight achieved over a 6-month period. Further weight loss may be attempted after a period of weight maintenance. Significant improvements in metabolic risk factors have been noted with modest weight loss (e.g., 5–10% of initial body weight).

20–D. Women are likely to be at risk for both calcium and iron deficiencies, because they tend to consume lower overall energy (kilocalories) than men, less dairy products (a good source of calcium), and less meat, chicken, or pork (high in iron).

21–C. Pasta would be found in the breads, rice, cereal, and pasta group, which makes up the base of the Food Guide Pyramid. These foods should comprise the majority of energy in a healthy diet, and whole-grain, higher-fiber choices should be emphasized. Oranges would be found in the fruit group; yogurt in the milk, yogurt, and cheese group; and olive oil in the fats, oils, and sweets group. Oils would be at the top of the pyramid and should be consumed the least, even though olive oil is considered to be a "healthy" fat.

22–B. Certain cancers (e.g., colon, pancreatic, and to a lesser extent, breast and prostate) are associated with obesity. Skin cancer is not. Obesity does increase the risk of developing both diabetes and all types of cardiovascular disease (e.g., coronary artery disease, stroke).

23–D. All fats, including stored body fat, contain energy in the amount of 3,500 kcal per pound. This energy deficit should be best reached by a combination of both elimination of foods in the diet and increased physical activity.

24–B. Vitamin D is essential to maintain blood calcium levels, which affect bone metabolism. Vitamin A is important for vision. Vitamin E is an antioxidant. Vitamin K is essential for blood clotting.

25–A. Body fat (in the form of stored triglycerides) represents the largest potential energy store in the body, because it is stored under the skin, in the abdominal cavity, and in the muscles. Fat also contains the highest amount of energy per gram (9 kcal/g). Muscle glycogen would represent the next largest potential energy source. Protein from muscle and tissue breakdown is not a significant energy source. Blood glucose is a short-term energy source from carbohydrates.

Program and Administration/Management

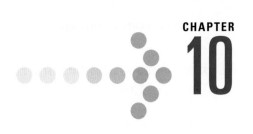

FREDERICK S. DANIELS AND GREGORY B. DWYER

I. General Description

A. Effective program administration creates safe, successful programs and services and reduces the risk of problems and legal situations.

B. The program director/manager ensures that the program meets the often-changing standards and practices for health/fitness and clinical exercise rehabilitation services.

C. The program director/manager needs to have knowledge of modern management and financial principles.

D. The program director/manager must coordinate many interrelated components and services.

E. The input of the facility's upper management (e.g., the institution's medical director, the fitness center's general manager) into program development and implementation is crucial and must be solicited by the program director/manager.

II. Characteristics of a Good Program Director/Manager

A good program director/manager:

A. **DESIGNS AND MONITORS THE IMPLEMENTATION OF EXERCISE PROGRAMS BY:**
   1. Organizing the required resources.
   2. Arranging the schedule.
   3. Guiding the staff or clients through the program.
   4. Purchasing equipment and supplies.

B. **ASSESSES PROGRAM AND CLIENT NEEDS BY:**
   1. Establishing goals for the program.
   2. Monitoring program and facility safety.
   3. Ensuring program evaluation.
   4. Implementing any changes warranted by evaluation.

C. **DEVELOPS AND MOTIVATES STAFF AND CLIENTS BY:**
   1. Demonstrating good communication skills with staff and clients.
   2. Coordinating staff and program development.
   3. Evaluating staff and programs.

D. **PROVIDES EDUCATION AND TRAINING, AS DEMONSTRATED BY:**
   1. Developing and implementing a staff training program.
   2. Possessing strong teaching skills.
   3. Soliciting feedback.

E. **PROVIDES A ROLE MODEL AS A LEADER BY:**
   1. Providing feedback.
   2. Being motivated and a good motivator.
   3. Controlling the situation, and assuming a position of leadership.

F. **MOTIVATES INDIVIDUALS BY:**
   1. Demonstrating strong communication skills.
   2. Being persuasive and influential.
   3. Demonstrating enthusiasm.
   4. Inciting action, and giving impetus to the program.

G. **ACTS AS A COUNSELOR BY:**
   1. Advising staff and clients.
   2. Practicing listening skills.
   3. Expressing opinions, but being willing to listen to those of others.
   4. Consulting with staff and clients.
   5. Suggesting changes and recommending action.

H. **POSSESSES THE ABILITY TO PROMOTE PROGRAMS, AS DEMONSTRATED BY:**
   1. Encouraging participation.
   2. Understanding the benefits of the program.
   3. Demonstrating the ability to communicate benefits to staff and clients.

III. Basic Responsibilities of a Program Director/Manager

A. Assesses client interest and satisfaction through surveys, client and staff feedback, and observation of programs.

B. **OBSERVES ALL ASPECTS OF THE PROGRAM, INCLUDING:**
   1. Staff performance.
   2. Efficiency of facility design.
   3. Efficiency of programs and services.
   4. Cleanliness and environmental condition of the facility.

C. **IMPLEMENT POLICIES AND PROCEDURES, INCLUDING:**
   1. Assisting staff in understanding and enforcing all rules and policies.
   2. Communicating emergency procedures clearly.
   3. Confirming understanding in the day-to-day operations of the facility.

D. **DETERMINES AVAILABILITY OF RESOURCES, INCLUDING:**
   1. Equipment.
   2. Supplies.
   3. Space.
   4. Staff.

E. **MANAGES THE FACILITY'S AND/OR PROGRAM FINANCIALS, INCLUDING:**
   1. Budget of costs and expected revenues.
   2. Cost/benefit analyses of specific programs.
   3. Containing costs within budgetary limits.

F. Promotes the program through marketing efforts, and designs promotions that attract participants.

G. **SCHEDULES CLASSES/PROGRAMS APPROPRIATELY, INCLUDING:**
   1. With target audience in mind.
   2. With consideration of other programs.

H. **MANAGES EMERGENCY PREPAREDNESS.**

I. **EVALUATES PROGRAMS USING OUTCOME EVALUATION TOOLS.**

J. **EVALUATES AND APPRAISES STAFF PERFORMANCE.**

IV. Organizational Structure and Staffing

A major challenge facing a program director/manager is to integrate the proper mix of staff into the program to provide the needed depth of knowledge and expertise. A program's organizational structure and staffing mix are closely tied to the program's goals and objectives, budgetary process, and outcome assessment.

A. **DELINEATION OF ROLES**
   1. Considerations for role assignment include:
      a. Individual staff expertise.
      b. Staffing levels and mix.
      c. Medicolegal issues.
      d. Certification/licensure.
   2. Important factors in the delineation of roles include:
      a. The needs of the clients served.
      b. The program's mission statement.
      c. The organizational structure.
   3. As a program grows and changes, the delineation of roles must be reviewed and altered as needed.

B. **JOB DESCRIPTIONS**
   1. Each staff position needs a specific, written job description that clearly details the **duties, responsibilities, and evaluation criteria** for the position.
   2. The job descriptions for all positions in the organization should be part of the policies and procedures (P&P) manual.
   3. The job description provides **criteria to evaluate** during the employee performance review.
   4. An effective job description is tailored to the specific needs and goals of the individual program.
   5. Because all possible duties and responsibilities cannot be detailed, some degree of **flexibility and adaptability** must be built into each job description.

C. **ORGANIZATIONAL FLOWCHART**
   1. A program's organizational flowchart specifies the **hierarchy of decision-making responsibility** and **lines of communication** in the program (*Figure 10-1*).
   2. The flowchart should clearly reflect the program's **mission statement, goals, staffing mix,** and other important aspects.
   3. The organizational chart should be readily accessible to all staff and be part of the P&P manual.

D. **STAFF COMPETENCY AND DEVELOPMENT**
   Maintaining staff competency is a major responsibility of the program director/manager.
   1. **Continuous professional development** is important for staff competency.
      a. The program director/manager must guide staff in seeking out opportunities for professional development.

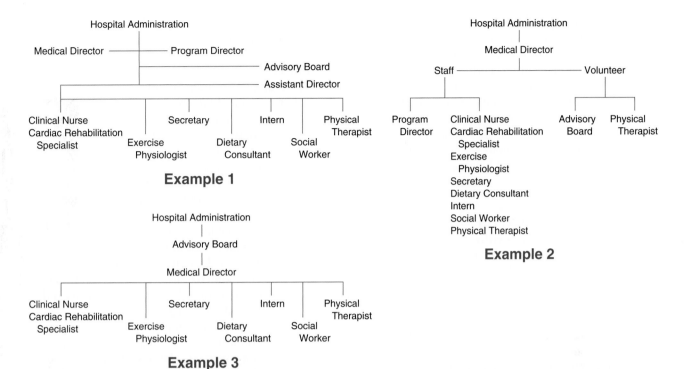

FIGURE 10-1. Organizational grids used for management of cardiopulmonary rehabilitation programs. (Redrawn with permission from Berra K, Hall LK: Administration of cardiac rehabilitation outpatient programs. In *Heart Disease and Rehabilitation.* Edited by Pollock ML, Schmidt DH. Champaign, IL, Human Kinetics, 1995, p 188.)

b. A typical staff is multidisciplinary.
  1) In a **clinical setting,** this may include:
    a) Nurses.
    b) Exercise physiologists.
    c) Respiratory therapists.
    d) Other health professionals.
  2) In a **fitness setting,** this may include:
    a) Exercise physiologists.
    b) Health/fitness instructors.
    c) Personal trainers.
    d) Massage therapists.
    e) Athletic trainers.
    f) Other health professionals.
  3) The various staff members will have varying needs and opportunities for professional development.
c. Staff meetings focused on professional development issues that can be aimed at a particular group of staff (e.g., operation of a new exercise machine) or that can encompass the entire staff (e.g., client service issues).
d. **In-service staff meetings are an excellent forum for professional development.** In-services can utilize staff skills or the knowledge and skills from outside professionals.

e. Encouraging staff to seek outside professional development will greatly enhance the skills and abilities of all staff members. Opportunities include:
  1) Continuing education.
  2) Attending professional conferences.
  3) Seeking additional certifications.
2. **Good communication** among staff members is an essential component of overall staff competency. **Strategies to foster staff communication** include:
  a. **Following lines of communication** depicted on the program's organizational flowchart.
  b. **Holding regular staff meetings,** both formal and informal, with the entire staff as well as with selected staff members involved in a particular program, project, or issue.
  c. Ensuring that **communication works in both directions,** thus creating an "open door" policy.
3. **Certification and licensure** of various staff members is another aspect of staff competency.
  a. Credentialing is relatively standardized for some staff (e.g., registered dietitians) but is less so for other positions (e.g., exercise physiologists).
  b. It is accepted that certified staff are more likely to be consistent in their care and

training and to possess a greater level of knowledge and abilities.

c. The health/fitness manager must be aware that many fitness certifications exists and that some do not follow the higher standards that organizations like the ACSM believe are necessary for safe and effective care of fitness clients. Understanding which certifications are acceptable is an important part of being a health/fitness manager.

E. PROGRAM CERTIFICATION

1. The move toward **certification of clinical exercise programs,** led by the American Association of Cardiovascular and Pulmonary Rehabilitation (AACVPR) and the International Health Club and Racquet Sports Association, is relatively recent.
2. The overall impact that program certification may have on the field is unknown.
3. For the clinical program, **certification might impact reimbursement** from insurance companies.
4. For the fitness program, **certification may help to standardize care** between various fitness companies and help potential members determine which facility is appropriate for them.

V. Program Development

A. NEEDS ASSESSMENT

1. Involves gathering data to determine if a program or service is needed within the community.
    a. These data may include **surveying** the community as well as members and staff within your own facility.
    b. Additional data might include **demographic and health data** as well as an understanding of similar programs offered by other facilities.
2. Includes a thorough market analysis for **financial considerations and an analysis of staffing and facility needs.**
3. Entails developing a **cost/benefit analysis** to help determine the financial impact of the program.

B. BUSINESS PLAN

1. The business plan is a detailed description of the mission statement, goals and objectives, program description, financial plan, and marketing plan.

2. The business plan also includes projections for program success.

C. PROGRAM PLANNING

1. **Scope Of Program Services**
    The scope of the program services depends on various factors, including the **needs of potential clients, the expertise of the staff** in certain areas, and the **market demand** for particular services.
    a. The **needs of potential clients** change with innovations in exercise. Thus, program directors/managers must be aware of the research literature and health care trends, and they must modify their program offerings based on this information.
    b. The **expertise of the staff** or contracted services available to the staff will shape the program offerings.
    c. An identified **market demand** is strong justification for offering a particular program or service, because it increases the likelihood of acceptance and financial success.
2. **Financial And Budgetary Considerations**
    a. Purposes of a budget include:
        1) To develop a financial plan for the program.
        2) To control costs.
        3) To evaluate program performance.
        4) To determine a program's viability.
        5) To identify financial difficulties early.
    b. Budget periods and goals should be established.
    c. Program revenue (income) includes:
        1) **Direct billing** for services, either to an individual client or to the client's health insurance carrier.
        2) **Contract for services** for a specific client group with a managed care organization.
        3) **Sale of merchandise** to clients, including:
            a) Clothing.
            b) Equipment.
            c) Supplies.
            d) Food/drink.
        4) **Grants for services or programs** from educational, governmental, or other foundations.
    d. **Expenses** of various types are defined in accounting:
        1) **Capital expenses** are those used for the purchase of equipment, buildings, and other tangible assets of the program.

2) **Fixed expenses** are those that are typically unchanged from month to month, including:
   a) Full-time salaries.
   b) Rent.
   c) Utilities.
3) **Variable expenses** are not as predictable, in that they may vary based on various factors, including:
   a) Disposable supplies.
   b) Part-time salaries.

e. Profit-and-loss analyses involve:
   1) The choice of the profit-and-loss model for a particular program, which is based on factors such as financial expectations and mission statement (e.g., for-profit vs. not-for-profit programs).
   2) **Two basic forms of profit and loss analyses**:
      a) The **break-even analysis** is designed around the function of the program such that the revenue generated is enough to pay for the expenses incurred, or the business venture is not-for-profit.
      b) The **profitability analysis** is an attempt to forecast future profits for the program based on potential revenue generation as well as on predicted fixed and variable expenses.

f. A **sample budget** for a clinical exercise program is given in *Table 10-1*.
g. A **sample budget** for a health/fitness program is given in *Table 10-2*.

3. **Marketing Plan**
   a. **Assesses competition**.
   b. Provides a detailed description of **marketing and promotional strategies**.
   c. Includes a **projection of marketing impact** on the business.

VI. Program Implementation

A. PROGRAM COMPONENTS
1. Client Care Plan and Exercise Prescription
   a. The foundation for any clinical exercise program, the client care plan, provides a **specific plan for rehabilitation and criteria for outcome assessment**.
   b. The foundation for any health/fitness exercise program, the exercise prescription, provides a **specific plan for improvement of specified fitness levels, health status, and attainment of client goals**.

c. The client care plan and exercise prescription should be **comprehensive, individualized, documented, reviewed and followed** by the entire staff, and modified and evaluated regularly.
d. The client care plan and exercise prescription should be reflected in, or be part of, **periodic progress reports** to the client's health care and fitness team.

2. Risk Stratification (Preparticipation Screening)
   a. Can be **modeled after published criteria,** including those from:
      1) The ACSM (clinical and health/fitness).
      2) The AACVPR (clinical).
      3) The YMCA (health/fitness).
      4) The American College of Physicians (clinical).
   b. **Can be useful for:**
      1) Participant entry criteria.
      2) Exercise testing guidelines
      3) Electrocardiogram (ECG) monitoring and supervision guidelines (clinical program).
   c. **Is important in:**
      1) Determining participant eligibility to an exercise program.
      2) Evaluating the need for physician clearance or examination.
      3) Developing of baseline fitness values.
      4) Designing a safe and effective exercise prescription (health/fitness program).
   d. May be tied to insurance reimbursement.

3. Other Program Components
   a. Participant referral categories:
      1) Participant was **self-referred** (chose to enter program voluntarily).
      2) Participant was referred by **primary care physician for general fitness** or weight loss.
      3) Participant was referred by **primary care physician or specialist for specific medical criteria.**
      4) Participant was referred by **case manager** for program maintenance.
   b. Participant inclusion/exclusion criteria.
   c. General exercise prescription guidelines.
   d. Home exercise plans.
   e. Medical supervision guidelines, including:
      1) Participant/staff ratios.
      2) ECG and other medical monitoring needs (clinical).
   f. Weight-training guidelines.
   g. Intensive risk factor monitoring/counseling guidelines (clinical).
   h. Periodic participant progress reports.

TABLE 10-1. Sample Budget for a Clinical Exercise Program

Enrollment Projections	Existing Clients	Monthly Fee ($)	New Clients	Average Fee ($)	Cancellations	Total Clients	Total Revenue ($)
Jan	700	45	0	150	0	750	42,120
Feb	750	45	75	150	23	803	44,320
March	803	45	75	150	24	853	46,640
Apr	853	45	65	150	26	893	47,380
May	893	45	55	150	27	921	47,620
June	921	45	50	150	28	943	48,110
July	943	45	50	150	28	965	49,100
Aug	965	45	50	150	29	986	50,060
Sept	986	45	60	150	30	1,017	52,480
Oct	1,017	45	65	150	30	1,051	54,580
Nov	1,051	45	70	150	32	1,090	56,850
Dec	1,090	45	50	150	33	1,107	55,540

TOTAL MEMBERSHIP REVENUE: 594,840

OTHER REVENUE ($)

Smoking Cessation	1,200
Massage	16,200
Guest Fees	35,000
1-To-1 Training	32,400
Weight Management	12,000
Pro-Shop	1,200
Rest	3,000
Wellness Programs	1,200
Miscellaneous	10,000
TOTAL OTHER REVENUE	112,200
MEMBER REVENUE	594,840
OTHER REVENUE	112,200
TOTAL REVENUE	707,040

PAYROLL PROJECTIONS ($)

General Manager	35,000
Sales 1	35,000
Administrator	20,000
Fitness Director	26,000
Full-Time Fitness 1	22,000
Full-Time Fitness 2	20,000
Part-Time Fitness	21,840
Receptionist	25,000
Aerobics	18,000
Nutrition	9,500
Cleaning	24,000
Bonus	8,000
TOTAL PAYROLL	264,340
TAXES	34,364
BENEFITS	18,240
TOTAL SALARIES	316,944

EXPENSE PROJECTIONS

TOTAL OPERATING EXPENSES ($)

Salaries, Tax, and Benefits	316,944
Marketing	48,000
Maintenance/Repair	
HVAC	1,500
Equipment	2,400
Exterminating	1,200
Other	500
TOTAL MAINTENANCE	5,600
Operating supplies	
Cleaning Supplies	1,200
Locker Room	3,000
Other Supplies	1,500
Towels	2,000
TOTAL SUPPLIES	7,700
Other Expenses	
Printing	3,600
Postage	3,000
Travel Seminars	2,000
Uniforms	6,000
Miscellaneous	1,000
Programs	500
Office Supplies	600
Telephone	7,200
TOTAL OTHER EXPENSES	10,800

TOTAL FIXED EXPENSES ($)

Cam	24,000
Debt	10,000
Insurance	18,000
Leasing	8,400
Management Fees	48,000
Rent	70,705
Utilities	
Electricity	36,000
Gas	4,800
Water	2,000
TOTAL UTILITIES	42,800
TOTAL FIXED EXPENSES	264,705
TOTAL EXPENSES	653,749
NET PROFIT/(LOSS)	53,299

(With permission from McCarthy J: Fund allocation has become critical. *Club Business International,* 1990.)

TABLE 10-2. Sample Budget for a Health/Fitness Program

ACSM Fitness Center	Existing Clients	Monthly Fee ($)	New Clients	Average Fee ($)	Cancellations	Total Clients	Total Revenue ($)
Jan	700	45	50	150	0	750	39,000
Feb	750	45	75	150	22	803	44,010
Mar	803	45	75	150	25	853	46,260
Apr	853	45	65	150	25	893	47,010
May	893	45	55	150	27	921	47,220
June	921	45	50	150	28	943	47,685
July	943	45	50	150	28	965	48,675
Aug	965	45	50	150	29	986	49,620
Sept	986	45	60	150	29	1,017	52,065
Oct	1,017	45	65	150	31	1,051	54,120
Nov	1,051	45	70	150	31	1,090	56,400
Dec	1,090	45	50	150	33	1,107	55,065
				TOTAL MEMBERSHIP REVENUE:			587,130

OTHER REVENUE ($)

Smoking Cessation	1,200
Massage	16,200
Guest Fees	35,000
1-to-1 Training	32,400
Weight Management	12,000
Pro-Shop	1,200
Rest	3,000
Wellness Programs	1,200
Miscellaneous	10,000
TOTAL OTHER REVENUE	112,200
MEMBERSHIP REVENUE	587,130
TOTAL REVENUE	699,330

PAYROLL PROJECTIONS ($)

General Manager	35,000
Sales 1	35,000
Administrator	20,000
Fitness Director	26,000
Full-Time Fitness 1	22,000
Full-Time Fitness 2	20,000
Part-Time Fitness	21,840
Receptionist	25,000
Aerobics	18,000
Nutrition	9,500
Cleaning	24,000
Bonus	8,000
TOTAL PAYROLL	264,340
TAXES	34,364
BENEFITS	18,240
TOTAL SALARIES	316,944

TOTAL OPERATING EXPENSES ($)

Salary, Tax, & Benefits	316,944
Marketing	48,000
Maintenance/Repair	
VAC	1,500
Equipment	2,400
Exterminate	1,200
Other	500
TOTAL MAINTENANCE	5,600
Operating Supplies	
Cleaning	1,200
Locker Room	3,000
Other	1,500
Towels	2,000
TOTAL SUPPLIES	7,700
Utilities	
Electric	36,000
Gas	4,800
Water	2,000
TOTAL UTILITIES	42,800
Rent	70,705
Other Expenses	
Printing	3,600
Postage	3,000
Travel	2,000
Uniforms	6,000
Programs	500
Office Supplies	600
Telephone	7,200
Miscellaneous	1,000
TOTAL OTHER EXPENSES	23,900
Corporate Expenses	
Amortization/Depreciation	24,000
Debt	
Insurance	
Leasing	
Management Fees	
TOTAL CORPORATE	108,400
TOTAL EXPENSES	624,049
NET PROFIT/(LOSS)	75,281

(With permission from McCarthy J. Fund Allocation has become critical. *Club Business International,* 1990.)

i. Communication with the client's health care team.

j. Emergency plans and postemergency physician referral procedures.

k. Graduation procedures and guidelines from various program components or phases (clinical).

l. Guidelines for referral to other services or providers (e.g., psychological counseling) (clinical).

m. Program data analyses and outcome assessment.

n. Continuing client education.

B. INTERACTION WITH THE MEDICAL COMMUNITY

1. Because a client's participation in a clinical exercise rehabilitation program generally depends on referral from a physician, the program director/manager (and medical director) should foster a good working relationship with the local medical community.

   a. This relationship can be fostered by:
      1) **Soliciting input** from physicians (and other health professionals, as applicable) on planning and implementation.
      2) **Maintaining regular communication** through consultation and progress reports.

   b. A program may even consider **establishing a medical advisory board** to ensure good communication with the medical community.

2. A client's participation in a health/fitness program often does not involve interaction or referral from a physician or health professional; however, an increasing number of fitness participants have medical issues that may require interaction with a health professional.

   a. The health/fitness program director/manager should also foster a good working relationship with the local medical community.

   b. This communication can be fostered by:
      1) **Soliciting input** from physicians (and other health professionals, as applicable) on prescription planning and implementation.
      2) **Maintaining regular communication** through consultation and progress reports.

   c. A program may even consider **establishing a medical advisory board** to ensure good

communication with the medical community.

C. PROGRAM MANAGEMENT

1. Program scheduling.

2. Staff scheduling, including vacation/sick coverage.

3. Facility and equipment maintenance and cleaning.

   a. All equipment must be safe and disinfected.

   b. All equipment should be in good repair and good working condition.

   c. All walkways need to have adequate clearance.

4. Incident management.

   a. Give immediate attention, and implement the emergency plan when necessary.

   b. Follow up in a timely manner (follow-up report).

   c. Deal with staff issues quickly and privately.

D. LEGAL AND ETHICAL CONSIDERATIONS

1. **Risk Assessment and Management**

   a. The program director/manager needs to **recognize all potential risk exposures** in the program and make the staff members are aware of these risks.

   b. Identified risks should be minimized through appropriate means, including:
      1) Procedures for dealing with malfunctioning equipment.
      2) Procedures for dealing with client injuries.

2. **Standards of Care**

   a. Applicable standards of care must be the basis of the program's policies and procedures.

   b. An example of an applicable standard of care is the sixth edition of the *ACSM's Guidelines for Exercise Testing and Prescription* (GETP), which may be used when performing various tasks in a clinical exercise rehabilitation program (e.g., exercise testing).

   c. A program affiliated with a hospital or other care facility must adhere to the standard of care set by that institution.

   d. A program that includes clinical exercise physiologists, nurses, respiratory therapists, and other health care professionals must take into account the standards of care for all involved professions.

   e. All professional staff (and most ancillary staff) should be certified in cardiopulmonary resuscitation, and all clinical staff should be certified in Advanced Cardiac Life Support (ACLS).

3. **Confidentiality**
   a. All client and staff records are considered to be confidential and are kept secure by the program director/manager as required by law.
   b. Individuals who do not have a legitimate, program-related need to see data should not have access to that data.

4. **Emergency Plans and Procedures**
   a. A plan for responding to emergency events should be outlined in the P&P manual. This **emergency response plan** must be well defined and well known to all staff members.
   b. **Emergency drills** should be carried out on a regular basis (at least quarterly), involve all staff members, and be documented. To increase the effectiveness of such drills, scenarios that reflect common or "most likely" emergency situations can be developed and practiced.
   c. **Emergency equipment should be calibrated and maintained** on a regular basis. Batteries should be tested and replaced to insure optimal working order.

5. **Accident/Injury Reporting**
   a. A process must be developed for the **timely reporting** of any and all accidents or injuries that may result from participation in a clinical exercise rehabilitation program.
   b. The accident/injury reporting process should be specified in the P&P manual.
   c. The form used to document accidents and injuries and the responses to these events must be kept in a secure location.

6. **Tort**
   a. A **tort** is a **type of civil wrongdoing**.
   b. **Negligence** is **failure to perform in a generally accepted standard**.

7. **Malpractice**
   a. **Malpractice** is a **specific type of negligence**.
   b. It involves **claims against a defined professional**.
   c. It is **usually limited to those with public authority to practice** arising from their responsibilities to a client.
   d. Charges usually claim a **breach of professional duties and responsibilities** toward a client.
   e. Generally, an injury has occurred, and a breach of duty preceded the injury

8. **State Laws and Regulations**
   The program director/manager must understand any written regulations or "practice acts" applicable to the programs and services offered.

E. **MARKETING AND PROMOTION**
   1. Develop both **internal** (within the facility) and **external** (outside the facility) marketing strategies
   2. **Promote the programs** and the benefits of a healthy lifestyle to various community and business organizations.
   3. **Follow the marketing plan** outlined in the business plan, and stay within the budget.

F. **PROGRAM EVALUATION**
   1. Careful evaluation of a program's effectiveness is an essential extension of program development and implementation.
   2. **Subjective evaluation** is accomplished through **surveys** of:
      a. Program participants.
      b. Program staff.
      c. Referring physicians.
      d. Any others who are involved.
   3. **Objective evaluation** can be based on **objective measures** such as **program statistics** (e.g., attendance, net income, goal attainment rates) or **client outcomes** as outlined in the plan of care or exercise prescription.
      a. Standardized tools can be used for outcome assessment.
      b. For example, in a clinical program, the outcome assessment and program resources manual of the AACVPR can be used.
   4. **Continuous quality improvement (CQI)**, also known as **quality assurance**, is a systematic process of evaluation and implementation designed to maximize program effectiveness.
   5. A program's evaluation criteria and process should be outlined in the P&P manual.
   6. As an aspect of overall program evaluation, the program director/manager needs to take into account **trends in health care** and to assess how well the program is adapting to these trends.

VII. Documentation

A. **THE MISSION STATEMENT**
   1. The **mission statement** is a simple **statement of the program's main purposes** (*Table 10-3*).

TABLE 10-3. Sample Mission Statements

Example 1	Example 2
The mission of the Maintenance Cardiac Rehabilitation Component (MCRC) of the _____ complements the Mission Statements of the _____ and _____. Specifically, the mission of the MCRC has several facets and targeted groups for intervention. One group that the MCRC addresses through its services are the undergraduate and graduate students of _____ through its opportunities in research, service, and academic training in the rehabilitation of individuals with chronic diseases. The other important targeted group for the MCRC are those members of the community who have Coronary Artery Disease and other chronic diseases, as defined by the participant inclusion criteria of the MCRC. The MCRC provides educational, research, and service opportunities for those individuals with Coronary Artery Disease in health and physical fitness assessment, exercise prescription and exercise programming components as well as in other lifestyle management areas (e.g., smoking, nutrition, etc.).	The mission of XYZ Health and Fitness Center is to provide high quality exercise, health, and wellness programs to the community with the ultimate goal of improving the health of our community. Our staff will continually work to develop innovative services and programs will enhance one's fitness, be cost-effective to the consumer, and maintain profitability.

2. This statement forms the **foundation of program planning, implementation, and evaluation.**
3. The statement should be:
   a. Worded clearly.
   b. Compatible with the parent organization's or institution's mission statement.
   c. Regularly reviewed and updated to reflect program changes.
4. A central aspect of CQI is the evaluation of how a program is meeting its goals based upon the mission statement.

B. GOALS AND OBJECTIVES

1. Goals are the essence of what the program should achieve in meeting its mission statement.
2. Goals are specific outcomes that the program wants to attain.
3. Objectives are the means by which a goal is achieved.

C. THE POLICY AND PROCEDURES (P&P) MANUAL

1. **Provides documentation** and dissemination of the program's specific policies and procedures.
2. **Describes in detail** how the programs and services work as well as the general rules and regulations of the program and facility.
3. Should **contain everything about a program,** from the organizational structure to the maintenance schedule for the facility and equipment.
4. Should be **readily accessible** to all staff members.
5. Is revised as the policies or procedures of a program are modified, and as such, should be viewed as a document in progress.

6. Must be **reviewed from a legal perspective,** written in close collaboration with the program's general managers and directors, and approved by the parent organization.
7. Should be **consistent with** the ever-changing **standards and practices of applicable national, regional, and local organizations.**

D. EMPLOYEE MANUAL

1. Provides specific rules and regulations for all staff positions.
2. Provides job descriptions and benefit descriptions.

E. PROGRAM DOCUMENTATION

A **written record** of agreements, waivers, releases, incidents, policies and procedures, and clearances is **critical for understanding of client activities and knowing who is protected** if problems occur.

1. **Agreements, Releases, and Consents**
   a. Clearly describe **client participation,** the **rights** of the client and the facility, and any **risks.**
   b. **Transfer some responsibility and risk** associated with participation **to the client** (see Chapter 7, Figure 7-2, for an example of a participant agreement).
   c. Often are created in clinical programs by the hospital or primary program management.
2. All fitness facilities are strongly encouraged to have **program/service agreements** and **informed consents drafted and/or reviewed by a lawyer** for their protection.
3. A client who does not meet the criteria for exercising or who wishes to break a policy to

exercise can sign a **waiver** to be allowed to participate, thus **accepting risk**.

4. A **"Physician Clearance"** requires a medical opinion of the client's risk with exercise. This document **places much of the risk on the medical professional** rather than on the fitness facility. A physician's clearance is recommended for:

   a. A client who has considerable risk with exercise, as indicated by a medical history questionnaire or Par-Q.

   b. A client who exhibits signs or symptoms during exercise that indicate increased risk if exercise continues.

5. **Incident reports** are used to document a problem or incident. These reports:

   a. Provide a **detailed description of the incident**.

   b. **List all witnesses.**

   c. Include **witness statements**, if possible.

   d. State the **results of the actions by the staff**.

   e. Include a **follow-up** status of clients and/or staff involved in the incident.

6. **Malpractice and liability insurance** are necessary to provide coverage for staff and facility in cases of litigation for malpractice and accidents.

VIII. Records

Records are important for the proper management of any program. Records are used for **program evaluation, client motivation, understanding the success of the business, liability protection, and marketing**. Types of records include:

A. **ATTENDANCE RECORDS**

B. **EVALUATION AND SCREENING RECORDS**

C. **WORKOUT AND TREATMENT RECORDS**

D. **MEDICAL TESTS AND MEDICAL RECORDS**

E. **SURVEYS**

F. **MAINTENANCE RECORDS**

G. **EXPENSE RECORDS**

Review Test

DIRECTIONS: Carefully read all questions, and select the BEST single answer.

1. In a budget for a clinical exercise rehabilitation program, all of the following are examples of variable expenses EXCEPT
   A) ECG electrodes.
   B) Temporary wages.
   C) Rental fees for the facility space.
   D) Consultant fees.

2. Which of the following statements about a clinical exercise rehabilitation program's mission statement is NOT correct?
   A) Perhaps the most important feature of the mission statement is its clarity or understandability.
   B) The mission statement should elucidate the program's goals.
   C) There should be a different mission statement for each program or, perhaps, even a different mission statement for each component of a program.
   D) A program's mission statement generally is fixed.

3. A program's policy and procedures manual should NOT
   A) Be stored away for safekeeping.
   B) Be revised as the program's policies and/or procedures are modified.
   C) Be viewed as a document in progress.
   D) Contain program information ranging from the organizational structure to the facility's maintenance schedule.

4. A comprehensive patient care plan is necessary for effective program management, because it
   A) Is required by federal law.
   B) Provides a "road map" for interventions.
   C) Is a requirement for insurance reimbursement.
   D) Provides raw data for analysis in CQI or outcomes assessment.

5. The process of risk stratification often is used for the criteria for clinical exercise rehabilitation program admission. Which of the following statements about risk stratification is NOT correct?
   A) Risk stratification can be modeled after the criteria published by the AACVPR.
   B) Risk stratification can be useful for participant entry criteria, exercise testing guide-

   lines, ECG monitoring, and supervision guidelines.
   C) Risk stratification can be tied to insurance reimbursement.
   D) Risk stratification often is used to determine the intensity of prescribed exercise.

6. Which of the following statements about confidentiality is NOT true?
   A) All records must be kept by the program director/manager under lock and key.
   B) Data must be available to all individuals who need to see it.
   C) Data should be kept on file for at least 1 year before being discarded.
   D) Sensitive information (e.g., participant's name) needs to be protected.

7. Which of the following statements about injury reporting is NOT correct?
   A) A process for injury reporting, backed up with a form, should be developed.
   B) The process to be used and the accompanying forms must be part of the P&P manual.
   C) Injury reporting forms must be kept under lock and key, just like data records.
   D) A physician should sign every injury report form that is filed.

8. One important aspect of staff competency is ensuring that staff members are well trained and kept up to date. Which of the following organizations has recently launched the Registry for Clinical Exercise Physiologists?
   A) AACVPR.
   B) American College of Physicians.
   C) American Heart Association.
   D) ACSM.

9. Informed consent is best described as
   A) A legal form.
   B) A process that is backed up by a form.
   C) Something that only a lawyer can provide to an exercise program.
   D) Being an informed consumer to ensure that one undertakes the proper exercise program.

10. Which of the following elements is NOT part of an emergency plan for a clinical exercise program?
    A) Annual practice sessions involving all staff.
    B) Emergency plan that constantly refers to national established guidelines (e.g., ACLS)

without addressing unique features of the
program.

C) Emergency drills carried out on a regular
basis and documented.

D) Scenarios developed to increase the applica-
bility of the emergency plan practice
sessions.

11. Which of the following is a fixed expense?
A) Office supplies.
B) Salaries.
C) Utilities (e.g., telephone).
D) Laboratory charge backs for blood work.

12. Which type of financial analysis would be appropriate for a not-for-profit program that wishes to
determine the amount of revenue from program
fees needed so that no other sources of revenue
are required to meet the program's expenses?
A) Break-down analysis.
B) Break-even analysis.
C) Profitability analysis.
D) Margin analysis.

13. Continuous quality improvement (CQI) is a sys-
tematic process of program evaluation that
involves all of the following steps EXCEPT
A) Data analysis.
B) Goals assessment.
C) Outcomes assessment.
D) Budget assessment.

14. Outcome assessment evaluates a program's effectiveness. Which of the following statements about
outcome assessment is NOT true?
A) The client care plan for each individual participant is not used in this process.
B) Data that are subjective or anecdotal in
nature can be used in the assessment.
C) Periodic progress reports are valuable and
should stimulate the need to collect objective data to support any subjective findings.
D) Standardized tools should be used for outcome assessment.

15. According to the AACVPR, elements of successful
adult education include all of the following
EXCEPT
A) Goal setting.
B) Rewards.
C) Contracts.
D) Knowledge testing.

16. Which one of the following statements concerning
a needs assessment is NOT true?
A) The needs and/or program assessment is a
useful tool for gathering data and support for
program implementation.

B) The needs and/or program assessment often
must be a creative tool developed in-house
to meet the program's specific needs.

C) Given that the needs assessment may be
developed in-house without the benefit of
external validity, generalizing the results may
be difficult.

D) Program planning is an essential step before
needs assessment can be performed.

17. A comprehensive clinical exercise rehabilitation
program
A) Is based on historical features of program
administration.
B) Adapts to trends in program services.
C) Is limited in scope and practice.
D) Is the same for the entire client population
served.

18. Do fitness instructors need management skills?
A) Only if they wish to become floor supervisors
or program managers.
B) Yes, because of the natural progression of
advancement into management.
C) Yes, because as instructors, they manage
client programs and manage the floor with
the clients.
D) No, because they will be trained in management if they become managers.

19. A fitness newsletter, fitness library, and bulletin
boards
A) Are part of staff news.
B) Are part of client and staff education.
C) Are part of the facility marketing.
D) Require considerable money and must be
budgeted carefully.

20. Why would a fitness facility be interested in public
relations?
A) To increase exposure for the facility and sell
its services.
B) To become involved in local politics.
C) To improve staff morale.
D) To make the staff work harder.

21. Why would a fitness instructor have an interest in
tort laws?
A) Negligence is breaking a tort law and can
ruin an instructor's career.
B) State taxes often are related to profit, which
is governed by tort laws.
C) Tort laws are related to worker's compensa-
tion regulations.
D) They relate to the Americans with
Disabilities Act (ADA).

22. What is the best way that an administrator can educate the fitness staff?
    A) Voicing his or her opinion.
    B) Joining fitness organizations, and subscribing to fitness journals.
    C) Buying fitness videos.
    D) Reading the newspaper.

23. What should the manager's involvement be in developing fitness programs?
    A) The manager should maintain a hands-off approach.
    B) The manager should be involved only in the budgeting and final approval.
    C) The manager should be the only person involved in program development.
    D) The manager should be active as a program developer as well as a resource, supporter, and critic for programs developed by other staff.

24. Budgets are designed to
    A) Make management happy.
    B) Determine if a program is viable.
    C) Save money.
    D) Teach managers about cost analysis.

25. The rules and regulations of a facility are commonly referred to as
    A) The law.
    B) The client rights statement.
    C) Policies and procedures.
    D) A check and balance for management and clients.

26. A physician's clearance
    A) Is not necessary if the client completes the medical history questionnaire.
    B) Is a communication tool with little exercise value.
    C) Provides information about the physician's attitude regarding your club.
    D) Provides a medical opinion about a client's risk with exercise.

27. Some of the duties in supervising a fitness staff include scheduling, implementing the policies and procedures, and
    A) Cleaning the equipment.
    B) Emergency procedures and evaluations.
    C) Marketing and promotions.
    D) Managing the fitness billing.

28. What is the primary reason why a manager or director should conduct a needs assessment?
    A) To determine the specific needs and interests of the target market.
    B) To determine the quality of potential fitness instructors who could be hired in the area.

C) To determine the needs of management before developing the budget.
D) To determine the need for new or different exercise equipment.

29. Policies and procedures are important in a fitness center, because they
    A) Explain how to use the fitness equipment properly.
    B) Clarify the rights of and risks in being a fitness member.
    C) Are general guidelines for operating a fitness program or department.
    D) Explain the employee insurance plans and how to use them.

30. What are some of the common sales "rules" in promoting your fitness program?
    A) Selling memberships at any cost is key.
    B) You know more than they do, so be aggressive.
    C) Honesty and an understanding of the needs of the potential member are always the best way.
    D) Long-term agreements make more money than short-term agreements.

31. Program description, resource availability, and client interest are examples of
    A) A business plan.
    B) A survey.
    C) Management factors.
    D) Budget categories.

32. What do effective program administration and management create and/or reduce?
    A) They create problems with staff egos.
    B) They reduce memberships.
    C) They create successful programs and reduce problems.
    D) They create more work for the staff and reduce feedback.

33. Incident reports are important, because
    A) They inform the manager which employees are performing poorly.
    B) They indicate which members are problematic and should be dismissed.
    C) They document and give details of any incident or problem that occurs.
    D) State laws often require them.

34. Why are records valuable to a fitness program?
    A) They help in evaluation of a program.
    B) They offer music not found on tapes or CDs.
    C) They help to provide facts in any legal issues.
    D) They help the front desk to monitor paid and unpaid clients.

35. Examples of program records include
    A) Client progress and outcomes.
    B) Member needs.
    C) Performance of clients on selected exercises.
    D) Member suggestions and any actions taken regarding them.

36. Which of the following is an example of participant interaction as part of the supportive role of a manager?
    A) Offering a shoulder on which to cry.
    B) Conducting surveys, and responding to client needs.
    C) Encouraging members to "let go" in exercise classes.
    D) Having members teach classes.

37. The manager's role in staff education is
    A) Valuable, because it looks good to the owners.
    B) To create many opportunities for educating the staff.
    C) To let the staff handle their own education but also to encourage it.
    D) Not very valuable, because member retention and sales are the key to any program.

38. Staff certification is
    A) Not important, because members do not care.
    B) Important, primarily because it adds spice to marketing materials.
    C) Not a good idea, because certified staff will increase your payroll.
    D) Important, primarily because it adds a standard of knowledge and credibility to your facility.

39. Capital budgets
    A) Reflect the costs of implementing a program.
    B) Reflect the costs to operate a program.
    C) Are not necessary with fitness programs.
    D) Are part of the balance sheet in financial reports.

40. What do budgets determine?
    A) Fitness equipment costs.
    B) If a company is making or losing money.
    C) Viability, identification of problems, and a plan for the future of a program.
    D) Assets and liabilities of the financial plan.

41. Why should a fitness operator be concerned with state practice laws?
    A) State laws help to identify illegal aliens who may apply for a job in your club.
    B) State laws may control the number of minority employees working at your club.
    C) State laws may affect how much can be charged for a membership.
    D) Many states have practice acts that control the behavior and actions of fitness instructors.

42. Why is public relations important to a fitness program?
    A) It helps to promote the program and staff to the public.
    B) It reduces the risk of legal action against your staff.
    C) It lowers your malpractice insurance premium by promoting quality.
    D) It makes sure that your clients are happy and getting what they want.

ANSWERS AND EXPLANATIONS

1–C. Rent is typically an agreed-on cost and, thus, is a fixed as opposed to a variable expense. Variable expenses vary based on program use; examples would include supplies (e.g., ECG electrodes) and any part-time or temporary wages.

2–D. The mission statement should be reviewed and revised as often as necessary as a program changes in character. Thus, the mission statement is not fixed but, rather, is a dynamic component of the P&P manual.

3–A. The P&P manual must be available to all staff and, thus, is kept in a readily accessible location and it not filed away. Also, the P&P manual is meant to be referred to and revised as needed.

4–B. A patient care plan is a thoughtfully produced document that plans for effective, individualized interventions. It should be used often in planning for any and all interventions.

5–D. Risk stratification is rarely, if ever, used to determine the intensity of prescribed exercise. However, risk stratification can be an important tool for patient inclusion/exclusion criteria, and it can be used for insurance reimbursement as well.

6–C. There is no accepted minimum or maximum amount of time that data should be stored. Clearly, however, data must be stored in a confidential (lock-and-key) manner, and discretion must be used when sharing data.

7–D. Legal advice suggests that the injury report form does not necessarily require a physician's signature. However, a process for injury reporting needs to be followed consistently and be described in the P&P manual.

8–D. The ACSM launched the Registry of Clinical Exercise Physiologists in 2000. The overall impact of this registry is hard to predict at present.

9–B. Informed consent is a process, backed up by a form, that among other things describes the risks and benefits of participation in certain activities (e.g., an exercise test). It is suggested that a legal expert be consulted regarding any informed consent procedures.

10–A. Practice sessions involving all staff members should be held at least quarterly. These sessions should be documented and may be most effective if scenarios are "played out" to mimic real emergencies.

11–B. Staff salaries usually are a fixed expense and not subject to change based on variable factors (e.g., number of program participants). However, as program use increases, so do expenses such as blood work charge backs, telephone expenses, and office supplies. Thus, these latter expenses are known as variable expenses.

12–B. A break-even analysis is ideal for not-for-profit organizations that wish to understand how to best meet all of their expenses, including payroll. The for-profit sector will use a profitability analysis to determine how much, if any, money can be earned in a period of time.

13–D. Budget assessment is not necessarily a part of the CQI process, although it is a valuable step in program evaluation. Generally, CQI is an outcomes assessment based on the program's goals using data analysis of various measures.

14–A. The client care plan is a vital component of outcomes assessment. Outcomes assessment is driven by goals established for each client or patient.

15–D. According to the AACVPR, adult education can involve many techniques to foster education and behavior change, including goal setting, contracts, rewards, and support. However, there is little justification for knowledge-based testing in promoting behavioral change.

16–D. Needs assessment should be done *before* the program planning and implementation phases to provide data on which to base these steps. However, needs assessment is not a one-time measure. Successful programs perform frequent formal or informal needs assessments as they grow.

17–B. The justification for a clinical exercise rehabilitation program is based on its ability to adapt to changing operating practices and procedures for rehabilitation services. Thus, whereas history is important and interesting, flexibility is needed to adapt to an ever-changing health care model.

18–C. The definition of a manager is someone who designs, implements, and monitors programs, which is what fitness instructors are responsible for as a natural part of their job. Managing a client's program fits the basic definition of a manager, so the skills of managing a person and his or her program fit the need for management training. A fitness instructor does not naturally become a manager.

19–B. Educating a fitness client on the principles of exercise, proper nutrition, and good health is important, and this information can be communicated in a variety of ways. Newsletters, libraries, and bulletin boards are some of the recommended ways to communicate with and educate members. Staff news should not necessarily be within the library or posted on a board. Marketing strategies often do not include the library or bulletin boards. These forms of education usually are inexpensive to develop and maintain.

20–A. Public relations, a common form of promotion, is important for any business. It is very important to "get your name out" and increase exposure, and these activities can help people to learn who you are and how good you are. Public relations has nothing to do with politics when it involves your facility. It may improve the morale of your staff, but the intent is to generate exposure for your club. Public relations should not be considered a strategy for making the staff work harder.

21–A. A tort law refers to a civil wrong, such as negligence (failure to perform at a generally accepted standard). Negligence in fitness often refers to the instructor giving bad instruction or advice that leads to an injury or accident. Clients often sue instructors for negligence, which can be very damaging. Tort laws do not involve state taxes, are not regulated by workers compensation insurance, and do not involve the ADA.

22–B. Fitness organizations and journals offer excellent opportunities for staff and management to learn about many aspects of fitness. Most fitness organizations and journals work with experts in fitness and provide accurate and up-to-date information. An administrator's opinion may not be an educated or unbiased one, which can make for poor education. Newspapers and videos often present misinterpreted or inaccurate information.

23–D. The manager's job is to manage programs by being a program developer, to act as a resource for staff and clients, to evaluate programs, and to provide constructive input to staff. A hands-off approach is not recommended, because it often leads to poor program implementation and problems. Managing program development, not just budgeting, is an important role for managers. It is important to involve the staff in the design and implementation of the programs; otherwise, the manager does all of the work.

24–B. One of the primary goals of a fitness business is to make a profit. Budgeting helps a manager and the owner to understand if a program can make money and be successful (i.e., viable). Budgets are not designed to save money; the programs are designed to save money. Management is only happy if the budgets show a profit. Managers must learn cost analysis before developing budgets so that they know how to create a budget that will make management happy.

25–C. Policies and procedures are essentially the rules and regulations of a facility, plus the means of conducting and implementing the regulations correctly. Regulations can be considered to be the law, but they are not often labeled as such. The client rights statement is a different document. Management monitors the rules and makes sure that staff and members follow them; however, these regulations are not considered to be a balance measurement.

26–D. A fitness instructor will request or require a physician's clearance when concern exists regarding the risk of a medical crisis with exercise. The clearance is a medical opinion that it is safe for the client to exercise. The medical history will indicate if a concern with exercise is evident, but it will not assure the fitness instructor that it is safe for the client to exercise. A physician's clearance is a very important tool for the safety of the exercising client and should not be an opinion statement about your facility.

27–B. Evaluating staff members and developing emergency procedures are common duties in supervising staff. It is important that your staff know how to implement emergency procedures, and the supervisor must train the staff. The staff, not the supervisors, handles the equipment cleaning. Marketing and billing are duties that are not involved with fitness staff supervision.

28–A. A needs assessment is designed to analyze your target market and determine what that market needs and wants. This assessment has nothing to do with assessing fitness staff, equipment, or management needs.

29–C. Policies and procedures provide general guidelines as well as how to enact those guidelines in implementing an exercise program. Policies and procedures help to establish control of the operations of programs. Use of fitness equipment may be a part of a P&P statement, but policies and procedures are much more than that. The rights and risks of a fitness member are written in the client rights statement. Insurance plans are presented in the employee handbook, not in the policies and procedures.

30–C. Honesty and understanding are always the best policy. It is very important to know what the client needs and wants. This information can help you to sell the programs that meet those needs and desires. Being honest enhances your reputation and client retention, because clients get what you told them they would get. Selling memberships at any cost often results in losing business over time, either because of dishonesty or because of giving away too much. Being aggressive and assuming the client does not know anything can alienate potential clients. Short-term agreements tend to improve client retention.

31–C. Managing involves many characteristics or factors. Developing programs, being a resource to staff and members, and monitoring client interest are some of the factors of management. A business plan explains the business in detail, the target market, and marketing strategies; it does not explain the resource availability. Surveys can assess client interest, but they do not assess program descriptions. These examples are not part of a budget.

32–C. Effective management should create a successful facility that meets the needs of the clients, staff, and owners. Problems should be reduced, membership should increase, and feedback and communication should be enhanced, not reduced.

33–C. Incident reports provide a detailed record of what happened in any incident at the fitness facility. These records may be critical for a physician or emergency medical unit if an accident occurs. The report also provides evidence, witnesses, and the results of actions taken by the staff. These reports are not intended to inform management of bad employees or members. State laws do not require incident reports, though they may recommend them.

34–A. Records help management in many ways, including in the evaluation of a program. Recording the workouts, client attendance, feedback, and more can help to determine if the program was successful. Records can help as evidence in a legal issue as well, but this value is not nearly as important as answer A. Records also help at the front desk, but they are not part of a fitness program. Instead, they are part of the facility management. Records, in this case, do not involve music.

35–A. Program records refer to the specific evaluation of an individual or group program. The progress of clients throughout the program and the outcomes following the program are very important factors to assess. Specific exercise records are part of the data in the program records, which are then used to chart progress and outcomes. Member needs and suggestions usually are not part of program recordings; these usually are recorded as part of a survey.

36–B. Fitness facilities constantly seek information on what their clients want, need, like, and dislike. Interacting with clients makes clients feel important and respected. Conducting surveys and responding to client input are two of the better ways to invite interaction. A shoulder to cry on is not a way to encourage interaction, nor do you want to increase the risk of a problem by letting clients "let go" or teach your classes.

37–B. Creating opportunities for educating the staff is very important, because it enhances their knowledge and provides a perk for them. A well-educated staff enhances the quality and safety of your programs, improves the facility's reputation, and increases the respect and acceptance of your clients. It is not valuable to provide education only for the purpose of looking good to the owners or to ignore the need for education.

38–D. Certification shows the clients that your staff members meet industry standards. The staff should have a certain level of skill and competency with certifications. Most members *do* care, and payroll should be a secondary factor to the choice of certifying staff. Certified staff should bring more members, which can justify the increased cost. The marketing also is secondary to the value to the clients and the program.

39–A. Capital budgets refer to the budgeting of program implementation or facility. How much does it cost to start the program and to implement the first stage? Capital budgets usually include equipment, staffing, initial marketing, and so on in the start-up. Operating a program is part of the operating budget, not the capital budget. Capital budgets are critical in determining whether to start a program. Capital budgets are not included in the balance sheet.

40–C. Budgets show what it will cost to run a program and whether the program will be profitable. Managers can review a budget and determine if the program has financial problems. Budgets are a future look at a program and should be developed with the idea of making money. Budgets also present only a part of the financial statement of the company. The company must include other financial information (e.g., assets, liabilities) to determine if it is making or losing money.

41–D. Each state may set its own laws in regulating fitness facilities and fitness staff. These laws differ from state to state. It is important to know these laws and to be sure that your facility and staff follow them. Issues regarding illegal aliens, discrimination, and membership fees are not addressed in the laws governing how fitness centers conduct programs.

42–A. Public relations is a way to promote your facility to various groups or communities. It shows the community who you are and what you offer. It also promotes quality. However, this is no guarantee that you will not be negligent or sued, so malpractice insurance is not affected by public relations. In addition, public relations is designed to make those people who have not yet joined familiar with you and to want to join your facility, not to make your current clients happy. Client participation programs (e.g., surveys, suggestion boxes, feedback opportunities) make clients happy and give them the opportunity to ask for what they want.

Metabolic Calculations

KHALID W. BIBI

CHAPTER 11

I. Overview

A. RATIONALE FOR USE OF THE ACSM METABOLIC FORMULAE

Fundamental to the application of proper exercise testing or prescription is the ability to measure or estimate energy expenditure.

1. **Direct Measurement of Oxygen Consumption ($\dot{V}O_2$) Is Impractical**

   Actual $\dot{V}O_2$, as determined using open-circuit spirometry, provides the best measure of the energy cost of physical activity. Oxygen uptake values obtained during maximal exercise ($\dot{V}O_2max$) are commonly used as the index of cardiopulmonary fitness. Unfortunately, accurate $\dot{V}O_2$ measurement is arduous and costly, making it impractical.

2. **$\dot{V}O_2$ Can Be Estimated using the ACSM Metabolic Formulae**

   The ACSM metabolic formulae were introduced to provide health and fitness practitioners with a practical method to estimate the oxygen cost of the most common exercises. **Practical uses for the ACSM metabolic formulae include the following:**

   a. Estimating the rate of oxygen uptake during exercise allows for an **estimate of the energy expenditure and, hence, the caloric consumption** from fat associated with exercise.

   b. An estimate of the rate of oxygen uptake during $\dot{V}O_2max$ indicates the maximal capacity for aerobic work, allowing **fitness categorization as well as inter- and intrasubject comparisons**. See Appendix D in the *ACSM's Guidelines for Exercise Testing and Prescription*, 7th ed., for more information about the estimation of $\dot{V}O_2max$.

   c. Calculating the appropriate exercise intensity (**work rate**) needed to elicit the desired $\dot{V}O_2$ will allow the health and fitness professional **to develop more effective exercise prescriptions**.

B. WHAT TO EXPECT ON THE ACSM WRITTEN EXAM

1. Expect from **6 to 10 metabolic calculation questions** on the ACSM written examination. A few of these questions will be simple, requiring straightforward algebraic calculations. Some may be classified as moderately difficult, requiring simple mathematic substitution. One or two questions may be classified as difficult, requiring additional algebraic manipulation of these formulae.

2. A copy of the ACSM metabolic formulae (*Table 11-1*) is included in the written examination packet. You should be familiar with these formulae before you sit for the exam.

3. The **unit conversion factors** and the **energy equivalency factors** will **not** be provided with the examination. **Commit these numbers to memory.**

4. The written examination might contain metabolic calculation questions that will not require use of the metabolic equations. However, a good understanding of energy expenditure and energy equivalency will be needed to arrive at the correct answer.

C. EXPRESSIONS OF ENERGY

Energy expenditure in humans can be expressed in many terms. Converting from one expression to another is simple. Be familiar with the following terms:

1. **Absolute $\dot{V}O_2$**

   This is the volume of oxygen consumed by the whole person, expressed in liters per minute ($L \cdot min^{-1}$) or milliliters per minute ($mL \cdot min^{-1}$).

   a. **Resting absolute $\dot{V}O_2$ for a 70-kg person is** approximately $0.245 \ L \cdot min^{-1}$.

   b. In highly trained subjects, **absolute $\dot{V}O_2max$** as high as $4.9 \ L \cdot min^{-1}$ may be expected.

   c. Absolute $\dot{V}O_2$ is useful, because it allows an easy **estimation of caloric expenditure. Each liter of oxygen consumed expends 5 kcal, or 20.9 kJ.**

TABLE 11-1. Summary of Metabolic Calculations[a]

Walking[a]
$\dot{V}o_2 = (0.1 \cdot S) + (1.8 \cdot S \cdot G) + 3.5$

Treadmill and Outdoor Running
$\dot{V}o_2 = (0.2 \cdot S) + (0.9 \cdot S \cdot G) + 3.5$

Leg Cycling[b]
$\dot{V}o_2 = (1.8 \cdot \text{Work Rate} \div \text{Body Weight}) + 3.5 + 3.5$

Arm Cycling[b]
$\dot{V}o_2 = (3 \cdot \text{Work Rate} \div \text{Body Weight}) + 3.5$

Stepping[c]
$\dot{V}o_2 = (0.2 \cdot f) + (1.33 \cdot 1.8 \cdot H \cdot f) + 3.5$

The above formulae yield gross $\dot{V}o_2$ values expressed in relative terms (mL·kg^{-1}·min^{-1}) and are presented without units for simplification purposes, where:

[a] (S = speed in **m·min^{-1}**, G = treadmill grade expressed as a **fraction**, e.g. 12% = 0.12)

[b] (Work Rate expressed in **kg·m·min^{-1}**, Body Weight expressed in **kg**)

[c] (f = stepping rate expressed as the **number** of steps·min^{-1}, H = step height in **meters**)

Modified from Table D-1 of the *ACSM'S Guidelines for Exercise Testing and Prescription*, 7th ed., LWW, Philadelphia, 2005, p. 289. **Candidates are encouraged to familiarize themselves with that table.**

2. **Relative $\dot{V}o_2$**

   This is the measure of **$\dot{V}o_2$ relative to body weight**, expressed in mL · kg^{-1} · min^{-1}—in other words, the **volume of oxygen consumed by the cells of each kilogram of body weight every minute.**

   a. **For the ACSM examination**, a given mass of lean body tissue requires the same amount of oxygen at rest and at any given work rate, regardless of gender, race, age, and level of fitness. The **resting relative $\dot{V}o_2$ is always assumed to be 3.5 mL · kg^{-1} · min^{-1}.**

   b. In highly trained aerobic athletes, a relative $\dot{V}o_2$max may be as high as 75 to 80 mL · kg^{-1} · min^{-1}.

   c. **Relative $\dot{V}o_2$** is commonly used to compare $\dot{V}o_2$ of individuals who vary in size. Because $\dot{V}o_2$max also is used as an index of cardiopulmonary fitness, **a higher value indicates greater aerobic fitness.**

   d. **All ACSM formulae provide $\dot{V}o_2$ values in gross relative terms.**

3. **Metabolic Equivalents (MET)**

   Physicians and clinicians commonly use the term **MET** as an expression of **energy expenditure or exercise intensity.** One MET is equivalent to the relative $\dot{V}o_2$ at rest. Therefore, **1 MET = 3.5 mL · kg^{-1} · min^{-1}.**

   a. **METs are calculated by dividing the relative $\dot{V}o_2$ by 3.5.** For example, an individual consuming 35 mL · kg^{-1} · min^{-1} during steady-state exercise is exercising at 10 MET.

   b. A MET is a useful expression, because it allows an easy **comparison of the amount of oxygen uptake during exercise with that at rest.**

4. **Calorie**

   This expression of energy intake and expenditure is commonly used to quantify the **amount of energy derived from consumed foods** as well as the **amount of energy expended at rest and during physical activity** (see Chapter 9 Section XA, for more information about this topic).

5. **Fat Stores**

   a. The human body stores the majority of excess energy intake as fat.

   b. It takes **3,500 calories** to make and store **1 pound of body fat.**

   c. Stated in reverse, **1 pound of fat can provide the body with 3,500 calories**—the amount of energy needed to **walk or run approximately 35 miles!**

6. **Net Versus Gross $\dot{V}o_2$**

   a. **Humans** require approximately **3.5 mL · kg^{-1} · min^{-1} (1 MET)** of oxygen at rest. This amount of oxygen uptake is **vital for survival of the body's cells, tissues, and systems.**

   b. **Physical activity elevates $\dot{V}o_2$** above the resting oxygen requirements.

   c. **Net $\dot{V}o_2$** is the difference between the $\dot{V}o_2$ value for exercise and the resting value. Net $\dot{V}o_2$ is used to assess the caloric cost of exercise.

   d. **Gross $\dot{V}o_2$** is the sum of the oxygen cost of physical activity and the resting component.

   e. Hence,

   Net $\dot{V}o_2$ = Gross oxygen uptake
       − Resting oxygen uptake

   f. Net and gross oxygen uptake **can be expressed in relative or absolute terms.**

   g. The **ACSM metabolic formulae** in *ACSM's Guidelines for Exercise Testing and Prescription*, 7th ed., and those described in this chapter were designed to provide you with **gross values.**

The ability to convert from one energy expression to another is fundamental. Do not proceed to the next section of this chapter until you master this task.

- Converting an expression merely requires the multiplication or division of that expression by a constant. For example, to convert from MET to relative oxygen consumption, multiply the MET value by 3.5. Conversely, to convert from relative oxygen consumption to MET, divide by 3.5 (*Figure 11-1*). Commit these constants to memory.
- *Figure 11-1*, the **Energy Equivalency Chart**, will help you to remember these conversions.
- *Figure 11-2* is a **practice sheet**. Duplicate this sheet, and practice completing it from memory. Then, answer the following questions.

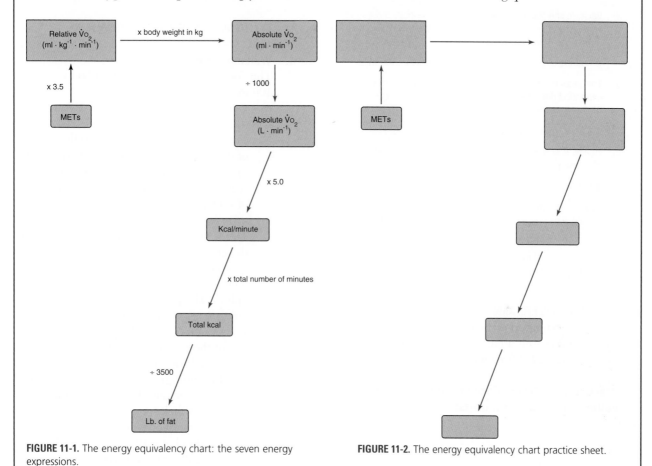

FIGURE 11-1. The energy equivalency chart: the seven energy expressions.

FIGURE 11-2. The energy equivalency chart practice sheet.

Practice Questions: Converting Energy Expressions

1. What is the MET equivalent to 8.75 mL · kg^{-1} · min^{-1}?
2. What is the absolute $\dot{V}_{O_2}$ equivalent to 10 METs for a 155-pound male?
3. What is the equivalent total caloric expenditure of 2.5 pounds of fat?
4. A 70-kg male expends 7.5 kcal · min^{-1} while exercising. What is the equivalent MET value?
5. How many pounds of fat will a 50-kg woman lose after 4 weeks of training if she exercises at a frequency of 3 days per week, a duration of 45 minutes per session, and an energy expenditure of 6.5 kcal · min^{-1}? Assume that no modifications occur in her eating habits during the 4 weeks of training.
6. Using the ACSM walking formula, you calculate a gross $\dot{V}_{O_2}$ of 13.0 mL · kg^{-1} · min^{-1}. What is the net oxygen uptake?

Solutions

1. To convert from mL · kg^{-1} · min^{-1} to MET, divide 8.75 by 3.5. The correct answer is **2.5 METs**.
2. To convert from MET to $\dot{V}_{O_2}$ in absolute terms, first multiply the MET value by 3.5 to convert to $\dot{V}_{O_2}$ in relative terms (mL · kg^{-1} · min^{-1}), and then multiply the product (35 mL · kg^{-1} · min^{-1}) by the body weight expressed in kilograms (155 pounds ÷ 2.2 = 70.5 kg). The correct answers are **2,467.5 mL · min^{-1}**, or **2.47 L · min^{-1}**.
3. To convert from pounds of fat to total kilocalories, multiply the fat weight (expressed in pounds) by 3,500. The correct answer is **8,750 kcal.**
4. To convert from kcal · min^{-1} to MET:
   a. First, convert the value to absolute $\dot{V}_{O_2}$ in L · min^{-1}:

   $$7.5 \text{ kcal} \cdot \text{min}^{-1} \div 5.0 = 1.5 \text{ L} \cdot \text{min}^{-1}$$

b. Then, convert to absolute $\dot{V}O_2$ in $mL \cdot min^{-1}$:

$1.5\ L \cdot min^{-1} \times 1{,}000 = 1{,}500\ mL \cdot min^{-1}$

c. Then, convert to relative $\dot{V}O_2$:

$1{,}500\ mL \cdot min^{-1} \div 70\ kg = 21.43\ mL \cdot kg^{-1} \cdot min^{-1}$

d. Finally, convert to METs:

$21.43\ mL \cdot kg^{-1} \cdot min^{-1} \div 3.5 = 6.12\ METS$

5. The first step to solving this conversion question is to calculate the total number of minutes spent exercising during the 4 weeks.

   a. Because she trained for 45 minutes per session, 3 days per week, she accumulated a total of 540 minutes of exercise during the 4 weeks:

   $45\ min/session \cdot 3\ sessions/week \cdot 4\ weeks = 540\ min$

   b. The second step is to calculate the total number of calories expended during exercise throughout the 4 weeks (540 minutes) of training:

   $6.5\ kcal \cdot min^{-1} \times 540\ min\ of\ exercise = 3{,}510\ kcal$

   c. Finally, find the fat weight equivalent to the expended calories:

   $3{,}510\ kcal \div 3{,}500 = 1.003\ pounds\ of\ fat$

   or approximately 1 pound of fat.

6. Because gross $\dot{V}O_2$ = net $\dot{V}O_2$ + resting $\dot{V}O_2$, then net $\dot{V}O_2$ = gross $\dot{V}O_2$ − resting $\dot{V}O_2$:

   Net $\dot{V}O_2 = 13.0\ mL \cdot kg^{-1} \cdot min^{-1} - 3.5\ mL \cdot kg^{-1} \cdot min^{-1}$
   Net $\dot{V}O_2 = 9.5\ mL \cdot kg^{-1} \cdot min^{-1}$

D. OTHER CONVERSION FACTORS

You must commit to memory some other important conversions as well. Practice writing out the conversions in *Table 11-2* from memory.

Practice Questions: Convert the following values to the desired units:

1. 1.5 m to centimeters.
2. 59.1 inches to meters.
3. 70 kg to pounds.
4. 6.0 mph to meters per minute.
5. 50 rpm on the Monark leg ergometer to meters per minute.

TABLE 11-2. Conversion Factors

To convert from	To	Do this
Centimeters (cm)	Meters (m)	÷ 100
Inches	Meters (m)	× 0.0254
Inches	Centimeters (cm)	× 2.54
$kg \cdot m \cdot min^{-1}$	Watts (W)	÷ 6.0
Liters (L)	Milliliters (mL)	× 1000
Miles per hour (mph)	Meters per minute ($m \cdot min^{-1}$)	× 26.8
Pounds	Kilograms (kg)	÷ 2.2
Revolutions per minute (rpm) on a	Meters per minute ($m \cdot min^{-1}$)	
Monark arm ergometer		× 2.4
Monark leg ergometer		× 6
Tunturi or BodyGuard cycle ergometer		× 3

Solutions

1. 1.5 meters $\cdot$ 100 = **150 cm**
2. 59.1 inches $\cdot$ 0.0254 = **1.5 m**
3. 70 kg $\cdot$ 2.2 = **154 pounds**
4. 6.0 mph $\cdot$ 26.8 = **160.8 m $\cdot$ min^{-1}**
5. 50 rpm $\cdot$ 6 = **300 m $\cdot$ min^{-1}**

II. The ACSM Metabolic Formulae

All ACSM formulae yield **gross** oxygen uptake in **relative** terms.

A. WALKING AND RUNNING FORMULAE (*FIGURE 11-3*)

1. Walking Formula

This formula applies to speeds of 50 to $100\ m \cdot min^{-1}$ (1.9–3.7 mph).

   a. **Gross $\dot{V}O_2$** is calculated in **relative terms** ($mL \cdot kg^{-1} \cdot min^{-1}$).

   b. The **horizontal component** is the product of the speed of the treadmill, expressed in $m \cdot min^{-1}$, multiplied by 0.1 (the oxygen cost of walking). The product, the $\dot{V}O_2$ of walking forward, is expressed in $mL \cdot kg^{-1} \cdot min^{-1}$.

   c. The **vertical component** is the product of the grade of the treadmill multiplied by the speed of the treadmill ($m \cdot min^{-1}$) multiplied by 1.8 (the oxygen cost of walking uphill). The product, the $\dot{V}O_2$ of walking uphill, is expressed in $mL \cdot kg^{-1} \cdot min^{-1}$.

      1) Do not confuse the percentage grade of the treadmill with the degree angle of inclination.

      2) **Percentage grade of the treadmill** is the amount of vertical rise for 100 units of belt travel.

      3) For example, a client walking on a treadmill at a 12% grade travels 12 m vertically for every 100 m of belt travel.

   d. The **resting component** is $3.5\ mL \cdot kg^{-1} \cdot min^{-1}$.

2. Running Formula

   a. This formula applies to treadmill and outdoor running speeds exceeding $134\ m \cdot min^{-1}$ (5.0 mph) and for true jogging speeds exceeding $80.4\ m \cdot min^{-1}$ (3.0 mph).

   b. This formula also may be used for off-the-treadmill level running, but it should not be used for running on a graded track.

   c. **Gross $\dot{V}O_2$** is calculated in **relative terms** ($mL \cdot kg^{-1} \cdot min^{-1}$).

   d. The **horizontal component** is the product of the speed of the treadmill, expressed in $m \cdot min^{-1}$, multiplied by 0.2 (the oxygen

General Structure: ACSM Walking and Running Formulae

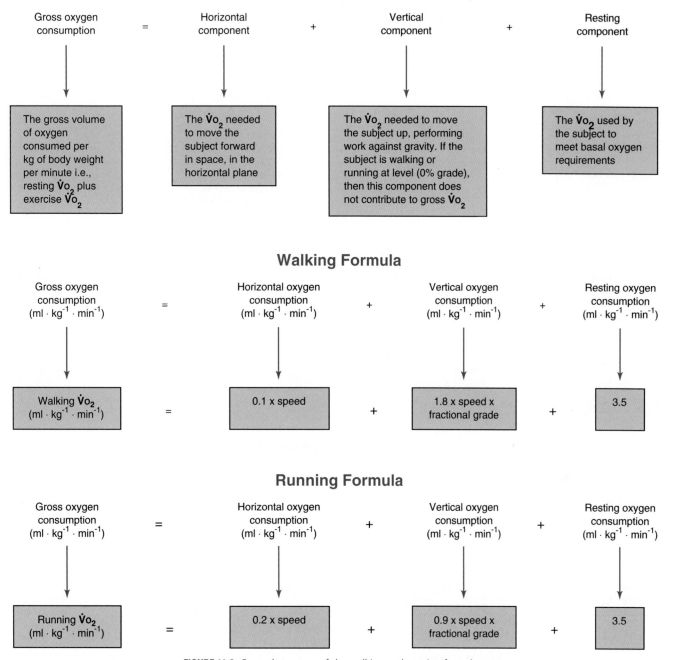

FIGURE 11-3. General structure of the walking and running formulae.

cost of running). The product, the $\dot{V}o_2$ of running forward, is expressed in $mL \cdot kg^{-1} \cdot min^{-1}$.

e. The **vertical component** is the product of the fractional grade (elevation) of the treadmill multiplied by the speed of the treadmill ($m \cdot min^{-1}$) multiplied by 0.9 (the oxygen cost of running uphill). The product, the $\dot{V}o_2$ of running uphill, is expressed in $mL \cdot kg^{-1} \cdot min^{-1}$.

f. The **resting component** is $3.5\ mL \cdot kg^{-1} \cdot min^{-1}$.

B. **LEG AND ARM ERGOMETRY FORMULAE** *(FIGURE 11-4)*

1. **Leg Cycling**

a. This formula applies to work rates between 300 and 1,200 $kg \cdot m \cdot min^{-1}$, or 50 to 200 watts (50–200 W).

b. **Gross oxygen** consumption is calculated in **relative terms** ($mL \cdot kg^{-1} \cdot min^{-1}$).

c. **Oxygen cost of loaded leg cycling** is the product of the cost of cycling (1.8) multiplied by the work rate ($kg \cdot m \cdot min^{-1}$) divided by the body weight (kg). The

General Structure: ACSM Leg and Arm Ergometry Formulae

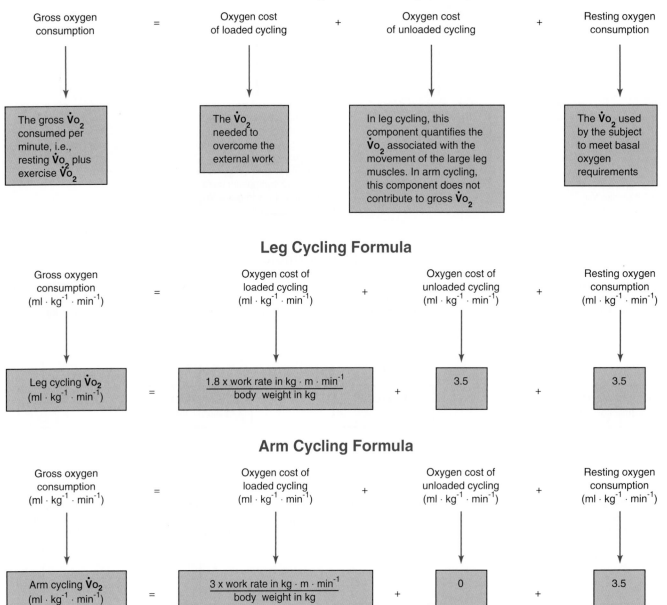

FIGURE 11-4. General structure of the leg and arm ergometry formulae.

oxygen cost of loaded leg cycling also may be calculated as:

$10.8 \cdot$ Work rate (W) $\div$ Body weight (kg)

d. **Oxygen cost of unloaded leg cycling** is the oxygen cost ($3.5 \text{ mL} \cdot \text{kg} \cdot \text{min}^{-1}$) for the movement of the legs in space.

e. The **resting oxygen** component is $3.5 \text{ mL} \cdot \text{kg}^{-1} \cdot \text{min}^{-1}$.

2. **Arm Cycling**

a. This formula applies to work rates between 150 and 750 kg $\cdot$ m $\cdot$ min^{-1} (25–125 W).

b. **Gross oxygen** consumption is calculated in relative terms (mL $\cdot$ kg^{-1} $\cdot$ min^{-1}).

c. **Oxygen cost of loaded arm cycling** is the product of the cost of cycling (3) multiplied by the work rate (kg $\cdot$ m $\cdot$ min^{-1}) divided by the body weight (kg). The oxygen cost of loaded arm cycling also may be calculated as:

$18 \cdot$ Work rate (W) $\div$ Body weight (kg)

d. **Oxygen cost of unloaded arm cycling** is not a factor, because arm cycling does not incur an oxygen cost of unloaded cycling.

e. The **resting component is** $3.5 \text{ mL} \cdot \text{kg}^{-1} \cdot \text{min}^{-1}$.

Exam Note: Work Rate–Leg Ergometer

The work rate may be provided to you in the question. You also may be expected to derive it from the **cadence** of the cycle ergometer and the **resistance** set on the flywheel.

- Work rate, also known as the **power output** or **workload**, is the product of the resistance set on the cycle ergometer and the speed of cycling (velocity):

  Work rate = Force (resistance set on the flywheel in kg) · Velocity $(m \cdot min^{-1})$

  The units for the resistance set on the flywheel, **kilogram-force (kgf) and kilopond (kp)**, can be used interchangeably (1 kgf = 1 kp).

- **Calculate velocity from revolutions per minute (RPM)** by multiplying the RPM value by **6 for a Monark cycle ergometer** or by **3 for a Tunturi or a BodyGuard.** For example, an individual cycling at 50 rpm on a Monark leg ergometer is pedaling at a velocity of 300 $m \cdot min^{-1}$. If the same individual works against a resistance of 2 kp, then the work rate will be 2 · 50 · 6 = 600 $kg \cdot m^{-1} \cdot min^{-1}$.

- **Work rate also can be expressed in watts:**

  1 W = 6.0 $kg \cdot m^{-1} \cdot min^{-1}$

Exam Note: Work Rate–Arm Ergometer

The work rate may be provided to you in the question. You also may be expected to derive it from the cadence of the cycle ergometer and the resistance set on the flywheel.

- Work rate, also known as the power output or workload, is the product of the resistance set on the flywheel and the speed of cycling (velocity):

  Work rate = Force (resistance set on the flywheel in kg) · Velocity $(m \cdot min^{-1})$

- Calculate velocity from rpm by multiplying the rpm value by **2.4 for a Monark arm ergometer.** The units for the resistance set on the flywheel, kilogram-force (kgf) and kilopond (kp), can be used interchangeably (1 kgf = 1 kp).

For example, an individual arm cycling at 50 rpm on a Monark arm ergometer is pedaling at a velocity of 120 $m \cdot min^{-1}$. If the same individual works against a resistance of 2 kp, then the work rate will be 2 · 50 · 2.4 = 240 $kg \cdot m^{-1} \cdot min^{-1}$.

- Work rate can also be expressed in watts:

  1 W = 6.0 · $kg \cdot m^{-1} \cdot min^{-1}$

C. **STEPPING FORMULA** *(FIGURE 11-5)*

1. This formula applies to stepping performed on a step box, a bleacher, or a similar stepping object where both concentric contractions (moving up against gravity) and eccentric contractions (moving down with gravity) are involved.

2. The formula is appropriate for stepping rates between 12 and 30 steps · min^{-1} and heights between 0.04 and 0.4 m (1.6–15.7 inches).

3. **Gross oxygen** consumption is calculated in **relative terms** $(mL \cdot kg^{-1} \cdot min^{-1})$.

4. The **horizontal component** is the product of the rate of stepping per minute multiplied by 0.2. The product is oxygen consumption in $mL \cdot kg^{-1} \cdot min^{-1}$.

5. The **vertical component** is the product of the height of each step (m) multiplied by the rate of stepping per minute multiplied by 1.33 multiplied by 1.8. The product is oxygen consumption in $mL \cdot kg^{-1} \cdot min^{-1}$.

6. The **resting component** is 3.5 $mL \cdot kg^{-1} \cdot min^{-1}$.

ACSM Stepping Formula

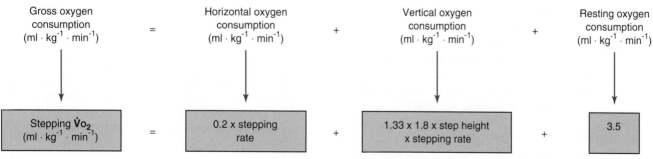

FIGURE 11-5. ACSM stepping formula.

III. Solving the ACSM Metabolic Formulae

A. USING A SYSTEMATIC APPROACH

The task of solving the ACSM formulae is much easier using a systematic approach, which will help you to avoid small but costly mistakes.

1. Read each question carefully, and do not proceed until you know what you are expected to calculate. Remember, some questions may be solved without the use of a metabolic formula.
2. Extract the required information. Do not be misled with extraneous information. If, for example, a question wants you to calculate the $\dot{V}O_2$ for walking on a treadmill, volunteered data about the height, age, or gender of the subject are irrelevant.
3. Select the correct metabolic equation. A common error committed by many candidates is choosing the wrong formula.
4. Write down each step. **Do not take shortcuts.** Going through all the steps once is faster than making two shortcut attempts!
5. On the top left corner of a clean sheet of paper, write the known values, and indicate what value is unknown.
6. When needed, convert all values to the appropriate units (see *Table 11-2*).
   a. Convert the treadmill speed or cycling cadence to $m \cdot min^{-1}$.
   b. Convert body weight to kilograms.
   c. Convert step height to meters.
   d. Convert work rate to $kg \cdot m \cdot min^{-1}$.
7. Write down the formula, and plug in the known values and constants. Write clearly, and place units after all variables.
8. Solve for the unknown value. If the unknown is on the left side of the equation (i.e., the $\dot{V}O_2$ value), simply calculate the sum of the three components of the appropriate equation. If the unknown is on the right side of the equation, substitute and solve for the unknown. (Solving linear equations will be discussed in more detail later.)
9. Examine the answer. Is the answer logical? Does it fall within expected "normal" values and human abilities?
10. Examine the choices. Make sure that your answer is in the same units as the answer on the examination, especially if a question does not specify what energy expression is needed (i.e., relative or absolute $\dot{V}O_2$, MET, kcal).

B. SOLVING LINEAR EQUATIONS

1. The ACSM metabolic formulae are simple linear regression equations.

To solve an equation with an unknown value on the right side of the equation, you must simplify the expression so that the unknown value stands by itself on one side of the equation and all the known numbers stand on the other.

---

2. The process of arriving at an answer to a metabolic calculation question is greatly simplified if the unknown is the $\dot{V}O_2$ value.
3. When the $\dot{V}O_2$ value is known, you might be expected to calculate an unknown value on the right side of the equation (e.g., resistance on the cycle ergometer, speed of the treadmill, height of the step bench).
   a. Example 1
      Solve for χ in the following equation:

      $\chi - 4 = 10$

      Solution: Add 4 to both sides of the equation:

      $\chi - 4 + 4 = 10 + 4$
      $\chi = 14$

   b. Example 2
      Solve for α in the following equation:

      $2\alpha + 7 = 3$

      Solution: Subtract 7 from both sides of the equation:

      $2\alpha = -4$

      Divide both sides by 2:

      $\alpha = -2$

   c. Example 3
      Solve for β in the following equation:

      $4\beta - 3/4 = 7/9$

      Solution: Add 3/4 to both sides of the equation:

      $4\beta = 55/36$

      Divide both sides by 4:

      $\beta = 55/144$

Helpful hint: Substitute your answer for the unknown value in the original equation. If the left side equals the right side after the substitution, then your answer is correct. For example, in the previous problem, plugging in 55/144 in place of β yields 7/9. Hence, 55/144 is the correct answer.

Math Reminder

Multiply and divide numbers **before** adding or subtracting. For example, in the following expression:

$$Y = 5 + 2 \cdot 5 + 7 \cdot 2$$

Multiply the 2 by the 5 (= 10), the 7 by the 2 (= 14), and then add the 10, the 14, and the 5 together. The correct answer is $Y = 29$, not $Y = 84$.

Solving Metabolic Calculations: Examples

1. What is the gross oxygen cost of walking on a treadmill at 3.5 mph and a 10% grade?

2. A 176-pound client set the treadmill at 3.0 mph and a 2% grade. While exercising, his heart rate was 140 bpm, and his blood pressure was 160/80 mm Hg. What was his estimated $\dot{V}_{O_2}$ in relative terms?

3. What resistance should you set a Monark leg cycle ergometer at to elicit a $\dot{V}_{O_2}$ value of 2,750 mL · min^{-1} while cycling at 50 rpm? The subject is 65 inches tall and weighs 110 pounds.

Solutions

1. Choose the walking equation.
   a. On the top left corner of a clean sheet of paper, write down the known values, and convert all numbers to the appropriate units:

   Speed (m · min^{-1}) = 3.5 mph · 26.8 = 93.8 m · min^{-1}

   b. Write down the ACSM walking formula:

   Walking (mL · kg^{-1} · min^{-1}) = (0.1 · speed)
   + (1.8 · speed · fractional grade) + 3.5 · kg^{-1} · min^{-1}

   c. Substitute the variable name with the **known values**:

   Walking (mL · kg^{-1} · min^{-1}) = (0.1 × **93.8** m · min^{-1})
   + (1.8 × **93.8** m · min^{-1} × **0.1**) + 3.5 mL · kg^{-1} · min^{-1}

   d. Multiply the values:

   Walking (mL · kg^{-1} · min^{-1}) = 9.38 mL · kg^{-1} · min^{-1}
   +16.88 mL · kg^{-1} · min^{-1} + 3.5 mL · kg^{-1} · min^{-1}

   e. Then, add the numbers:

   Gross walking $\dot{V}_{O_2}$ = **29.76 mL · kg^{-1} · min^{-1}**

2. The question is clearly asking for $\dot{V}_{O_2}$ in relative terms (mL · kg^{-1} · min^{-1}).
   a. Extract the information you need (speed and elevation of the treadmill) and ignore extraneous information (heart rate and blood pressure).
   b. Choose the walking equation.
   c. On the top left corner of a clean sheet of paper, write down the known values, and convert all numbers to the appropriate units:

   Weight = 176 pounds ÷ 2.2 = 80.0 kg
   Speed = 3.0 mph · 26.8 = **80.4 m · min^{-1}**
   Treadmill elevation = 2% grade = 2/100 = **0.02**

   d. Plug the known values into the formula, and calculate the answer:

   Walking (mL · kg^{-1} · min^{-1}) = (0.1 × **80.4** m · min^{-1}) +
   (1.8 × **0.02** × 80.4 m · min^{-1}) + 3.5 mL · kg^{-1} · min^{-1}
   Walking (mL · kg^{-1} · min^{-1}) = 8.04 mL · kg^{-1} · min^{-1}
   + 2.89 mL · kg^{-1} · min^{-1} + 3.5 mL · kg^{-1} · min^{-1}
   Relative $\dot{V}_{O_2}$ = **14.43 mL · kg^{-1} · min^{-1}**

3. Read the question carefully; know what the question is asking for. The question is providing you with the absolute $\dot{V}_{O_2}$ (2,750 mL · min^{-1}), but it expects you to calculate the resistance (F) to be set on the cycle ergometer.
   a. Extract the information you need. Only the weight of the subject and the speed of the cycle are needed.
   b. Convert the known units:

   110 pounds = **50.0 kg**

   c. Select the leg ergometer equation
   d. Calculate the gross **relative $\dot{V}_{O_2}$** from the given information:

   $\dot{V}_{O_2}$ (mL · kg^{-1} · min^{-1}) = 2,750 mL · min^{-1} ÷ **50.0 kg**
   = **55.0** mL · kg^{-1} · min^{-1}

   e. Now, write out the leg ergometer formula

   Leg cycling (mL · kg^{-1} · min^{-1}) = 1.8 · Work rate
   ÷ body weight + 3.5 mL · kg^{-1} · min^{-1}
   + 3.5 mL · kg^{-1} · min^{-1}

   f. Note that the unknown (resistance in kg) is part of the work rate. Write out the work rate as force (kg) · speed (m · min^{-1}):

   55.0 mL · kg^{-1} · min^{-1} = 1.8 · F · Speed ÷ Body weight
   + 3.5 (mL · kg^{-1} · min^{-1}) + 3.5 (mL · kg^{-1} · min^{-1})

   g. From the given information, we also know that the speed of cycling is 300 m · min^{-1} (50 rpm · 6). Plug all the known values into the equation:

   55.0 mL · kg^{-1} · min^{-1} = 1.8 · F · 300 (m · min^{-1})
   ÷ 50 (kg) + 3.5 (mL · kg^{-1} · min^{-1})
   + 3.5 (mL · kg^{-1} · min^{-1})

   h. Move the unknown F to one side of the equation, all the known values to the other side, and calculate for the unknown:

   55.0 mL · kg^{-1} · min^{-1} = 1.8 · F · 300 (m · min^{-1})
   ÷ 50 (kg) + 3.5 (mL · kg^{-1} · min^{-1})
   + 3.5 (mL · kg^{-1} · min^{-1})

   55.0 mL · kg^{-1} · min^{-1} − 3.5 mL · kg^{-1} · min^{-1}
   − 3.5 mL · kg^{-1} · min^{-1} = 1.8 · F · 300 m/min ÷ 50 kg

   48 mL · kg^{-1} · min^{-1} = 1.8 · F · 300 m/min ÷ 50 kg

   (48 · 50)/(1.8 · 300) = F

   4.44 kp = F

Review Test

DIRECTIONS: Carefully read all questions, and select the BEST single answer.

1. What is the relative $\dot{V}o_2$ of walking on a treadmill at 3.5 mph and a 0% grade?
   A) 9.38 mL · kg^{-1} · min^{-1}
   B) 12.88 mL · kg^{-1} · min^{-1}
   C) 18.76 mL · kg^{-1} · min^{-1}
   D) 22.26 mL · kg^{-1} · min^{-1}

2. A client is walking on a treadmill at 3.4 mph and a 5% grade. What is her $\dot{V}o_2$ in relative terms?
   A) 9.11 mL · kg^{-1} · min^{-1}
   B) 11.9 mL · kg^{-1} · min^{-1}
   C) 24 mL · kg^{-1} · min^{-1}
   D) 20.81 mL · kg^{-1} · min^{-1}

3. A 70-kg client is running on a treadmill at 5 mph and a 5% grade. What is his caloric expenditure rate?
   A) 12.7 kcal · min^{-1}
   B) 1.271 kcal · min^{-1}
   C) 3.633 kcal · min^{-1}
   D) 36.33 kcal · min^{-1}

4. What is the relative $\dot{V}o_2$ of walking on a treadmill at 3.5 mph and a 10% grade?
   A) 181.72 mL · kg^{-1} · min^{-1}
   B) 18.17 mL · kg^{-1} · min^{-1}
   C) 29.76 mL · kg^{-1} · min^{-1}
   D) 27.96 mL · kg^{-1} · min^{-1}

5. What is the MET equivalent to level walking on a treadmill at 3.0 mph?
   A) 5.59 MET.
   B) 3.30 MET.
   C) 2.30 MET.
   D) 3.02 MET.

6. What is the relative $\dot{V}o_2$ of running on a treadmill at 6.5 mph and a 0% grade?
   A) 34.84 mL · kg^{-1} · min^{-1}
   B) 34.48 mL · kg^{-1} · min^{-1}
   C) 38.34 mL · kg^{-1} · min^{-1}
   D) 43.83 mL · kg^{-1} · min^{-1}

7. What is the relative $\dot{V}o_2$ of running on a treadmill at 5.5 mph and a 12% grade?
   A) 29.48 mL · kg^{-1} · min^{-1}
   B) 45.4 mL · kg^{-1} · min^{-1}
   C) 47.2 mL · kg^{-1} · min^{-1}
   D) 48.9 mL · kg^{-1} · min^{-1}

8. A 150-pound male sets the treadmill speed at 5.0 mph and a 5.2% grade. Calculate his MET value.
   A) 36.57 METs.
   B) 10.45 METs.

C) 12.25 METs.
D) Not enough information to answer the question.

9. What is a subject's work rate in watts if he pedals on a Monark cycle ergometer at 50 rpm at a resistance of 2.0 kiloponds?
   A) 50 W.
   B) 100 W.
   C) 200 W.
   D) 300 W.

10. A 110-pound female pedals a Monark cycle ergometer at 50 rpm against a resistance of 2.5 kiloponds. Calculate her absolute $\dot{V}o_2$.
    A) 300 mL · min^{-1}
    B) 750 mL · min^{-1}
    C) 1.25 L · min^{-1}
    D) 1.7 L · min^{-1}

11. How many calories will a 110-pound woman expend if she pedals on a Monark cycle ergometer at 50 rpm against a resistance of 2.5 kiloponds for 60 minutes?
    A) 12.87 calories.
    B) 31.28 calories.
    C) 510 calories.
    D) 3,500 calories.

12. A 55-kilogram woman trains on a cycle ergometer by pedaling at 60 rpm against a resistance of 1.5 kiloponds. What is her absolute $\dot{V}o_2$?
    A) 1.36 L · min^{-1}
    B) 2.47 L · min^{-1}
    C) 3.62 L · min^{-1}
    D) 3600 mL · min^{-1}

13. The same 55-kilogram woman (from question 12) also trains on a Monark arm ergometer at 60 rpm against a resistance of 1.5 kiloponds. What is her absolute $\dot{V}o_2$?
    A) 1.52 L · min^{-1}
    B) 773.0 mL · min^{-1}
    C) 0.840 L · min^{-1}
    D) 0.774 L · min^{-1}

14. If a 70-kg man runs on a treadmill at 8 mph and a 0% grade for 45 minutes, what is his caloric expenditure?
    A) 1,067.07 calories.
    B) 392.18 calories.
    C) 730.48 calories.
    D) Not enough information to answer the question.

15. What is the relative oxygen cost of bench stepping at a rate of 24 steps per minute up a 10-inch stepping box? The individual weighs 140 pounds.
    A) $12.91 \text{ mL} \cdot \text{kg}^{-1} \cdot \text{min}^{-1}$
    B) $14.61 \text{ mL} \cdot \text{kg}^{-1} \cdot \text{min}^{-1}$
    C) $16.41 \text{ mL} \cdot \text{kg}^{-1} \cdot \text{min}^{-1}$
    D) $22.89 \text{ mL} \cdot \text{kg}^{-1} \cdot \text{min}^{-1}$

16. What stepping rate should a client use if she wishes to exercise at 5 METs? The step box is 6 inches high, and the client weighs 50 kg.
    A) 12 steps per minute.
    B) 32 steps per minute.
    C) 25 steps per minute.
    D) 96 steps per minute.

17. A 143-pound woman regularly exercises on a treadmill at a speed of 5.5 mph and a 2% elevation. What is her caloric expenditure?
    A) $6.78 \text{ kcal} \cdot \text{min}^{-1}$
    B) $11.58 \text{ kcal} \cdot \text{min}^{-1}$
    C) $20.85 \text{ kcal} \cdot \text{min}^{-1}$
    D) $25.47 \text{ kcal} \cdot \text{min}^{-1}$

18. A 143-pound woman regularly exercises on a treadmill at a speed of 5.5 mph and a 2% elevation. How much weight will she lose weekly if she exercises for a duration of 45 minutes per session, with a frequency of three sessions per week?
    A) 1.5 kg.
    B) 2.07 kg.
    C) 0.25 pounds.
    D) 0.45 pounds.

19. What resistance would you set a cycle ergometer at if your 80-kg client needs to train at 6 METs? Assume a 50 rpm cycling cadence.
    A) 1.5 kg.
    B) 2.07 kg.

C) 0.25 pounds.
D) 0.45 pounds.

20. At what running speed would you set a level treadmill at to elicit an $\dot{V}O_2$ of $40 \text{ mL} \cdot \text{kg}^{-1} \cdot \text{min}^{-1}$?
    A) 5.0 mph
    B) 6.8 mph
    C) $18.25 \text{ m} \cdot \text{min}^{-1}$
    D) 18.25 mph

21. If a healthy young man exercises at an intensity of $45 \text{ mL} \cdot \text{kg}^{-1} \cdot \text{min}^{-1}$ three times per week for 45 minutes each session, how long would it take him to lose 10 pounds of fat?
    A) 4 weeks.
    B) 7.14 weeks.
    C) 16.5 weeks.
    D) 19 weeks.

22. A 35-year-old woman reduces her caloric intake by 1,200 kcal per week. How much weight will she lose in 26 weeks?
    A) 8.9 pounds.
    B) 12.0 pounds.
    C) 26.0 pounds.
    D) 34.3 pounds.

23. How much weight will the woman (from question 22) lose in 26 weeks if she integrates a 1-mile walk, taken three times per week, into her weight loss program?
    A) 3 pounds.
    B) 6 pounds.
    C) 11 pounds.
    D) 15 pounds.

ANSWERS AND EXPLANATIONS

1–B. The steps are as follows:

a. Choose the ACSM walking formula.

b. Write down your known values, and convert the values to the appropriate units:

$3.5 \text{ mph} \times 26.8 \text{ m} \cdot \text{min}^{-1} = 93.8 \text{ m} \cdot \text{min}^{-1}$
$0\% \text{ grade} = 0.0$

c. Write down the ACSM walking formula:

Walking = $(0.1 \cdot \text{Speed}) + (1.8 \cdot \text{Speed} \cdot \text{Fractional grade}) + 3.5 \text{ (mL} \cdot \text{kg}^{-1} \cdot \text{min}^{-1})$

d. Substitute the known values for the variable name:

$\text{mL} \cdot \text{kg}^{-1} \cdot \text{min}^{-1} = (0.1 \cdot 93.8)$
$+ (1.8 \cdot 93.8 \cdot 0) + 3.5$
$\text{mL} \cdot \text{kg}^{-1} \cdot \text{min}^{-1} = 9.38 + 0 + 3.5$

e. Solve for the unknown:

$\text{mL} \cdot \text{kg}^{-1} \cdot \text{min}^{-1} = 9.38 + 3.5$
Gross walking $\dot{V}O_2 = 12.88 \text{ mL} \cdot \text{kg}^{-1} \cdot \text{min}^{-1}$

2–D. The steps are as follows:

a. Choose the ACSM walking formula.

b. Write down your known values, and convert the values to the appropriate units:

3.4 mph $\times$ 26.8 m $\cdot$ min^{-1} = 91.12 m $\cdot$ min^{-1}
5% grade = 0.05

c. Write down the ACSM walking formula:

Walking = (0.1 $\cdot$ Speed) + (1.8 $\cdot$ Speed $\cdot$ Fractional grade) + 3.5 (mL $\cdot$ kg^{-1} $\cdot$ min^{-1})

d. Substitute the known values for the variable name:

mL $\cdot$ kg^{-1} $\cdot$ min^{-1} = (0.1 $\cdot$ 91.12) + (1.8 $\cdot$ 91.12 $\cdot$ 0.05) + 3.5
mL $\cdot$ kg^{-1} $\cdot$ min^{-1} = 9.112 + 8.2008 + 3.5

e. Solve for the unknown:

mL $\cdot$ kg^{-1} $\cdot$ min^{-1} = 9.112 + 8.2008 + 3.5
Gross walking $\dot{V}o_2$ = 20.81 mL $\cdot$ kg^{-1} $\cdot$ min^{-1}

3–A. The steps are as follows:

a. Choose the ACSM running formula.

b. Write down your known values, and convert the values to the appropriate units:

5 mph $\cdot$ 26.8 = 134 m $\cdot$ min^{-1}
5% grade = 0.05

c. Write down the ACSM running formula:

Running = (0.2 $\cdot$ Speed) + (0.9 $\cdot$ Speed $\cdot$ Fractional grade) + 3.5 (mL $\cdot$ kg^{-1} $\cdot$ min^{-1})

d. Substitute the known values for the variable name:

mL $\cdot$ kg^{-1} $\cdot$ min^{-1} = (0.2 $\cdot$ 134) + (0.9 $\cdot$ 134 $\cdot$ 0.05) + 3.5
mL $\cdot$ kg^{-1} $\cdot$ min^{-1} = 26.8 + 6.03 + 3.5

e. Solve for the unknown:

mL $\cdot$ kg^{-1} $\cdot$ min^{-1} = 26.8 + 6.03 + 3.5
Gross running $\dot{V}o_2$ = 36.33 mL $\cdot$ kg^{-1} $\cdot$ min^{-1}

f. The question is asking you to find the client's caloric expenditure rate, which means that you need to first determine his oxygen consumption in absolute terms: (refer to Figure 11-1)

Absolute $\dot{V}o_2$ (mL $\cdot$ min^{-1}) = relative $\dot{V}o_2$ (mL $\cdot$ kg^{-1} $\cdot$ min^{-1}) $\cdot$ Body weight (kg)
mL $\cdot$ min^{-1} = 36.33 mL $\cdot$ kg^{-1} $\cdot$ min^{-1} $\times$ 70 kg
Absolute $\dot{V}o_2$ (mL $\cdot$ min^{-1}) = 2,543.1 mL $\cdot$ min^{-1}

Now, divide by 1,000 to convert to L $\cdot$ min^{-1}:

2,543.1 ÷ 1,000 = 2.54 L $\cdot$ min^{-1}

g. Multiply absolute $\dot{V}o_2$ by 5.0 to determine his caloric expenditure rate:

2.54 L $\cdot$ min^{-1} $\times$ 5.0 = 12.7 kcal $\cdot$ min^{-1}

4–C. The steps are as follows:

a. Choose the ACSM walking formula.

b. Write down your known values, and convert the values to the appropriate units:

3.5 mph $\cdot$ 26.8 = 93.8 m $\cdot$ min^{-1}
10% grade = 0.10

c. Write down the ACSM walking formula:

Walking = (0.1 $\cdot$ Speed) + (1.8 $\cdot$ Speed $\cdot$ Fractional grade) + 3.5 (mL $\cdot$ kg^{-1} $\cdot$ min^{-1})

d. Substitute the known values for the variable name:

mL $\cdot$ kg^{-1} $\cdot$ min^{-1} = (0.1 $\cdot$ 93.8) + (1.8 $\cdot$ 93.8 $\cdot$ 0.1) + 3.5
mL $\cdot$ kg^{-1} $\cdot$ min^{-1} = 9.38 + 16.884 + 3.5

e. Solve for the unknown:

mL $\cdot$ kg^{-1} $\cdot$ min^{-1} = 9.38 + 16.884 + 3.5
Gross walking $\dot{V}o_2$ = 29.76 mL $\cdot$ kg^{-1} $\cdot$ min^{-1}

5–B. The steps are as follows:

a. Choose the ACSM walking formula.

b. Write down your known values, and convert the values to the appropriate units:

3.0 mph $\cdot$ 26.8 = 80.4 m $\cdot$ min^{-1}
0% grade (level walking) = 0.0

c. Write down the ACSM walking formula:

Walking (mL $\cdot$ kg^{-1} $\cdot$ min^{-1}) = (0.1 $\cdot$ Speed) + (1.8 $\cdot$ Speed $\cdot$ Fractional grade) + 3.5

d. Substitute the known values for the variable name:

mL $\cdot$ kg^{-1} $\cdot$ min^{-1} = (0.1 $\cdot$ 80.4) + (1.8 $\cdot$ 80.4 $\cdot$ 0) + 3.5

e. Solve for the unknown:

mL $\cdot$ kg^{-1} $\cdot$ min^{-1} = 8.04 + 0 + 3.5
Gross walking $\dot{V}o_2$ = 11.54 mL $\cdot$ kg^{-1}min^{-1}

f. Because this question wants you to find the MET equivalent, we must divide our gross walking $\dot{V}o_2$ by 3.5:

MET = Relative $\dot{V}o_2$ (mL $\cdot$ kg^{-1} $\cdot$ min^{-1}) ÷ 3.5
MET = 11.54 mL $\cdot$ kg^{-1} $\cdot$ min^{-1} ÷ 3.5
MET = 3.30

6–C. The steps are as follows:

a. Choose the ACSM running formula.

b. Write down your known values, and convert the values to the appropriate units:

6.5 mph $\cdot$ 26.8 = 174.2 m $\cdot$ min^{-1}
0% grade = 0.0

c. Write down the ACSM running formula:

Running = (0.2 $\cdot$ Speed) + (0.9 $\cdot$ Speed $\cdot$ Fractional grade) + 3.5 (mL $\cdot$ kg^{-1} $\cdot$ min^{-1})

d. Substitute the known values for the variable name:

$mL \cdot kg^{-1} \cdot min^{-1} = (0.2 \cdot 174.2)$
$+ (0.9 \cdot 174.2 \cdot 0) + 3.5$

e. Solve for the unknown:

$mL \cdot kg^{-1} \cdot min^{-1} = 34.84 + 0 + 3.5$
Gross running $\dot{V}O_2 = 38.34 \ mL \cdot kg^{-1} \cdot min^{-1}$

7–D. The steps are as follows:

a. Choose the ACSM running formula.

b. Write down your known values, and convert the values to the appropriate units:

$5.5 \ mph \cdot 26.8 = 147.4 \ m \cdot min^{-1}$
$12\% \ grade = 0.12$

c. Write down the ACSM running formula:

Running = $(0.2 \cdot Speed) + (0.9 \cdot Speed \cdot Fractional$
grade$) + 3.5 \ (mL \cdot kg^{-1} \cdot min^{-1})$

d. Substitute the known values for the variable name:

$mL \cdot kg^{-1} \cdot min^{-1} = (0.2 \cdot 147.4)$
$+ (0.9 \cdot 147.4 \cdot 0.12) + 3.5$

e. Solve for the unknown:

$mL \cdot kg^{-1} \cdot min^{-1} = 29.48 + 15.92 + 3.5$
Gross running $\dot{V}O_2 = 48.9 \ mL \cdot kg^{-1} \cdot min^{-1}$

8–B. The steps are as follows:

a. Choose the ACSM running formula.

b. Write down your known values, and convert the values to the appropriate units:

$5.0 \ mph \cdot 26.8 = 134 \ m \cdot min^{-1}$
$5.2\% \ grade = 0.052$

c. Write down the ACSM running formula:

Running = $(0.2 \cdot Speed) + (0.9 \cdot Speed \cdot Fractional$
grade$) + 3.5 \ (mL \cdot kg^{-1} \cdot min^{-1})$

d. Substitute the known values for the variable name:

$mL \cdot kg^{-1} \cdot min^{-1} = (0.2 \cdot 134)$
$+ (0.9 \cdot 134 \cdot 0.052) + 3.5$

e. Solve for the unknown:

$mL \cdot kg^{-1} \cdot min^{-1} = 26.8 + 3.5$
Gross running $\dot{V}O_2 = 36.57 \ mL \cdot kg^{-1} \cdot min^{-1}$

f. This question asks us for his MET value, so we must divide his gross running $\dot{V}O_2$ (mL $\cdot$ $kg^{-1} \cdot min^{-1}$) by the constant 3.5 (we can ignore his weight, which is extraneous information):

MET = Relative $\dot{V}O_2$ (mL $\cdot kg^{-1} \cdot min^{-1}$) $\div$ 3.5
MET = $36.57 \ mL \cdot kg^{-1} \cdot min^{-1} \div 3.5$
MET = 10.45

9–B. This question does not require the use of a metabolic formula. The steps are as follows:

a. Write down your known values, and convert the values to the appropriate units:

$50 \ rpm \cdot 6 \ m = 300 \ m \cdot min^{-1}$
(Each revolution on a Monark cycle ergometer = 6 m)
$2.0 \ kp = 2.0 \ kg$

b. Write down the formula for work rate:

Work rate = Force $\cdot$ Distance $\div$ Time

c. Substitute the known values for the variable name:

Work rate = $2.0 \ kg \times 300 \ m \cdot min^{-1}$
Work rate = $600 \ kg \cdot m \cdot min^{-1}$

d. The question asks for work rate in watts, so we must divide the work rate $(kg \cdot m \cdot min^{-1})$ by 6:

W = $600 \ kg \cdot m \cdot min^{-1} \div 6$
W = 100

10–D. The steps are as follows:

a. Choose the ACSM leg cycling formula.

b. Write down your known values, and convert the values to the appropriate units:

$110 \ pounds \div 2.2 = 50 \ kg$
$50 \ rpm \cdot 6 \ m = 300 \ m \cdot min^{-1}$
$2.5 \ kp = 2.5 \ kg$

c. Write down the ACSM leg cycling formula:

Leg cycling $(mL \cdot kg^{-1} \cdot min^{-1})$
$= (1.8 \cdot Work \ rate \div Body \ weight) + 3.5 + 3.5$

d. Calculate the work rate:

Work rate = $kg \cdot m \cdot min$
Work rate = $2.5 \ kg \times 300 \ m \cdot min^{-1}$
$= 750 \ kg \cdot m \cdot min^{-1}$

e. Substitute the known values for the variable name:

$mL \cdot kg^{-1} \cdot min^{-1} = (1.8 \cdot 750 \div 50) + 3.5 + 3.5$

f. Solve for the unknown:

$mL \cdot kg^{-1} \cdot min^{-1} = 27 + 3.5 + 3.5$
Gross leg cycling $\dot{V}O_2 = 34 \ mL \cdot kg^{-1} \cdot min^{-1}$

g. This question is asking for her absolute $\dot{V}O_2$, so we must multiply her gross $\dot{V}O_2$ (in relative terms) by her body weight:

Absolute $\dot{V}O_2$ = Relative $\dot{V}O_2 \cdot$ Body weight
Absolute $\dot{V}O_2$ = $34 \ mL \cdot kg^{-1} \cdot min^{-1} \times 50 \ kg$
$= 1,700 \ mL \cdot min^{-1}$

h. To get L $\cdot min^{-1}$, divide by 1,000:

$1,700 \ mL \cdot min^{-1} \div 1,000 = 1.7 \ L \ min^{-1}$

11–C. The steps are as follows:

a. Choose the ACSM leg cycling formula.

b. Write down your known values, and convert the values to the appropriate units:

110 pounds ÷ 2.2 = 50 kg
50 rpm · 6 m = 300 m · min^{-1}
2.5 kp = 2.5 kg
60 minutes of cycling

c. Write down the ACSM formula:

Leg cycling (mL · kg^{-1} · min^{-1})
= (1.8 · Work rate ÷ Body weight)
+ 3.5 (mL · kg^{-1} · min^{-1})
+ 3.5 (mL · kg^{-1} · min^{-1})

d. Calculate the work rate:

Work rate = kg · m ÷ min = 2.5 kg · 300 m · min^{-1}
= 750 kg · m^{-1} · min^{-1}

e. Substitute the known values for the variable name:

mL · kg^{-1} · min^{-1} = (1.8 · 750 ÷ 50) + 3.5 + 3.5

f. Solve for the unknown:

Gross leg cycling $\dot{V}\text{o}_2$ = 34 mL · kg^{-1} · min^{-1}

g. To find out how many calories she expends, we must first convert her $\dot{V}\text{o}_2$ to absolute terms:

Absolute $\dot{V}\text{o}_2$ = relative $\dot{V}\text{o}_2$ · body weight
Absolute $\dot{V}\text{o}_2$ = 34 mL · kg^{-1} · min^{-1} × 50 kg
= 1,700 mL · min^{-1}

h. Convert mL · min^{-1} to L · min^{-1} by dividing by 1,000:

1,700 mL · min^{-1} ÷ 1,000 = 1.7 L · min^{-1}

i. Next, we must see how many calories she expends per minute by multiplying her absolute $\dot{V}\text{o}_2$ (L · min^{-1}) by the constant 5.0:

1.7 L · min^{-1} × 5.0 = 8.5 kcal · min^{-1}

j. Finally, multiply the number of calories she expends per minute by the number of minutes that she cycles:

8.5 kcal · min^{-1} × 60 min = 510 total calories

12–A. The steps are as follows:

a. Choose the ACSM leg cycling formula.

b. Write down your known values, and convert the values to the appropriate units:

55 kg = body weight
60 rpm · 6 m = 360 m · min^{-1}
1.5 kp = 1.5 kg

c. Write down the ACSM formula:

Leg cycling (mL · kg^{-1} · min^{-1})
= (1.8 · Work rate ÷ body weight) + 3.5 + 3.5

d. Calculate work rate:

Work rate = kg · m · min
= 1.5 kg × 360 m · min^{-1}
= 540 kg · m · min^{-1}

e. Substitute the known values for the variable name:

mL · kg^{-1} · min^{-1} = (1.8 · 540 ÷ 55) + 3.5 + 3.5

f. Solve for the unknown:

mL · kg^{-1} · min^{-1} = 17.67 + 3.5 + 3.5
Gross leg cycling $\dot{V}\text{o}_2$ = 24.67 mL · kg^{-1} · min^{-1}

g. To get her absolute $\dot{V}\text{o}_2$, multiply by her body weight:

Absolute $\dot{V}\text{o}_2$ = Relative $\dot{V}\text{o}_2$ · Body weight
Absolute $\dot{V}\text{o}_2$ = 24.67 mL · kg^{-1} · min^{-1} × 55 kg
= 1,356.85 mL · min^{-1}

h. To get absolute $\dot{V}\text{o}_2$ in L · min^{-1}, divide mL · min^{-1} by 1,000:

1,356.85 mL · min^{-1} ÷ 1,000 = 1.36 L · min^{-1}

13–C. The steps are as follows:

a. Choose the ACSM arm cycling formula.

b. Write down your known values, and convert the values to the appropriate units:

55 kg = body weight
60 RPM · 2.4 m = 144 m · min^{-1}
(Each revolution on a Monark arm ergometer = 2.4 m)
1.5 kp = 1.5 kg

c. Write down the ACSM formula:

Arm cycling (mL · kg^{-1} · min^{-1})
= (3 · Work rate ÷ Body weight)
+ 0 + 3.5 (mL · kg^{-1} · min^{-1})

d. Calculate the work rate:

Work rate = kg · m ÷ min
Work rate = 1.5 kg × 144 m · min^{-1}
= 216 kg · m^{-1} · min^{-1}

e. Substitute the known values for the variable name:

mL · kg^{-1} · min^{-1} = (3 · 216 ÷ 55) + 0 + 3.5

f. Solve for the unknown:

mL · kg^{-1} · min^{-1} = 11.78 + 0 + 3.5
Gross arm cycling $\dot{V}\text{o}_2$ = 15.28 mL · kg^{-1} · min^{-1}

g. To get her absolute $\dot{V}O_2$, multiply her relative $\dot{V}O_2$ by her body weight:

Absolute $\dot{V}O_2$ = Relative $\dot{V}'O_2$ · Body weight
Absolute $\dot{V}O_2$ = 15.28 mL · kg^{-1} · min^{-1} × 55 kg
= 840.4 mL · min^{-1}

h. To get her absolute $\dot{V}O_2$ in L · min^{-1}, divide mL · min^{-1} by 1,000:

840.4 mL · min^{-1} ÷ 1,000 = 0.8404 L · min^{-1}

14–C. The steps are as follows:

a. Choose the ACSM running formula.

b. Write down your known values, and convert the values to the appropriate units:

8 mph · 26.8 = 214.4 m · min^{-1}
70 kg = body weight
45 minutes of running
0% grade

c. Write down the ACSM running formula:

Running = (0.2 · Speed) + (0.9 · Speed
· Fractional grade) + 3.5 (mL · kg^{-1} · min^{-1})

d. Substitute the known values for the variable name:

mL · kg^{-1} · min^{-1} = (0.2 · 214.4)
+ (0.9 · 214.4 · 0) + 3.5

e. Solve for the unknown:

mL · kg^{-1} · min^{-1} = 42.88 + 0 + 3.5
Gross running $\dot{V}O_2$ = 46.38 mL · kg^{-1} · min^{-1}

f. To find out his total caloric expenditure, we must first put his gross running $\dot{V}O_2$ in absolute terms by multiplying by his body weight:

Absolute $\dot{V}O_2$ = Relative $\dot{V}'O_2$ · Body weight
Absolute $\dot{V}O_2$ = 46.38 mL · kg^{-1} · min^{-1} × 70 kg
= 3,246.6 mL · min^{-1}

g. Next, we must convert mL · min^{-1} to L · min^{-1} by dividing by 1,000:

3,246.6 mL · min^{-1} ÷ 1,000 = 3.2466 L · min^{-1}

h. We then multiply L · min^{-1} by the constant 5.0 to get kcal · min^{-1}:

3.2466 L · min^{-1} × 5.0 = 16.233 kcal · min^{-1}

i. Finally, we multiply kcal · min^{-1} by the total number of minutes to get the total caloric expenditure:

16.233 kcal · min^{-1} × 45 min = 730.48 calories

15–D. The steps are as follows:

a. Choose the ACSM stepping formula.

b. Write down your known values, and convert the values to the appropriate units:

Rate = 24 steps per minute
Step height = 10 inches · 0.0254 = 0.254 m
(Body weight is irrelevant in this problem.)

c. Write down the ACSM stepping formula:

Stepping = (0.2 · Stepping rate)
+ (1.33 · 1.8 · Step height · Stepping rate)
+ 3.5 (mL^{-1} · kg^{-1} · min^{-1})

d. Substitute the known values for the variable name:

mL · kg^{-1} · min^{-1} = (0.2 · 24)
+ (1.33 · 1.8 · 0.254 · 24) + 3.5

e. Solve for the unknown:

mL · kg^{-1} · min^{-1} = 4.8 + 14.59 + 3.5
Gross stepping $\dot{V}O_2$ = 22.89 mL · kg^{-1} · min^{-1}

16–C. The steps are as follows:

a. Choose the ACSM stepping formula.

b. Write down your known values, and convert the values to the appropriate units:

5 MET · 3.5 = 17.5 mL · kg^{-1} · min^{-1}
(This gives us the relative $\dot{V}O_2$ equivalent,
which we will need for the stepping formula.)
6 inches · 0.0254 = 0.1524 m
(Body weight is irrelevant in this problem.)

c. Write down the ACSM stepping formula:

Stepping = (0.2 · Stepping rate)
+ (1.33 · 1.8 · Step height · Stepping rate)
+ 3.5 (mL^{-1} · kg^{-1} · min^{-1})

d. Substitute the known values for the variable name:

17.5 = (0.2 · Stepping rate)
+ (1.33 · 1.8 · 0.1524 · Stepping rate) + 3.5

e. Move all the known values to one side of the equation, and keep the unknown on the other:

17.5 − 3.5 = (0.2 · Stepping rate)
+ (0.365 · Stepping rate)
14 = 0.565 · Stepping rate

f. Divide by 0.565 to get the stepping rate:

24.78 = stepping rate
Approximately 25 steps per minute = stepping rate

17–B. The steps are as follows:

a. Choose the ACSM running formula.

b. Write down your known values, and convert the values to the appropriate units:

143 pounds ÷ 2.2 = 65 kg
5.5 mph = 147.4 m · min^{-1}
2% grade = 0.02

c. Write down the ACSM running formula:

Running (mL · kg^{-1} · min^{-1}) = (0.2 · Speed) + (0.9 · Speed · Fractional grade) + 3.5

d. Substitute the known values for the variable name:

mL · kg^{-1} · min^{-1} = (0.2 · 147.4) + (0.9 · 147.4 · 0.02) + 3.5

e. Solve for the unknown:

mL · kg^{-1} · min^{-1} = 29.48 + 2.65 + 3.5
Gross running $\dot{V}O_2$ = 35.63 mL · kg^{-1} · min^{-1}

f. To find out how many calories per minute she is expending, we must first convert her gross running $\dot{V}O_2$ (in relative terms) to an absolute $\dot{V}O_2$ by multiplying by her body weight:

Absolute $\dot{V}O_2$ = relative $\dot{V}O_2$ · Body weight
Absolute $\dot{V}O_2$ = 35.63 mL · kg^{-1} · min^{-1} × 65 kg
= 2,315.95 mL · min^{-1}

g. Convert mL · min^{-1} to L · min^{-1} by dividing by 1,000:

2,315.95 mL · min^{-1} ÷ 1,000 = 2.31595 L · min^{-1}

h. Finally, we can find out how many calories she is expending per minute by multiplying 2.31595 by the constant 5.0:

2.31595 L · min^{-1} × 5.0 = 11.58 kcal · min^{-1}

18–D. This problem expands on problem 17. We established that she is expending 11.58 kcal per minute. The steps are as follows:

a. Multiply 11.58 kcal per minute by the total number of minutes that she exercises (45 min · 3 sessions per week = 135 total min):

11.58 kcal · min^{-1} × 135 total min
= 1563.3 total calories expended

b. To find out how many pounds of fat she will lose per week, divide the total calories expended by 3,500 (because 1 pound of fat contains 3,500 kcal):

1563.3 kcal ÷ 3,500
= 0.4466 pounds of fat per week of exercise

19–B. The steps are as follows:

a. Choose the ACSM leg cycling formula.

b. Write down your known values, and convert the values to the appropriate units:

6 MET · 3.5 = 21 mL · kg^{-1} · min^{-1}
80 kg = body weight

c. Write down the ACSM leg cycling formula:

Leg cycling (mL · kg^{-1} · min^{-1})
= (1.8 · Work rate ÷ Body weight) + 3.5 + 3.5

d. Substitute the known values for the variable name:

21 = (1.8 · Work rate ÷ 80) + 7

Assuming that he cycles at 50 rpm (or 300 m · min^{-1}):

21 = [(1.8 · 300 · F) ÷ 80] + 7

e. Move all of the known values to one side of the equation, and solve for the unknown.

21 − 7 = 540F
14 · 80 = 540F
1,120 ÷ 540 = F
2.07 kg = F

About 2.0 kg of force (F) are needed

20–B. The steps are as follows:

a. Choose the ACSM running formula.

b. Write down your known values, and convert the values to the appropriate units:

40 mL · kg^{-1} · min^{-1} = Relative $\dot{V}O_2$
0% grade

c. Write down the ACSM running formula:

Running (mL · kg^{-1} · min^{-1}) = (0.2 · Speed) + (0.9 · Speed · Fractional grade) + 3.5

d. Substitute the known values for the variable name:

40 = (0.2 · Speed) + 0 + 3.5

e. Solve for the unknown:

36.5 = 0.2(Speed)
182.5 m · min^{-1} = Speed

f. Convert m · min^{-1} to mph by dividing m · min^{-1} by 26.8:

182.5 m · min^{-1} ÷ 26.8 = 6.8 mph

21–C. The steps are as follows:

a. Convert relative $\dot{V}O_2$ to absolute $\dot{V}O_2$ by multiplying relative $\dot{V}O_2$ (mL · kg^{-1} · min^{-1}) by his body weight. We are not given his body weight, so we cannot finish this problem.

b. Assuming that he is an average, 70-kg man:

Absolute $\dot{V}O_2$ = Relative $\dot{V}O_2$ · Body weight
= 45 mL · kg^{-1} · min^{-1} × 70 kg
= 3,150 mL · min^{-1}

c. To get L · min^{-1}, divide mL · min^{-1} by 1,000:

3,150 mL · min^{-1} ÷ 1,000 = 3.15 L · min^{-1}

d. Multiply 3.150 L · min^{-1} by the constant 5.0 to get kcal · min^{-1}:

3.15 L · min^{-1} × 5.0 = 15.75 kcal · min^{-1}

e. Multiply 15.75 kcal per minute by the total number of minutes that he exercises (45 min · 3 times per week = 135 total min) to get the total caloric expenditure:

15.75 kcal per min · 135 min
    = 2,126.25 total kcal per week

f. Divide by 3,500 to get pounds of fat:

2,126.25 kcal ÷ 3,500
    = 0.6075 pounds of fat per week

g. Divide 10 pounds by 0.6075 pounds of fat per week to get how many weeks it will take him to lose 10 pounds of fat:

10 ÷ 0.6075 = 16.46 weeks (~16.5 weeks)

22–A. No metabolic formula is needed. The steps are as follows:

a. Multiply the number of calories per week that she is eliminating by the number of weeks:

1,200 kcal per week · 26 weeks = 31,200 total kcal

b. Now, divide by 3,500 to get the total pounds she will lose:

31,200 ÷ 3,500 total kcal
    = 8.9 (~9 pounds) over 26 weeks

23–C. No metabolic formula is needed for this question either. The steps are as follows:

a. One mile of walking or running expends approximately 100 kcal. Because she walks 1 mile three times per week, she expends approximately 300 kcal per week. Multiply 300 kcal by 26 weeks to determine the total amount of calories she expends by walking:

300 kcal per week · 26 weeks = 7,800 kcal

b. Divide 7,800 kcal by 3,500 to see how many pounds of fat this represents:

7,800 kcal ÷ 3,500 = 2.22 pounds (~2 pounds)

So, she would lose approximately 11 pounds over 26 weeks if she incorporated walking into her weight loss program.

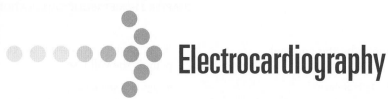

CHAPTER
12

Electrocardiography

THEODORE J. ANGELOPOULOS, DIANA LAHUE, AND ROBERT TUNG

I. Electrical Activity of the Heart and Basic Electrocardiogram (ECG) Waves

The ECG records differences in electrical potential (voltage) between two electrodes placed on the skin. The electrical conduction system is shown in *Figure 12-1*.

A. PRINCIPLES OF ELECTROPHYSIOLOGY

1. Myocardial cells can be excited in response to external electrical, chemical, and mechanical stimuli.

2. The myocardium comprises **ordinary contractile cells in the atria and ventricles as well as specialized cells** that conduct electrical impulses.

3. Cardiac impulses normally **arise in the sinoatrial (SA) or sinus node,** which is located in the right atrium near the opening of the superior vena cava.

4. From the SA node, impulses travel through the right atrium into the left atrium. Thus, the **SA node functions as the normal pacemaker.**

5. The **first phase of cardiac activation** involves electrical stimulation of the right and left atria. This in turn signals the atria to contract and to pump blood simultaneously through the tricuspid and mitral valves into the right and left ventricles.

6. The **electrical stimulus then spreads** to specialized conduction tissues in the atrioventricular (AV) junction, which includes the AV node and the bundle of His, and then into the left and right bundle branches, which transmit the stimulus to the ventricular muscle cells.

7. During the **resting period of the myocardial cell,** the inside of the cell membrane is negatively charged, and the outside of the cell membrane is positively charged. As such, the term **polarized cell** is reserved for the normal resting myocardial cell and describes the presence of electrical potential across the cell membrane because of the separation of electrical charges.

8. When an electrical impulse is generated in a particular area in the heart, the outside of the cell in this area becomes negative, and the inside of the cell in the same area becomes positive. This excited state of the cell caused by a change in polarity is called **depolarization**.

   a. Cardiac impulses originate in the SA node and spread to both atria, causing **atrial depolarization**, which is represented on the ECG by a P wave.

   b. **Ventricular depolarization** is represented on the ECG by the QRS complex.

9. **Repolarization** is the return of the stimulated myocardial cells to their resting state.

   a. **Atrial repolarization** is not usually seen on an ECG, because it is obscured by ventricular potentials.

   b. **Ventricular repolarization** is represented on the ECG by the ST segment, T wave, and U wave.

B. PRINCIPLES OF ELECTROCARDIOGRAPHY

1. The movement of ions inside and across the membrane of myocardial cells constitutes a flow of electrical charge (ionic current) that is recorded on the ECG.

2. Cardiac electrical potentials are recorded on special ECG graph paper that, under standard conditions, travels at a speed of 25 mm/s.

   a. **Horizontally, the ECG measures duration**.

      1) Each small square is 0.04 second in duration.

      2) Each large square is 0.20 second in duration.

   b. **Vertically, the ECG measures voltages.** Because ECGs are standardized, 1 mV of electrical potential registers a deflection of 10 mm in amplitude.

C. ELEMENTS OF ECG WAVEFORMS (FIGURE 12-2)

1. The **P wave** is a small positive (or negative) deflection preceding the QRS complex.

2. A **QRS complex** may be composed of a Q wave, an R wave, and an S wave.

   a. A **Q wave** is a negative deflection of the QRS complex preceding an R wave.

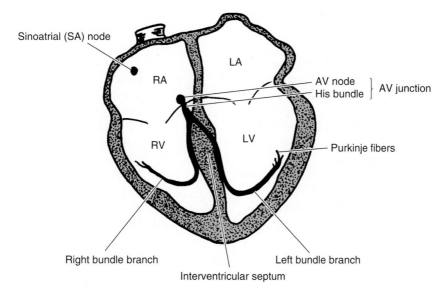

FIGURE 12-1. Conduction system of the heart. Normally, the cardiac stimulus is generated in the sinoatrial (SA) node, which is located in the right atrium (RA). The stimulus then spreads through the RA and left atrium (LA). Next, it spreads through the atrioventricular (AV) node and the bundle of His, which comprise the AV junction. The stimulus then passes into the left ventricle (LV) and right ventricle (RV) by way of the left and right bundle branches, which are continuations of the bundle of His. Finally, the cardiac stimulus spreads to the ventricular muscle cells through the Purkinje fibers. (From Goldberger AL: *Clinical Electrocardiography: A Simplified Approach,* 6th ed. St. Louis, Mosby, 1999, p 4.)

b.   An **R wave** is the first positive deflection of the QRS complex.

c.   An **S wave** is a negative deflection of the QRS complex following an R wave.

3.   The **ST segment** is that portion of the ECG from the point where the S wave of the QRS complex ends (the **J point**) to the beginning of the T wave.

a.   The ST segment should be isoelectric.

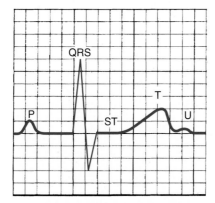

FIGURE 12-2. Basic ECG complexes. The P wave represents atrial depolarization. The PR interval is the time from initial stimulation of the atria to initial stimulation of the ventricles. The QRS represents ventricular depolarization. The ST segment, T wave, and U wave are produced by ventricular repolarization. (From Goldberger AL: *Clinical Electrocardiography: A Simplified Approach,* 6th ed. St. Louis, Mosby, 1999, p 8.)

b.   The ST segment is considered to be a **sensitive indicator of myocardial ischemia or infarction.**

4.   The **PR interval** is measured from the beginning of the P wave to the beginning of the QRS complex, and it reflects the time needed for the impulse to spread through the atria and pass through the AV junction.

a.   The normal PR interval is 0.12 to 0.20 second.

b.   A PR interval prolonged for longer than 0.20 second with all P waves being conducted and all PR intervals the same indicates **first-degree AV block.**

5.   The **QRS interval** is measured from the beginning of the first wave of the QRS complex to the end of the last wave of the QRS complex. The normal range is 0.04 to 0.11 second.

6.   The **QT interval** is measured from the beginning of the QRS complex to the end of the T wave.

a.   Normal QT intervals depend on the heart rate (HR).

b.   A prolonged QT interval may be related to certain drugs, electrolyte disturbances, and myocardial ischemia and infarction.

7.   The **T wave** represents ventricular repolarization.

a.   Normal T waves lack symmetry.

b. **Prominent peaked T waves** may indicate myocardial infarction (MI) or hyperkalemia.

c. Deep, symmetrically **inverted T waves** suggest myocardial ischemia.

8. The **U wave** represents the last phase of ventricular repolarization.

a. The U wave frequently is hard to detect in a normal ECG, but it may appear as a small deflection after the T wave.

b. U waves are prominent in hypokalemia and left ventricular hypertrophy (LVH).

c. Inverted U waves suggest ischemia.

D. THE 12-LEAD ECG

The 12-lead ECG represents 12 electrically different views of the heart recorded on special ECG paper.

1. The 12 leads can be subdivided into three groups (*Figure 12-3*).

a. **Bipolar standard leads I, II, and III**.

b. **Unipolar augmented leads aVR, aVL, and aVF**.

c. **Unipolar precordial leads V₁ through V₆**.

2. Leads I, II, III, aVR, aVL, and aVF are collectively called **limb leads**, because they record potential differences through electrodes placed on limbs.

a. **Lead I** records the difference in electrical potential between the left-arm (positive) and right-arm (negative) electrodes.

b. **Lead II** records the difference in electrical potential between the left-leg (positive) and right-arm (negative) electrodes.

c. **Lead III** records the difference in electrical potential between the left-leg (positive) and left-arm (negative) electrodes.

d. The **augmented unipolar leads** record electrical potentials at one site relative to zero potential. Electrical potentials are augmented electronically by the ECG.

1) For **lead aVR**, the positive electrode is placed on the right arm.

2) For **lead aVL**, the positive electrode is placed on the left arm.

3) For **lead aVF**, the positive electrode is placed on the left foot.

3. The six **unipolar precordial leads** view electrical activity of the heart in the horizontal

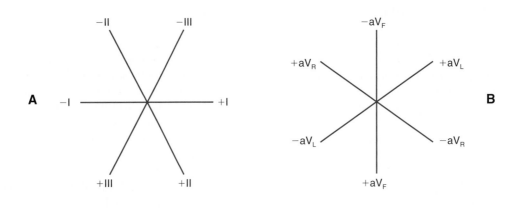

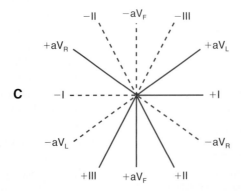

FIGURE 12-3. Derivation of hexaxial lead diagram. A. Triaxial diagram of the bipolar leads (I, II, and III). B. Triaxial diagram of the unipolar leads (aVR, aVL, and aVF). C. The two triaxial diagrams can be combined into a hexaxial diagram that shows the relationship of all six extremity leads. The negative pole of each lead is now indicated by a dashed line. (From Goldberger AL: *Clinical Electrocardiography: A Simplified Approach,* 6th ed. St. Louis, Mosby, 1999, p 26.)

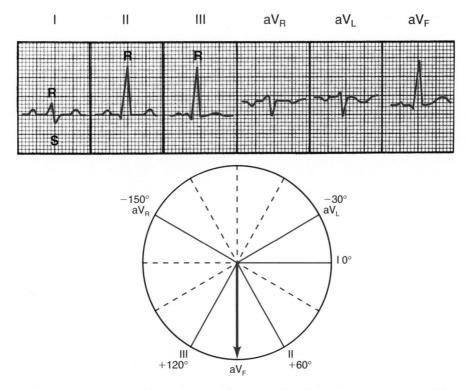

FIGURE 12-4. Mean QRS axis of +90°. (From Goldberger AL: *Clinical Electrocardiography: A Simplified Approach,* 6th ed. St. Louis, Mosby, 1999, p 46.)

plane. An electrode is placed on six different positions on the chest.

  a. **Lead V_1**: at the fourth intercostal space on the right sternal border.

  b. **Lead V_2**: at the fourth intercostal space on the left sternal border.

  c. **Lead V_3**: at the midpoint of a straight line between leads V_2 and V_4.

  d. **Lead V_4**: at the fifth intercostal space, on the left midclavicular line.

  e. **Lead V_5**: on the anterior axillary line and horizontal to lead V_4.

  f. **Lead V_6**: on the midaxillary line and horizontal to leads V_4 and V_5.

4. The **mean QRS axis** represents the average direction of depolarization as it travels through the ventricles, resulting in excitation and contraction of myocardial fibers. The mean QRS axis can be calculated simply by inspecting leads I, II, III, aVR, aVL, and aVF and then applying the following general rules:

  a. The mean QRS axis is directed midway between two leads that register tall R waves of equal amplitude.

  b. The mean QRS axis is directed at right angles (90°) to any extremity lead that registers a biphasic isoelectric complex

(e.g., in *Figure 12-4*, the mean QRS axis is +90°).

  1) Axes between −30° and +100° are normal.

  2) An axis more negative than −30° is considered to be **left-axis deviation**.

  3) An axis more positive than +100° is considered to be **right-axis deviation**.

5. **Heart rate** is the number of times that the myocardium depolarizes and contracts (beats) in 1 minute. Several techniques are available for determining HR.

  a. If the HR is regular, then the constant, 300, is divided by the number of large boxes between two consecutive QRS complexes.

  b. If the HR is irregular, then the number of cardiac cycles (one cardiac cycle is the unit between two consecutive R waves) over a 6-second period is multiplied by 10 (e.g., in *Figure 12-5*, the HR is 100 bpm).

II. Arrhythmias and Conduction Disturbances

A. SINUS ARRHYTHMIAS *(FIGURE 12-6)*

1. **Sinus bradycardia** is characterized by a normal sinus rhythm but an HR of less than 60 bpm.

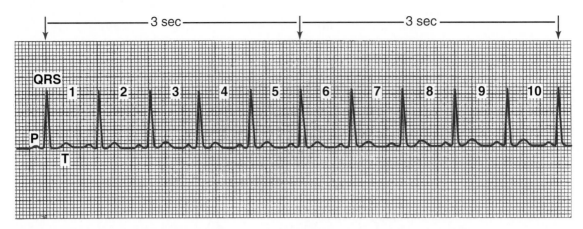

FIGURE 12-5. Measurement of heart rate (bpm) by counting the number of cardiac cycles in a 6-second interval and multiplying this number by 10. In this example, 10 cardiac cycles occur in 6 seconds. Therefore, the heart rate is 10 · 10 = 100 bpm. The arrows point to 3-second markers. (From Goldberger AL: *Clinical Electrocardiography: A Simplified Approach,* 6th ed. St. Louis, Mosby, 1999, p 16.)

2. **Sinus tachycardia** is characterized by a normal sinus rhythm but an HR of 100 to 180 bpm.
3. Under certain circumstances, the SA node does not maintain a regular sinus rate from beat to beat. This condition is called **sinus arrhythmia (respiratory arrhythmia)**.
4. The SA node may fail to depolarize the atria for pathological reasons. This condition, which is differentiated by the absence of a P wave or a QRS complex, is termed **sinus pause**, or **sinus arrest**. This condition may lead to cardiac arrest unless the AV node or some other focus assumes the role as pacemaker.

B. ATRIAL ARRHYTHMIAS
   1. Atrial Flutter and Atrial Fibrillation *(Figure 12-7)*
   a. In these arrhythmias, the atria are stimulated not from the SA node but, rather, from some ectopic focus or foci.
   b. The rate of atrial contraction varies from 250 to 350 bpm for atrial flutter and from 400 to 600 bpm for atrial fibrillation.
   c. With either atrial flutter or atrial fibrillation, the rate of ventricular depolarization depends on the rate at which the AV node conducts the supraventricular stimuli.

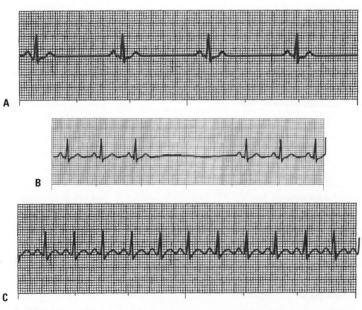

FIGURE 12-6. A. Sinus bradycardia. B. Sinus arrest. C. Sinus tachycardia. (From Aehlert B: *ECGs Made Easy Pocket Reference.* St. Louis, Mosby, 1995, p 25, 26, 29.)

carotid massage begins

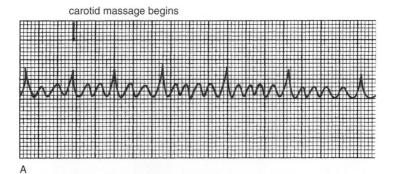

A

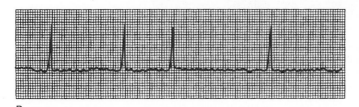

B

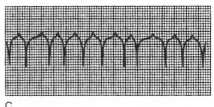

C

FIGURE 12-7. A. Atrial flutter. Carotid massage increases the block from 3:1 to 5:1. B. Atrial fibrillation with a slow, irregular ventricular rate. C. Another example of atrial fibrillation. In the absence of a clearly fibrillating baseline, the only clue that this rhythm is atrial fibrillation is the irregularly irregular appearance of the QRS complex. (From Thaler MS: *The Only EKG Book You'll Ever Need,* 3rd ed. Philadelphia, Lippincott Williams & Wilkins, 1999, pp 125–126.)

d. The presence of characteristic **"sawtooth" waves differentiates atrial flutter,** and the absence of P waves and irregular ventricular response characterizes atrial fibrillation.

e. Atrial flutter and atrial fibrillation can occur in otherwise healthy people as well as in those with heart disease.

2. **Supraventricular Tachycardia** *(Figure 12-8)*
   a. Supraventricular ectopic rhythm with an HR of 140 to 250 bpm.
   b. Distinguishing features:
      1) Regular HR.
      2) Ectopic P waves.
      3) A PR interval that may be normal.
      4) A QRS complex that typically is normal.

C. **JUNCTIONAL ARRHYTHMIA** *(FIGURE 12-9)*
   1. Supraventricular ectopic rhythm that results from a **focus of automaticity located in the bundle of His.**
   2. ECG waveform characteristics:
      a. A regular rhythm.
      b. HR of 100 to 140 bpm.
      c. Normal QRS interval.
      d. P waves (when present) possibly appearing upright or retrograde.

D. **VENTRICULAR ARRHYTHMIAS**
   1. **Premature Ventricular Complexes (PVCs)**
      a. Premature ventricular depolarizations that occur in one of the ventricles and spread to the other ventricle, with some delay

because of slow conduction through the ventricular myocardial fibers.
      1) The ventricles are not depolarized simultaneously.
      2) The duration of the QRS is 0.12 second.
   b. Cases of PVCs are **common in both apparently healthy individuals and in patients** with pathological heart disease. Common causes include emotional stress, electrolyte abnormalities, drug therapy, and myocardial ischemia and/or infarction.
   c. Decreased ectopy during exercise testing may be benign. However, **increased ectopy or onset of ventricular tachycardia** may be related to underlying pathology or other cardiac disorder.
   d. Sometimes, PVCs linked to acute MI are the forerunners of ventricular tachycardia and ventricular fibrillation.
   e. PVCs may occur with varying frequency:
      1) Two PVCs occurring in a row are referred to as a **ventricular couplet**.
      2) Three or more PVCs in a row constitute **ventricular tachycardia** *(Figure 12-10)*
      3) The repetitive pattern of one normal beat and one PVC is called **ventricular bigeminy**.
      4) The repetitive pattern of two normal beats and a PVC is called **ventricular trigeminy**.

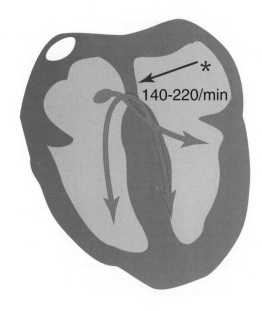

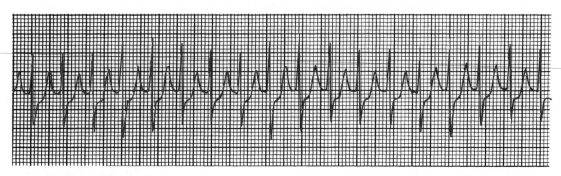

FIGURE 12-8. Atrial tachycardia. (From Davis D: *Quick and Accurate 12-Lead ECG Interpretation,* 3rd ed. Philadelphia, Lippincott Williams & Wilkins, 2001, p 412.)

5) Short, frequent bursts of nonsustained ventricular tachycardia are called **salvos**.

6) **Monomorphic ventricular tachycardia** produces ventricular beats of similar morphology (appearance).

7) **Polymorphic tachycardia** is defined by multiple forms of ventricular beats. Polymorphic tachycardias often are related to electrolyte imbalance or myocardial ischemia.

2. **Ventricular Escape**
   Ventricular beats occurring late in relation to the normal R-R cycle with a wide QRS complex.

3. **Ventricular Fibrillation**
   a. Often **triggered by the simultaneous conduction of ischemic ventricular**

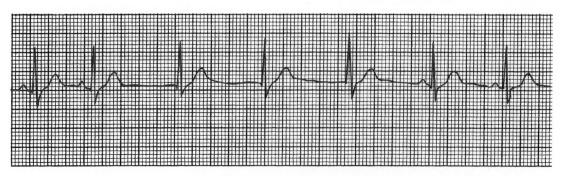

FIGURE 12-9. Sinus rhythm with three junctional escape beats. (From Davis D: *Quick and Accurate 12-Lead ECG Interpretation,* 3rd ed. Philadelphia, Lippincott Williams & Wilkins, 2001, p 408.)

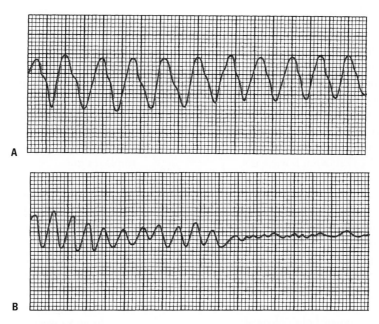

FIGURE 12-10. A. Ventricular tachycardia. The rate is approximately 200 bpm. B. Ventricular tachycardia degenerates into ventricular fibrillation. (From Thaler MS: *The Only EKG Book You'll Ever Need,* 3rd ed. Philadelphia, Lippincott Williams & Wilkins, 1999, p 132–133.)

cells with enhanced automaticity in multiple locations of the ventricles.

b. Distinguishing features:
1) Regular rhythm.
2) Ventricular rate of 150 to 500 bpm
3) Fibrillatory waves
4) Absence of a distinct QRS complex.

c. Ventricular fibrillation may occur spontaneously in patients with pathological heart disease and is considered to be the **most common cause of sudden cardiac death** in patients during an acute MI.

d. Treatment of ventricular fibrillation requires defibrillation.

E. AV BLOCKS *(FIGURE 12-11)*
Result when **supraventricular impulses are delayed or blocked in the AV node or intraventricular conduction system.**

1. First-Degree AV Block
a. Is characterized by a delay in conduction of the impulse through the AV junction to the ventricles.
b. Does not impair cardiac function.
c. Has a PR interval of longer than 0.20 seconds.
d. Causes:
1) Hyperkalemia.
2) Quinidine

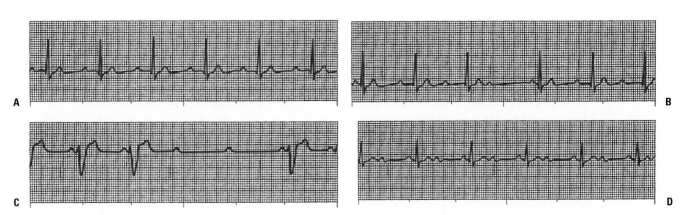

FIGURE 12-11. A. Sinus rhythm (borderline sinus bradycardia) at 60 bpm with a first-degree atrioventricular (AV) block. B. Second-degree AV block type I. C. Second-degree AV block type II. D. Second-degree AV block, 2:1 conduction, probably type I. (From Aehlert B: *ECGs Made Easy Pocket Reference.* St. Louis, Mosby, 1995, p 61– 64.)

3) Digitalis
4) Ischemic heart disease.

2. **Second-Degree AV Block**
   a. **Mobitz I (Wenckebach AV) Block**
      1) Impulse conduction through the AV junction becomes increasingly more difficult, causing a **progressively longer PR interval, until finally, a P wave is not conducted.**
         a) The ECG shows a P wave not followed by a QRS complex, which indicates that the AV junction failed to conduct the impulse from the atria to the ventricles.
         b) This pause allows the AV node to recover, and the following P wave is conducted with a normal or slightly shorter PR interval.
      2) This may be a normal physiological finding in a young athlete, and it usually disappears with the onset of exercise.
      3) Causes:
         a) Certain drugs (e.g., digitalis, calcium-channel blockers).
         b) Ischemic heart disease.
         c) Inferior wall MI.
   b. **Mobitz II Block**
      1) Is a delay in AV conduction at the level of the bundle branches.
      2) Is characterized by **fixed, normal PR intervals; broad QRS complexes; and nonconducted P waves (dropped beats).**
      3) Causes:
         a) Anterior wall MI.
         b) Severe conduction system disease.
      4) Patients may be considered as candidates for a pacemaker.

3. **Third-Degree AV Block**
   a. Also called **complete heart block,** because **no conduction of impulses occurs from the atria to the ventricles.**
   b. The PR interval changes continually, because no relationship exists between the P waves and the QRS complexes.
   c. The atria usually are under the control of the sinus node, so P waves are present with a normal atrial rate.
   d. The ventricles are paced by a pacemaker located below the point of blockage in the AV junction, so QRS complexes are seen with a ventricular rate of 30 to 60 bpm. These QRS complexes are of normal or

prolonged duration, depending on the pacemaker location.
   e. Causes:
      1) Advanced age.
      2) Digitalis intoxication.
      3) MI.
   f. Patients with third-degree AV block that is not transient (i.e., caused by digitalis intoxication) are good candidates for pacemaker implantation.

4. **Bundle Branch Blocks**
   a. **Right Bundle Branch Block (RBBB)**
      1) Represents a **delay in impulse conduction through the right bundle branch** (*Figure 12-12*).
      2) The QRS complex is widened (>0.12 second) as a result of delayed depolarization of the right ventricle.
      3) An **rSR' with a wide R wave in lead V_1** is a characteristic ECG change associated with RBBB.
      4) Although RBBB may be caused by heart disease, it also can be present in the absence of heart disease.
   b. **Left Bundle Branch Block (LBBB)**
      1) Represents a **delay in impulse conduction through the left bundle branch** (*Figure 12-13*).
      2) The impulse travels through the right bundle branch, then across the septum and depolarizes the left ventricle.
      3) The QRS complex is widened (>0.12 second) as a result of delayed depolarization of the left ventricle.
      4) **A wide negative deflection (QS) is present in lead V_1, and lead V_6 shows a wide, tall R wave.**
      5) Commonly, LBBB is associated with heart disease (e.g., coronary artery disease, hypertension, cardiomyopathy, LVH).

5. **Hemiblocks**
   Blocks involving the anterior or posterior fascicle of the main left bundle branch of the bundle of His.
   a. **Left Anterior Fascicular Block**
      1) **Blocked conduction through the anterior fascicle** of the main left bundle branch so that the impulse continues down the posterior fascicle.
      2) A mean **QRS axis of greater than −45° with a QRS duration of less than 0.12 second** suggests left anterior hemiblock.

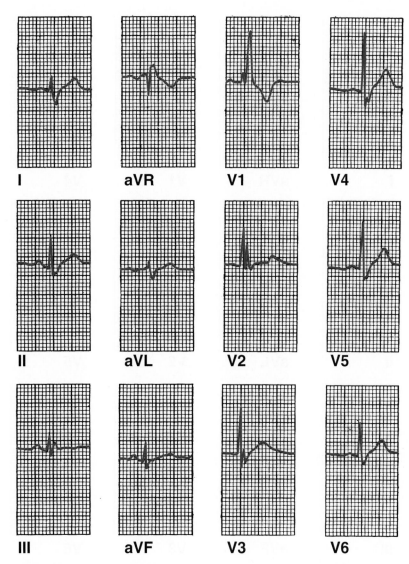

FIGURE 12-12. Right bundle branch block. (From Davis D: *Quick and Accurate 12-Lead ECG Interpretation,* 3rd ed. Philadelphia, Lippincott Williams & Wilkins, 2001, p 155.)

b. **Left Posterior Fascicular Block**
   1) **Blocked conduction through the posterior fascicle of the main left bundle branch** so that the impulse continues to travel down the posterior fascicle of the main left bundle branch.
   2) **A mean QRS axis of greater than +120° with a QRS duration of less than 0.12 second** suggests left posterior hemiblock.

III. ECG Patterns in Selected Disorders

A. CORONARY ARTERY DISEASE
In exercise ECG, which usually is performed on a treadmill or cycle ergometer, a horizontal or down-sloping ST-segment depression of at least 1 mm lasting for 0.08 second is considered to be an abnormal test finding and **may signify coronary artery disease.** T-wave abnormalities also may be seen in patients with coronary artery disease.

B. MYOCARDIAL ISCHEMIA AND INFARCTION
Myocardial ischemia may occur transiently and be limited to the inner myocardial layer (subendocardial ischemia) or affect the entire ventricular wall (transmural ischemia). If the myocardial oxygen supply remains inadequate, injury (necrosis) will occur. **Myocardial infarction is myocardial injury caused by severe or prolonged ischemia.** *Table 12-1* summarizes the ECG leads associated with various areas of myocardial injury.

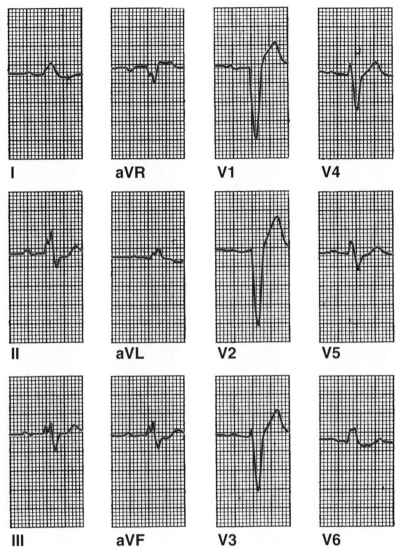

FIGURE 12-13. Left bundle branch block. (From Davis D: *Quick and Accurate 12-Lead ECG Interpretation,* 3rd ed. Philadelphia, Lippincott Williams & Wilkins, 2001, p 159.)

Figures 12-14 and *12-15* illustrate anterior and inferior infarction, respectively.

1. **Transmural Ischemia with MI**

   Transmural MI (also called STEMI) is associated with changes in both the QRS and ST-T complexes.

   a. **ST-segment elevation or tall, upright T waves are the earliest sign of transmural MI.**

   b. ST-segment elevations may persist for a few hours to a few days. During this period, Q waves form in leads with ST-segment elevations.

   c. During the evolving phase, ST-segment elevations may return to baseline, and T waves may become inverted.

   d. **Q waves may persist for years** following a transmural MI. However, their amplitude decreases, and in some cases, they may disappear.

   e. In most cases, inverted T waves persist indefinitely over the infarcted area following a transmural MI.

      1) Transmural MIs are localized to a specific portion of the left ventricular wall supplied by one of the coronary arteries:

         a) Left anterior descending artery.

         b) Right coronary artery.

         c) Left circumflex artery.

TABLE 12-1. Localization of MIs

Anterior infarction:	Q waves in leads V_1, V_2, V_3, and V_4
Inferior infarction:	Q waves in leads II, III, and aVF
Lateral infarction:	Q waves in leads I, aVL, V_5, and V_6
Posterior infarction:	Tall R waves in leads V_1 and V_2

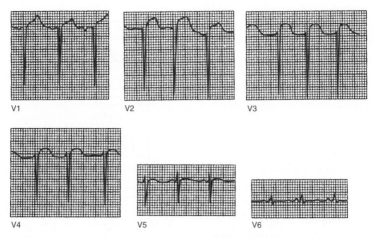

FIGURE 12-14. An anterior infarction with poor R-wave progression across the precordium. (From Thaler MS: *The Only EKG Book You'll Ever Need,* 3rd ed. Philadelphia, Lippincott Williams & Wilkins, 1999, p 221.)

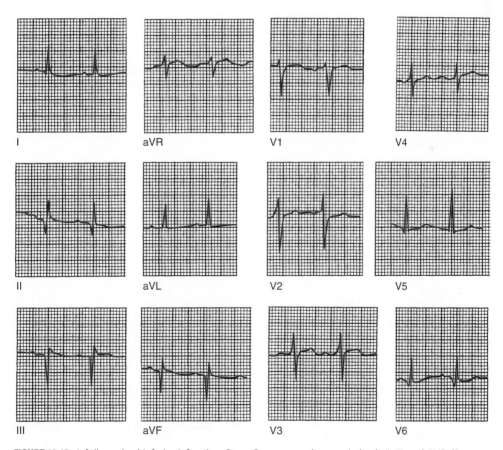

FIGURE 12-15. A fully evolved inferior infarction. Deep Q waves can be seen in leads II, III, and AVF. (From Thaler MS: *The Only EKG Book You'll Ever Need,* 3rd ed. Philadelphia, Lippincott Williams & Wilkins, 1999, p 219.)

2) A transmural MI can be diagnosed by the presence of abnormal Q waves (>0.04 second and at least 25% of the height of the R wave).

3) Q waves in leads V_1 and V_2 should be examined carefully, because they may be a normal variant or may signify anteroseptal MI.

4) MI can be determined and localized by viewing certain ECG leads (e.g., tall R waves in leads V_1 and V_2 may suggest posterior wall MI or right ventricular hypertrophy).

2. Subendocardial Ischemia and Infarction

a. **Subendocardial ischemia usually produces ST-segment depression in anterior leads, inferior leads, or both,** commonly during attacks of typical angina pectoris.

b. A horizontal or down-sloping ST-segment depression of 1 mm or greater lasting 0.08 second is considered to be an abnormal response during exercise ECG and constitutes a positive exercise test.

c. Severe subendocardial ischemia may lead to **subendocardial infarction** (also called non-STEMI) marked by persistent ST-segment depression, possible T-wave inversion, and usually, normal Q waves.

3. Ischemia or Infarction Location

The location of ischemia or the area of infarction can be identified by previously mentioned ECG changes as follows:

a. Inferior infarction: leads II, III, and aVF.

b. Anteroseptal infarction: leads V_1 and V_2.

c. Anterior infarction: leads V_2 through V_5.

d. Anterolateral infarction: leads V_2 through V_6, aVL, and I.

e. Lateral infarction: I and aVL.

4. Differentiation Between Q-Wave and Non-Q-Wave MI (NQWMI)

a. NQWMI is a clinical syndrome of acute chest pain, enzyme evidence of infarction, but lack of Q waves on the surface ECG.

b. Q-wave MI is demonstrated and diagnosed by Q-waves on the surface ECG.

c. Also called STEMI and non-STEMI.

C. ATRIAL ENLARGEMENT

1. **Left atrial enlargement** is best demonstrated in lead V_1.

a. A wide P wave of longer than 0.12 second is seen (*Figure 12-16B*).

b. P wave voltage is normal or slightly increased.

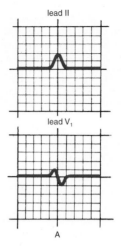
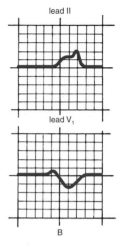

FIGURE 12-16. A. The normal P wave in leads II and V_1. B. Left atrial enlargement. Note the increased amplitude and duration of the terminal, left atrial component of the P wave. (From Thaler MS: *The Only EKG Book You'll Ever Need,* 3rd ed. Philadelphia, Lippincott Williams & Wilkins, 1999, p 80.)

c. Sometimes, the terminal portion of the P wave, which represents left atrial depolarization, shows a distinct, wide, negative deflection. As such, lead V_1 may show a biphasic P wave.

d. Wide P waves often are referred to as **P mitrale**, because they often are seen in patients with rheumatic mitral valve disease.

2. **Right atrial enlargement** is best detected in lead II (*Figure 12-17B*).

a. P-wave amplitude may be increased to greater than 2.5 mm.

b. P-wave duration may be normal.

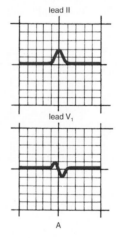
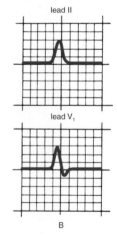

FIGURE 12-17. A. The normal P wave in leads II and V_1. B. Right atrial enlargement. Note the increased amplitude of the early, right atrial component of the P wave. The terminal left atrial component (and, hence, the overall duration of the P wave) is essentially unchanged. (From Thaler MS: *The Only EKG Book You'll Ever Need,* 3rd ed. Philadelphia, Lippincott Williams & Wilkins, 1999, p 79.)

c. The tall P wave seen in right atrial enlargement is called **P pulmonale**, because it is common in patients with pulmonary disease.

D. VENTRICULAR HYPERTROPHY

An increase in the size of either ventricular wall may produce high voltages in the leads over the hypertrophied area.

1. **Left Ventricular Hypertrophy (Figure 12-18)**
   a. Usually associated with abnormally **tall R waves in the left chest leads** and abnormally **deep S waves in the right chest leads.**
   b. Voltage criteria for the diagnosis of LVH:
      1) S wave in lead V_1 plus R wave in lead V_5 or V_6 of greater than 35 mm.
      2) R wave in lead aVL of greater than 11 mm.
   c. ST-segment changes and T-wave inversions usually are present in leads with tall R waves.
   d. Commonly, LVH is associated with conditions such as aortic stenosis and systemic hypertension.

2. **Right Ventricular Hypertrophy (RVH) (Figure 12-19)**
   a. Associated with high voltages in leads V_1 and V_2 and, possibly, an R wave greater than the S wave in these leads.

b. RVH also causes right-axis deviation as well as ST-segment changes and T-wave inversions in right chest leads.

E. PERICARDITIS

Acute pericarditis (inflammation of the pericardium) is associated with **diffuse ST-segment elevation** (in contrast to the localized ST-segment elevation seen in acute MI), possibly followed by T-wave inversion (*Figure 12-20*).

F. PULMONARY DISEASE

Patients with emphysema (chronic lung disease) often exhibit ECG changes, such as:
1. Low voltage.
2. Poor R-wave progression in chest leads.
3. A vertical or rightward QRS axis.

G. HYPERTENSIVE HEART DISEASE

1. Commonly causes LVH that eventually leads to left atrial enlargement.
2. Patients with long-standing hypertensive disease often develop LBBB and, in some cases, atrial fibrillation.

H. HYPERVENTILATION

1. Fast, deep breathing for approximately 20 seconds.

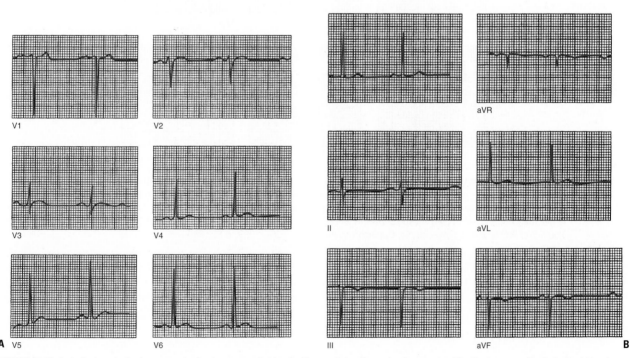

FIGURE 12-18. A. Left ventricular hypertrophy in the precordial leads. Three of the four criteria are met: The R-wave amplitude in lead V_5 plus the S-wave amplitude in lead V_1 exceeds 35 mm, the R-wave amplitude in lead V_6 exceeds 18 mm, and the R-wave amplitude in lead V_6 slightly exceeds the R-wave amplitude in lead V_5. The only criterion not met is for the R wave in lead V_5 to exceed 26 mm. B. Left ventricular hypertrophy in the limb leads. Criteria 1, 3 and 4 are met; only criterion 2, regarding the R-wave amplitude in lead AVF, is not met. (From Thaler MS: *The Only EKG Book You'll Ever Need,* 3rd ed. Philadelphia, Lippincott Williams & Wilkins, 1999, p 85, 86.)

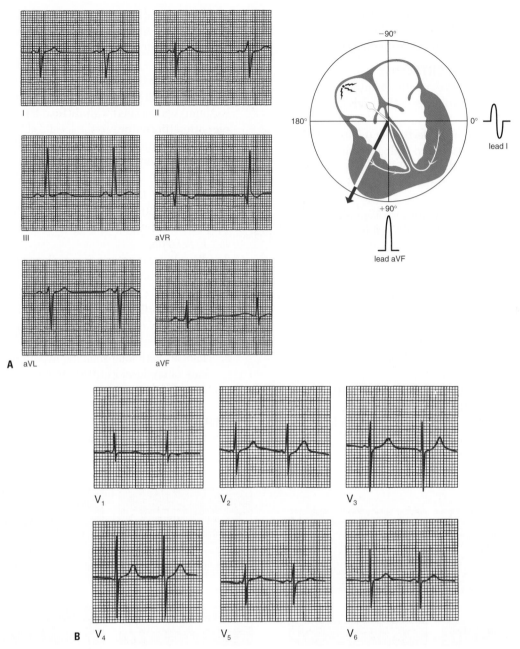

FIGURE 12-19. A. Right ventricular hypertrophy shifts the axis of the QRS complex to the right. The EKG tracings confirm right-axis deviation. In addition, the QRS complex in lead I is slightly negative, a criterion that many believe is essential for properly establishing the diagnosis of right ventricular hypertrophy. B. In lead V_1, the R wave is larger than the S wave. In lead V_6, the S wave is larger than the R wave. (From Thaler MS: *The Only EKG Book You'll Ever Need*, 3rd ed. Philadelphia, Lippincott Williams & Wilkins, 1999, p 82, 83.)

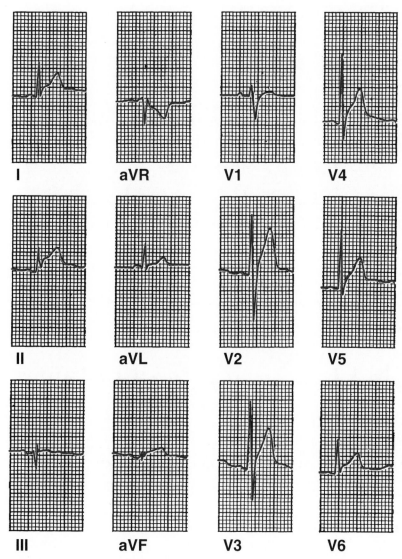

I	aVR	V1	V4

II	aVL	V2	V5

III	aVF	V3	V6

FIGURE 12-20. Pericarditis. (From Davis D: *Quick and Accurate 12-Lead ECG Interpretation,* 3rd ed. Philadelphia, Lippincott Williams & Wilkins, 2001, p 248.)

2. This procedure is performed before or after a stress test, and any ECG changes are noted.

3. Typical ECG changes may include **ST-segment and T-wave abnormalities in all leads** (*Figure 12-21*).

I. ELECTROLYTE ABNORMALITIES

1. **Hypokalemia** produces ST-segment depression with prominent U waves and flattened T waves (*Figure 12-22*).

2. **Hyperkalemia** produces predictable ECG changes depending on severity (*Figure 12-23*).
   a. Mild hyperkalemia causes narrowing and peaking of T waves.
   b. Moderate hyperkalemia is marked by prolonged PR intervals and small or, sometimes, absent P waves.

   c. Severe hyperkalemia produces wide QRS complexes and asystole.

3. **Hypocalcemia** produces prolonged QT intervals (*Figure 12-24*).

4. **Hypercalcemia** shortens ventricular repolarization and, thus, shortens the QT interval (*Figure 12-24*).

J. DRUG THERAPY

1. **Digitalis**, which is used to treat heart failure and arrhythmias, can produce a shortened QT interval and scooped ST-T complex (*Figure 12-25*). Digitalis toxicity often results in arrhythmias and conduction disturbances.

2. **Quinidine, procainamide**, and **disopyramide**, which are used to treat arrhythmias, can produce prolonged QT intervals and flattened T waves.

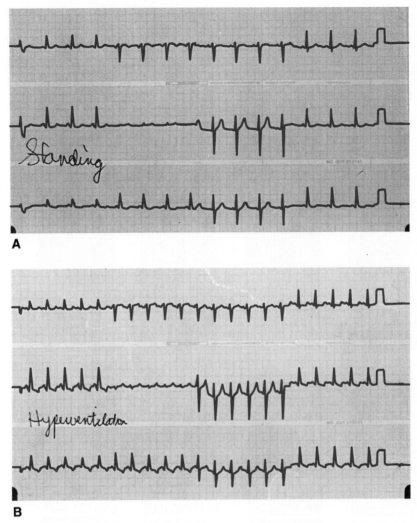

FIGURE 12-21. A. Resting ECG. B. ECG showing results of hyperventilation (inverted T waves).

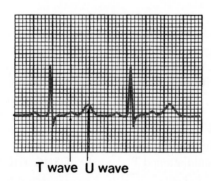

T wave U wave

FIGURE 12-22. Hypokalemia. The U waves are even more prominent than the T waves. (From Thaler MS: *The Only EKG Book You'll Ever Need,* 3rd ed. Philadelphia, Lippincott Williams & Wilkins, 1999, p 247.)

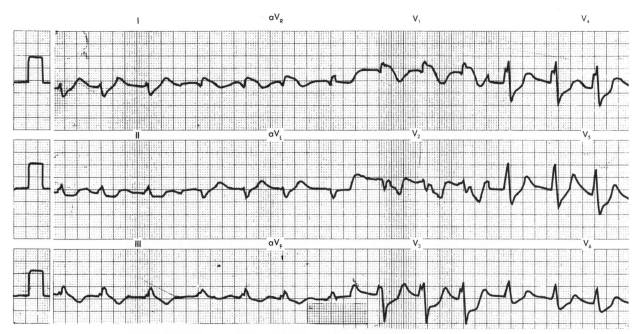

FIGURE 12-23. Marked hyperkalemia. The ECG is of a patient with a serum potassium concentration of 8.5 mEq/L. Note the absence of P waves and the presence of bizarre, wide QRS complexes. (From Goldberger AL: *Clinical Electrocardiography: A Simplified Approach,* 6th ed. St. Louis, Mosby, 1999, p 118.)

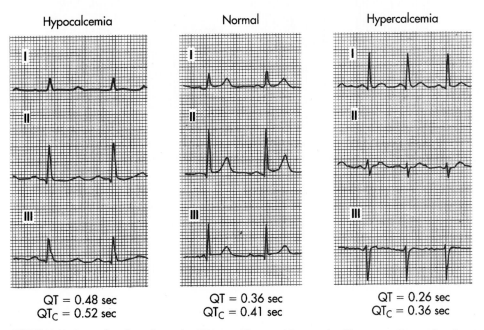

Hypocalcemia	Normal	Hypercalcemia
QT = 0.48 sec	QT = 0.36 sec	QT = 0.26 sec
QT$_C$ = 0.52 sec	QT$_C$ = 0.41 sec	QT$_C$ = 0.36 sec

FIGURE 12-24. Hypocalcemia prolongs the QT interval by stretching out the ST segment. Hypercalcemia decreases the QT interval by shortening the ST segment so that the T wave seems to take off directly from the end of the QRS complex. (From Goldberger AL: *Clinical Electrocardiography: A Simplified Approach,* 6th ed. St. Louis, Mosby, 1999, p 120.)

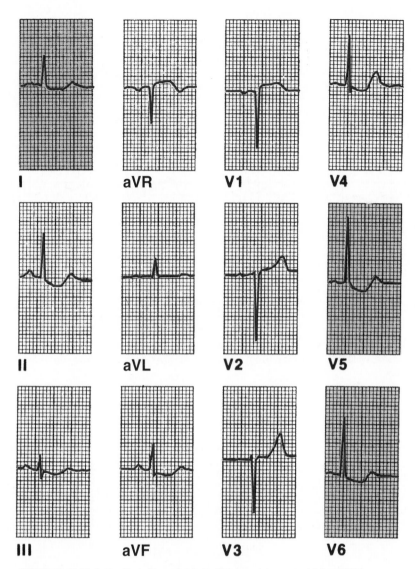

FIGURE 12-25. Digitalis effect. (From Davis D: *Quick and Accurate 12-Lead ECG Interpretation,* 3rd ed. Philadelphia, Lippincott Williams & Wilkins, 2001, p 263.)

Review Test

DIRECTIONS: Carefully read all questions, and select the BEST single answer.

1. Slow conduction in the AV node is associated with
    A)   Prolonged PR interval.
    B)   Prolonged QRS interval.
    C)   Shortened QT interval.
    D)   Elevated ST segment.

2. Examine the six extremity leads shown in the figure below. What is the appropriate mean QRS axis?
    A)   −30°.
    B)   60°.
    C)   90°.
    D)   120°.

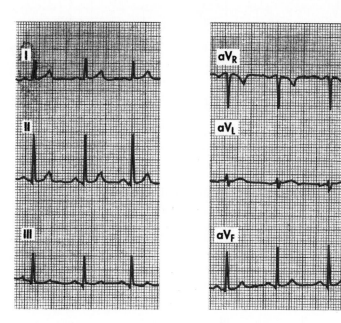

(From Goldberger AL: *Clinical Electrocardiography: A Simplified Approach,* 6th ed. St. Louis, Mosby, 1999, p 55.)

3. In the ECG shown on the following page, which of the following conduction abnormalities is indicated?
    A)   RBBB.
    B)   Third-degree AV block.
    C)   First-degree AV block.
    D)   Mobitz I.

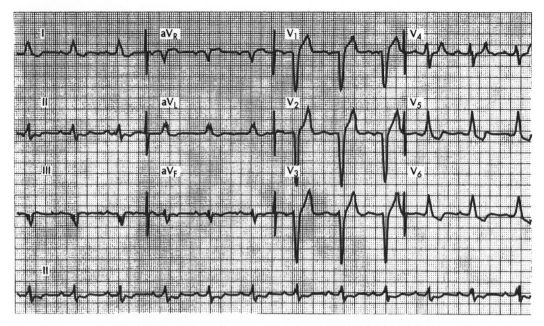

(From Goldberger AL: *Clinical Electrocardiography: A Simplified Approach,* 6th ed. St. Louis, Mosby, 1999, p 80.)

4. What condition can cause ST-segment elevation?
    A) Digitalis toxicity.
    B) Hypocalcemia.
    C) Hypokalemia.
    D) Acute pericarditis.

5. In the ECG strip shown below, what disorder is indicated?
    A) Acute pericarditis.
    B) Inferior MI.
    C) Posterior MI.
    D) Anterior MI.

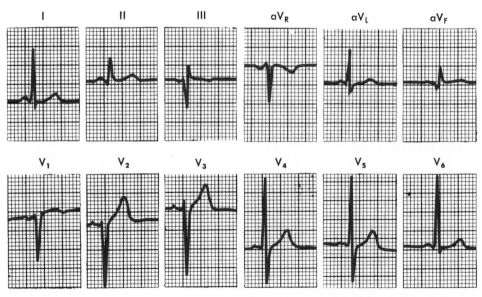

(From Goldberger AL: *Clinical Electrocardiography: A Simplified Approach,* 6th ed. St. Louis, Mosby, 1999, p 91.)

6. In the ECG strip shown below, what disorder is indicated?
   A) Subendocardial ischemia.
   B) Transmural ischemia.
   C) Acute inferior MI.
   D) Posterior MI.

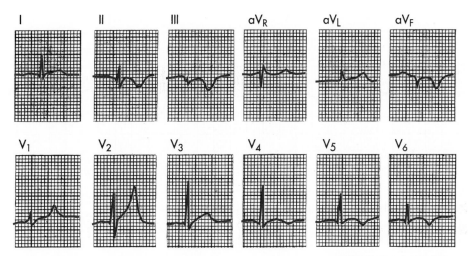

(From Goldberger AL: *Clinical Electrocardiography: A Simplified Approach,* 6th ed. St. Louis, Mosby, 1999, p 91.)

7. In the ECG strip shown below, what abnormality is indicated?
   A) LBBB.
   B) Posterior wall MI.
   C) RBBB.
   D) LVH.

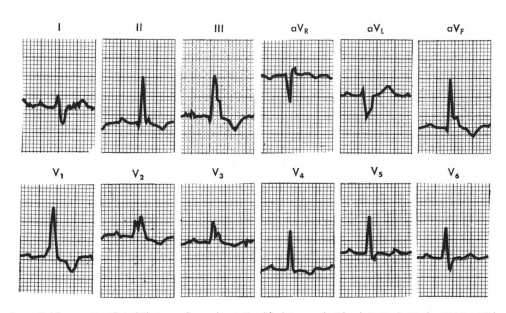

(From Goldberger AL: *Clinical Electrocardiography: A Simplified Approach,* 6th ed. St. Louis, Mosby, 1999, p 70.)

8. Subendocardial ischemia usually produces
   A) ST-segment elevation.
   B) ST-segment depression.
   C) Q waves.
   D) U waves.

9. In the ECG strip shown below, which arrhythmia is present?
    A) Premature ventricular contractions.
    B) Ventricular tachycardia.
    C) Ventricular trigeminy.
    D) Ventricular bigeminy.

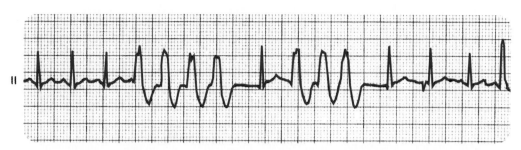

(From Goldberger AL: *Clinical Electrocardiography: A Simplified Approach,* 6th ed. St. Louis, Mosby, 1999, p 167.)

10. In the ECG strip shown below, which arrhythmia is indicated?
    A) Atrial flutter.
    B) Atrial fibrillation.
    C) Premature atrial contractions.
    D) Atrial tachycardia.

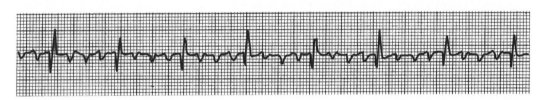

(From Goldberger AL: *Clinical Electrocardiography: A Simplified Approach,* 6th ed. St. Louis, Mosby, 1999, p 164.)

11. Abnormally tall and peaked T waves suggest which of the following?
    A) Hyperkalemia.
    B) Acute pericarditis.
    C) Acute MI.
    D) Hypokalemia.

12. Which of the following conditions can prolong the QT interval?
    A) Hypokalemia and hypercalcemia.
    B) Hyperkalemia and hypercalcemia.
    C) Hypocalcemia and hypokalemia.
    D) Hypocalcemia and hyperkalemia.

13. Differentiation between supraventricular and ventricular rhythm is made on the basis of the
    A) Duration (width) of the QRS complex and the presence or absence of P waves.
    B) Appearance of the ST segment.
    C) Amplitude of the U wave.
    D) Duration of the PR interval.

14. Which of the following is one cause of a wide QRS complex?
    A) Hypokalemia.
    B) Defective intraventricular conduction.
    C) Right atrial enlargement.
    D) Abnormal ST segment.

15. In response to various stimuli, movements of ions occur, causing the rapid loss of the internal negative potential. This process is known as
    A) Polarization.
    B) Repolarization.
    C) Automaticity.
    D) Depolarization.

16. Digitalis effect refers to
    A) Scooped-out depression of the ST segment produced by digitalis.
    B) Elevation of the PR interval produced by digitalis.
    C) Shortening of the QT interval produced by digitalis.
    D) Prolongation of the QRS complex produced by digitalis.

17. Tall, positive T waves may be caused to all of the following EXCEPT
    A) Hyperacute phase of MI.
    B) LVH.
    C) Acute pericarditis.
    D) Hypocalcemia.

18. In the ECG strip shown below, what abnormalities are indicated?
    A) Left atrial enlargement and LVH.
    B) Right atrial enlargement and right ventricular hypertrophy.
    C) Left anterior fascicular block and left posterior fascicular block.
    D) Subendocardial ischemia and infarction.

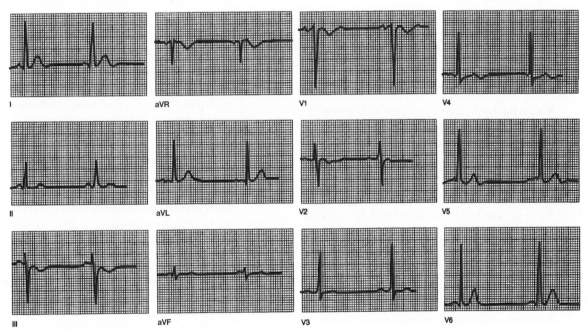

(From Thaler MS: *The Only EKG Book You'll Ever Need,* 3rd ed. Philadelphia, Lippincott Williams & Wilkins, 1999, p 87.)

19. Right-axis deviation may be caused by
    A) Acute pericarditis.
    B) Right atrial enlargement.
    C) Chronic obstructive pulmonary disease.
    D) Cardiomyopathy.

20. In atrial flutter, the stimulation rate is approximately
    A) 75 bpm.
    B) 125 bpm.
    C) 200 bpm.
    D) 300 bpm.

21. Myocardial cells can be excited in response to all
    of the following stimuli EXCEPT
    A) Electrical.
    B) Chemical.
    C) Mechanical.
    D) Emotional.

22. The P wave on the ECG can be
    A) Negative.
    B) Positive.
    C) Isoelectric.
    D) Either positive or negative.

ANSWERS AND EXPLANATIONS

1–A. The PR interval represents the time that it takes for the stimulus to spread through the atria and pass through the AV junction. As such, slow conduction in the AV node affects the PR interval. Slow conduction through the AV node is not associated with the duration of the QRS complex or the QT interval.

2–B. The mean QRS axis is 60°. Note the biphasic QRS complex in lead aVL. As such, the mean QRS axis must point at a right angle to −30°. Obviously, it points at 60°, because leads II, III, and aVF show positive QRS complexes.

3–C. Notice the QS in lead V_1 and the wide R wave in lead V_6. The PR interval is prolonged (>0.20 second). As such, first-degree AV block is present. There is no progressive PR prolongation with a nonconducted P wave; therefore, Mobitz I is not present.

4–D. Acute pericarditis is associated with ST-segment elevations. Digitalis produces scooping of the ST-T complex. Hypokalemia produces ST-segment depression, and hypocalcemia prolongs the QT interval.

5–B. Note the Q waves in leads II, III, and aVF. Posterior infarction produces tall R waves in leads V_1 and V_2. Anterior MI results in the loss of R-wave progression in the precordial leads and pathological waves in one or more of the chest leads. Acute pericarditis produces diffuse ST-segment elevations.

6–D. Note the tall R waves in leads V_1 and V_2. Also, note the Q waves in leads III and aVF. Acute inferior MI produces ST-segment elevation in leads II, III, and aVF.

7–C. Note the wide, notched R wave in lead V_2 and the secondary T-wave inversions in leads V_1, V_2, II, III, and aVF. Left bundle branch block produces a wide QS in lead V_1 and a wide R wave in lead V_6. Posterior wall MI produces tall R waves in leads V_1 and V_2 with ST-segment depression in the same leads. Left ventricular hypertrophy produces high voltages, marked by tall R waves in lead V_5 or V_6 and deep S waves in lead V_1 or V_2.

8–B. Subendocardial ischemia usually produces ST-segment depression. ST-segment elevations usually appear in transmural ischemia, pericarditis, and acute MI. Q waves appear following transmural MI, and U waves often are seen in hypokalemia.

9–B. Ventricular tachycardia is defined as a run of three or more consecutive premature ventricular contractions (PVCs). In ventricular bigeminy, each normal sinus impulse is followed by a PVC. In ventricular trigeminy, a PVC is seen after every two sinus impulses.

10–A. Atrial flutter is characterized by "sawtooth" flutter waves instead of P waves and a constant or variable ventricular rate. Atrial fibrillation shows fibrillatory waves instead of P waves and an irregular ventricular rate. Atrial tachycardia is defined as three or more consecutive premature atrial beats.

11–A. Moderate hyperkalemia is often accompanied by abnormally tall and peaked T waves. Hypokalemia often produces ST-segment depression with prominent U waves.

12–D. Hypokalemia often produces low-amplitude T waves and, sometimes, large U waves, which merge and result in a prolonged QT interval.

Hypocalcemia primarily prolongs the ST segment, resulting in a prolonged QT interval. Hyperkalemia causes narrowed and peaked T waves.

13–A. A narrow QRS complex (<0.1 second) indicates that the entire ventricular myocardium was depolarized quickly. This can occur only if electrical activation spreads along the ventricular conduction system. A wide QRS complex (>0.10 second) suggests that electrical activation required considerable time to spread. As such, the impulse did not use the ventricular conduction system to travel. The duration of the PR interval is an indication of the time required for the impulse to travel from the SA node down to the AV node. The ST segment represents the beginning of ventricular repolarization, and U waves are characteristic of hypokalemia or drug therapy.

14–B. A lesion in the ventricular conduction system will cause a slower spread of activation throughout the ventricles, leading to a wide QRS complex. Hypokalemia does not affect the duration of the QRS complex. Hypokalemia produces ST-segment depressions and prominent U waves. The ST segment represents the beginning of ventricular repolarization and is not related to the duration of the QRS complex.

15–D. In response to various stimuli, cations (mainly sodium) move inward, causing rapid loss of the internal negative potential. This process is known as depolarization. Polarization refers to the resting state of cardiac muscle cells where the interior of a cell is more negative compared to the exterior. Repolarization is the return of cardiac muscle cells to their resting negative potential. Automaticity refers to the ability of the heart to initiate its own beat.

16–A. Digitalis effect refers to the characteristic scooped-out depression of the ST segment produced by therapeutic doses of digitalis. A therapeutic dose of digitalis does not produce ST-segment elevation. ST-segment elevations often are observed in myocardial ischemia or infarction, acute pericarditis, hyperkalemia, and LVH. Hypercalcemia often is associated with shortening of the QT interval caused by shortening of the ST segment.

17–D. The hyperacute phase of a MI often produces tall, positive T waves. Tall, positive T waves also are seen in LVH (left precordial leads). Acute pericarditis is occasionally associated with tall T waves.

18–A. Left atrial enlargement is manifested by P-wave duration of greater than 0.11 second, P-wave notching, and negative P-wave deflection in lead V_1. Left ventricular hypertrophy is demonstrated by large R waves (>27 mm) in lead V_5 and deep waves in lead V_1. Left anterior hemiblock is associated with a mean QRS axis of $-45°$ and a QRS width of less than 0.12 second.

19–C. Chronic obstructive pulmonary disease causes right-axis deviation because of right ventricular overload. Any cause of right ventricular hypertrophy (e.g., pulmonic stenosis, primary pulmonary hypertension) also is associated with right-axis deviation. Cardiomyopathy is associated with dilation and, usually, with diffuse fibrosis.

20–D. With atrial flutter, the atrial stimulation rate is approximately 300 bpm, and the ventricular rate varies depending on the ability of the AV junction to transmit stimuli from the atria to the ventricles. In atrial flutter, the ventricular rate may not vary.

21–D. All myocardial cells can be stimulated by external electrical, chemical, and mechanical stimuli. The myocardium comprises ordinary contractile cells located in the atria and ventricles as well as specialized cells that conduct the impulses.

22–D. The P wave on the ECG can be either positive or negative, depending on the lead. For example, the P wave is always negative in a normal aVR lead and always positive in a normal V_6 lead.

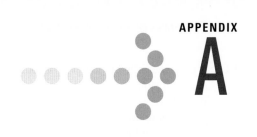
Health and Fitness Comprehensive Exam

DIRECTIONS: Each of the numbered items or incomplete statements in this section is followed by answers or by completions of the statement. Select the ONE lettered answer or completion that is BEST in each case.

1. Which of the following exercise modes allows buoyancy to reduce the potential for musculoskeletal injury and even allows an injured person an opportunity to exercise without further injury?
   A) Cycling.
   B) Walking.
   C) Skiing.
   D) Water exercise.

2. In the first 2 seconds of a 100-m race, on which of the following energy systems does skeletal muscle rely most heavily?
   A) ATP/PC.
   B) Anaerobic glycolysis.
   C) Oxidative phosphorylation.
   D) Free fatty acid metabolism.

3. Which of the following types of medications is designed to control blood lipids, especially cholesterol?
   A) Nitrates.
   B) α-Blockers.
   C) Antihyperlipidemics.
   D) β-Blockers.

4. Which of the following represents more than 90% of the fat stored in the body and is composed of a glycerol molecule connected to three fatty acids?
   A) Phospholipids.
   B) Cholesterol.
   C) Triglycerides.
   D) Free fatty acids.

5. Limited flexibility of which of the following muscle groups increases the risk of low back pain?
   A) Quadriceps.
   B) Hamstrings.
   C) Hip flexors.
   D) Biceps femoris.

6. Calcium, phosphorus, magnesium, potassium, sulfur, sodium, and chloride are examples of
   A) Macrominerals.
   B) Microminerals.
   C) Proteins.
   D) Vitamins.

7. Which of the following terms represents an imaginary horizontal plane passing through the midsection of the body and dividing it into upper and lower portions?
   A) Sagittal.
   B) Frontal.
   C) Transverse.
   D) Superior.

8. Which of the following is a function of bone?
   A) Provides structural support for the entire body.
   B) Serves as a lever that can change the magnitude and direction of forces generated by skeletal muscles.
   C) Protects organs and tissues.
   D) All of the above.

9. An elevation of either the systolic or diastolic blood pressure is classified as hypertension. This elevation must be measured on two different days, preferably several days apart. To be classified as hypertension, the blood pressure should be more than
   A) 100/60 mm Hg.
   B) 110/70 mm Hg.
   C) 120/80 mm Hg.
   D) 140/90 mm Hg.

10. The term **risk stratification** refers to
    A) The ability of the client to take airplane rides.
    B) The ability of the client to perform high-intensity exercise.
    C) The placing of clients into risk categories based on disease identification.
    D) The identification of latent or overt coronary artery disease.

11. Uncoordinated gait, headache, dizziness, vomiting, and elevated body temperature are signs and symptoms of
    A) Acute exposure to the cold.
    B) Hypothermia.
    C) Heat exhaustion and heat stroke.
    D) Acute altitude sickness.

12. A movement that decreases the joint angle is called
    A) Flexion.
    B) Extension.
    C) Abduction.
    D) Adduction.

13. Which of the following energy systems is capable of using all three fuels (carbohydrates, fats, and proteins)?
    A) Anaerobic glycolysis.
    B) Lactic acid system.
    C) Phosphagen system.
    D) Aerobic system.

14. How many calories will a 116.6-pound woman expend if she pedals on a Monark cycle ergometer at 50 rpm against a resistance of 2.5 kp for 30 minutes?
    A) 226.7 calories.
    B) 258.3 calories.
    C) 512 calories.
    D) 216 calories.

15. Relative proportions of fat and fat-free (lean) tissue can be assessed and reported as
    A) Percentage body fat.
    B) Relative composition.
    C) Hydrodensitometry.
    D) Near-infrared interactance.

16. Which of the following is/are characteristic(s) of an effective exercise leader or health/fitness instructor?
    A) The health/fitness instructor should be a resource for up-to-date, accurate information regarding health and fitness.
    B) The health/fitness instructor should be able to dispel myths and quackery regarding exercise.
    C) The health/fitness instructor is able to create an atmosphere and an opportunity for learning.
    D) All of the above.

17. The interconnected sacs and tubes surrounding each myofibril in which calcium ions are stored are referred to as
    A) Terminal cisternae.
    B) Sarcomeres.
    C) Myofilaments.
    D) Sarcoplasmic reticulum.

18. Anaerobic glycolysis also is known as the
    A) Phosphagen system.
    B) Aerobic metabolism.
    C) Lactic acid system.
    D) None of the above

19. Which of the following is true regarding changes in cardiac output during submaximal exercise at the same workload as a result of regular, chronic exercise?
    A) Cardiac output increases.
    B) Cardiac output decreases.
    C) Cardiac output stays the same.
    D) Cardiac output increases only during dynamic exercise.

20. Which of the following conditions is characterized by a decrease in bone mass and density, producing bone porosity and fragility?
    A) Osteoarthritis.
    B) Osteomyelitis.
    C) Epiphyseal osteomyelitis.
    D) Osteoporosis.

21. Studies designed to measure the success of a program based on some quantifiable data that can be analyzed examine
    A) Incomes.
    B) Outcomes.
    C) Client progress notes.
    D) Attendance records.

22. The Rating of Perceived Exertion (RPE) scale is considered to be an adjunct to using heart rate as a guide to exercise intensity. In general, when using the original Borg scale for the general public, intensity should be maintained between
    A) 7 and 10.
    B) 12 and 16.
    C) 16 and 20.
    D) 18 and 21.

23. Muscle fibers that can produce a large amount of tension in a very short period of time but fatigue quickly are referred to as
    A) Slow-twitch glycolytic.
    B) Fast-twitch glycolytic.
    C) Fast-twitch oxidative.
    D) Slow-twitch oxidative.

24. Rotation of the anterior surface of a bone toward the midline of the body is called
    A) Medial rotation.
    B) Lateral rotation.
    C) Supination.
    D) Pronation.

25. As each primary bronchus enters the lung, secondary bronchi branch off, with smaller and smaller branches continuing to branch off until the smallest narrow passage is formed, which is called the
    A) Lobes.
    B) Trachea.
    C) Bronchiole.
    D) Nasopharynx.

26. Cardiac output can be calculated by multiplying
    A) Heart rate and stroke volume.
    B) Stroke volume and the difference between the oxygen-carrying capacity of the arterial blood and venous blood.
    C) Oxygen consumption and heart rate.
    D) Heart rate and blood volume.

27. The initial cause of coronary artery disease is thought to be an irritation of, or an injury to, the tunica intima (innermost of the three layers in the wall) of the blood vessel. A source or sources of this initial injury may be
    A) Dyslipidemia.
    B) Hypertension.
    C) Turbulence of blood flow within the vessel.
    D) All of the above.

28. Which of the following is NOT considered to be an independent risk factor in the development of cardiovascular disease?
    A) Age (>55 years).
    B) Cigarette smoking.
    C) Being overweight.
    D) Hypertension.

29. Individuals with no signs and/or symptoms of cardiopulmonary disease but with more than two risk factors for the development of coronary artery disease, are in the
    A) Low-risk category.
    B) Moderate-risk category.
    C) High-risk category.
    D) All of the above.

30. Which of the following is NOT a contraindicated, high-risk exercise?
    A) Lateral neck stretches.
    B) Full squats.
    C) Hurdler's stretch.
    D) Full sit-ups.

31. Which of the following vitamins function(s) to maintain bone and teeth health and has/have a dietary source of dairy products?
    A) Vitamin A.
    B) Vitamin D.
    C) Vitamin K.
    D) Thiamine.

32. Each cusp of the atrioventricular (AV) valves in the heart is braced by tendinous fibers called chordae tendinae, which, in turn, are connected to special muscles on the inner surface of the ventricle, which are called
    A) Myocardial muscles.
    B) Papillary muscles.
    C) Endocardial muscles.
    D) Epicardial muscles.

33. An individual's maximal oxygen consumption ($\dot{V}O_2$max) is a measure of the power of the aerobic energy system. This value is generally regarded as the best indicator of aerobic fitness. What is the average $\dot{V}O_2$max of college-age males and females, respectively?
    A) 35 and 45 mL $\cdot$ kg^{-1} $\cdot$ min^{-1}.
    B) 45 and 35 mL $\cdot$ kg^{-1} $\cdot$ min^{-1}.
    C) 55 and 65 mL $\cdot$ kg^{-1} $\cdot$ min^{-1}.
    D) 45 mL $\cdot$ kg^{-1} $\cdot$ min^{-1} for both.

34. Cardiac muscle tissue is similar to skeletal muscle except for its ability to
    A) Summate.
    B) Tetanize.
    C) Contract.
    D) Relax.

35. Which of the following is NOT true regarding the psychological benefits of regular exercise in the elderly?
    A) Older people who exercise regularly have a more positive attitude toward their work and generally are in better health than sedentary persons.
    B) Strong correlations have been reported between the activity level of older adults and self-reported happiness.
    C) Older persons taking part in exercise programs commonly report that they find everyday tasks to be more difficult than before they began the exercise program.
    D) Older adults improve their score on self-concept questionnaires following participation in an exercise program.

36. A condition resulting from temporary or permanent reduction in blood flow in one or more coronary arteries may cause
    A) Pectoralis excavatum.
    B) Angina pectoris.
    C) Pectoralis reductum.
    D) Dysrhythmia.

37. To determine program effectiveness, psychological theories provide a conceptual framework for assessment and
    A) Development of programs or interventions.
    B) Application of cognitive-behavioral or motivational principles.
    C) Evaluation.
    D) All of the above.

38. Information gathered by way of an appropriate health screening allows the health/fitness instructor to develop specific exercise programs that are appropriate to the individual needs and goals of the client. This is called the
    A) Exercise prescription.
    B) Heart rate.

C)   Blood pressure.

D)   Graded exercise test.

39.   To maximize safety during a physical fitness assessment, which of the following items should be addressed?

A)   Hospital emergency room services.

B)   Emergency plan.

C)   Client financial status.

D)   All of the above.

40.   Some externally applied forces, such as exercise pulleys, do not act in a vertical direction as do weights attached to the body because

A)   A distractive force sometimes is used to promote normal joint movement.

B)   The angle of application changes in different parts of the range of motion, causing a change in the magnitude of the rotary component of the force and, thus, the torque.

C)   Weights applied to the body behave as weights of body segments, thus changing the torque and altering the difficulty of an exercise when weight is applied.

D)   By shifting the mass of the weight more proximally up the arm, less effort by the stabilizing muscles is required, so the torque that is produced at the glenohumeral joint is reduced.

41.   What will happen to a motor unit if it is rapidly stimulated without adequate time for relaxation?

A)   Tetanus.

B)   Repolarization.

C)   Twitch.

D)   None of the above.

42.   Heart rate can be measured by counting the number of pulses in a specified time period at one of several locations, including the radial, femoral, and carotid arteries. Which of the following is a special precaution when taking the carotid pulse?

A)   When the heart rate is measured by palpation, the first two fingers should be used and not the thumb, because the thumb has its own pulse.

B)   Heart rates taken during exercise sometimes exceed 200 bpm, making it too difficult to feel at the carotid artery.

C)   If the heart rate is taken at the carotid artery, do not press too hard, or a reflex slowing of the heart may occur and cause dizziness.

D)   The heart rate should never be taken at the carotid artery.

43.   As a result of regular exercise training, which of the following is NOT affected during maximal exercise?

A)   Cardiac output.

B)   Stroke volume.

C)   Heart rate.

D)   None of the above.

44.   When exercise testing children

A)   Most ergometers used in adult exercise testing can be used for children, with the treadmill generally being preferred to cycle ergometers.

B)   Only strength should be measured.

C)   Flexibility should be stressed.

D)   Use only the heart rate as an indicator of cardiovascular fitness.

45.   Which of the following risk factors for the development of coronary artery disease has the greatest likelihood of being influenced by regular exercise?

A)   Smoking.

B)   Cholesterol.

C)   Type I diabetes.

D)   Hypertension.

46.   At minimum, professionals performing fitness assessments on others should possess which combination of the following?

A)   Cardiopulmonary resuscitation (CPR) and ACSM Health/Fitness Instructor.

B)   Advanced Cardiac Life Support and ACSM Program Director.

C)   Advanced Cardiac Life Support and ACSM Health/Fitness Director.

D)   Only physicians can perform fitness assessments.

47.   For an exercise prescription, which of the following combinations work inversely with each other?

A)   Intensity and duration.

B)   Mode and intensity.

C)   Mode and duration.

D)   Mode and frequency.

48.   Which of the following types of muscle stretching alternates contraction and relaxation of both agonist and antagonist muscle groups, may cause residual muscle soreness, is time consuming, and typically requires a partner?

A)   Static stretching.

B)   Ballistic stretching.

C)   Proprioceptive neuromuscular facilitation stretching.

D)   All of the above.

49.   Glucose, fructose, and sucrose commonly are referred to as

A)   Proteins.

B)   Complex carbohydrates.

C) Simple carbohydrates.

D) Fats.

50. Failure of a health/fitness instructor to perform in a generally acceptable standard is called
    A) Malpractice.
    B) Malfeasance.
    C) Negligence.
    D) None of the above.

51. All energy for muscular contraction must come from the breakdown of a chemical compound called
    A) ATP.
    B) STP.
    C) NADH + H^+.
    D) $FADH_2$.

52. Actin is a muscle protein (sometimes called the thin filament) that can be visualized as looking like a twisted strand of beads. Actin also contains which two other proteins?
    A) Epimysium and perimysium.
    B) Perimysium and endomysium.
    C) Troponin and tropomyosin.
    D) Myosin and troponin.

53. From rest to maximal exercise, the systolic blood pressure should _____ with an increasing workload.
    A) Increase.
    B) Decrease.
    C) Stay the same.
    D) Decrease with isometric or increase with isotonic contractions.

54. The majority of sedentary people are not motivated to initiate exercise programs, and if exercise is initiated, they are likely to stop within
    A) 1 to 2 days.
    B) 3 to 6 weeks.
    C) 1 month.
    D) 3 to 6 months.

55. Reasons for fitness testing of the older adult include
    A) Evaluation of progress.
    B) Exercise prescription.
    C) Motivation.
    D) All of the above.

56. A body weight of 15 percent less than expected, a morbid fear of fatness, a preoccupation with food, and an abnormal body image are symptoms of
    A) Bulimia nervosa.
    B) Dieting.
    C) Anorexia nervosa.
    D) Obesity.

57. If a motor unit receives a second stimulation before it is allowed to relax, then the two impulses are added, and the tension developed is greater. This is called
    A) Twitch.
    B) Tetanus.
    C) Summation.
    D) Motor unit.

58. What is the energy cost of running at 6.5 mph up a grade of 5%?
    A) 13.2 MET.
    B) 15.2 MET.
    C) 10.2 MET.
    D) 8.2 MET.

59. Feeling good about being able to perform an activity or skill, such as finally being able to run a mile or to increase the speed of walking a mile, is an example of
    A) Extrinsic rewards.
    B) Intrinsic rewards.
    C) External stimulus.
    D) Internal stimulus.

60. Albuterol, terbutaline, glucocorticosteroids, cromolyn sodium, and theophylline are effective drugs to prevent or reverse
    A) Coronary artery disease.
    B) Emphysema.
    C) Asthma.
    D) Cancer.

61. Safety in the fitness center is very important to the welfare of the client. Specifically, exercise equipment should be
    A) Flexible enough to allow for different body sizes.
    B) Large enough to accommodate small and large clients.
    C) Inexpensive enough to allow for changing out equipment periodically.
    D) Placed on the floor with wheels so that it can be moved easily.

62. The ACSM recommendation for intensity, duration, and frequency of physical activity for apparently healthy individuals includes
    A) Intensity of 60% to 90% maximal heart rate, duration of 20 to 60 minutes, and frequency of 3 to 5 days a week.
    B) Intensity of 85% to 90% maximal heart rate, duration of 30 minutes, and frequency of 3 days a week.
    C) Intensity of 50% to 70% maximal heart rate, duration of 15 to 45 minutes, and frequency of 5 days a week.
    D) Intensity of 60% to 90% maximal heart rate reserve, duration of 20 to 60 minutes, and frequency of 7 days a week.

63. A method of strength and power training that involves an eccentric loading of muscles and tendons followed immediately by an explosive concentric contraction is called
    A) Plyometrics.
    B) Periodization.
    C) Super-sets.
    D) Isotonic reversals.

64. Which of the following are characteristics of a good manager?
    A) Designs programs, and monitors the implementation of the program.
    B) Guides staff or clients through the program.
    C) Is a strong communicator.
    D) All of the above.

65. Agreements, releases, and consents are documents that clearly describe
    A) What the client is participating in, the risks involved, and the rights of the client and the facility.
    B) What the client can and cannot do in your facility.
    C) The relationship between the facility operator and the health/fitness instructor.
    D) The rights and responsibilities of the club owner to reject an application by a prospective client.

66. Enough ATP is stored in a given skeletal muscle to fuel how much activity?
    A) 2 to 3 seconds.
    B) 5 to 10 seconds.
    C) 10 to 20 seconds.
    D) 1 hour.

67. The sliding filament theory of muscle contraction depends on the interaction of actin and myosin. At rest, no interaction occurs. When called on to contract, these two create an interdigitation, and the muscle then contracts. This process is dependent on the presence of
    A) Magnesium.
    B) Manganese.
    C) Creatine.
    D) Calcium.

68. After 30 years of age, skeletal muscle strength begins to decline, primarily because of
    A) A gain in fat tissue.
    B) A gain in lean tissue.
    C) A loss of muscle mass caused by a loss of muscle fibers.
    D) Myogenic precursor cell inhibition.

69. The rate of an acute cardiovascular event occurring during exercise in men is
    A) 1 in 20,000 hours.
    B) 1 in 57,000 hours.

C) 1 in 187,500 hours.
D) 1 in 1 million hours.

70. Which of the following is a complex carbohydrate that is not digestible by the body and passes straight through the digestive system?
    A) Fats.
    B) Proteins.
    C) Sugars.
    D) Fiber.

71. The Health Belief Model assumes that people will engage in a behavior, such as exercise, when
    A) There is a perceived threat of disease.
    B) There is a belief of susceptibility to disease.
    C) The threat of disease is severe.
    D) All of the above.

72. The informed consent document
    A) Is a legal document.
    B) Provides immunity from prosecution.
    C) Provides an explanation of the test to the client.
    D) All of the above.

73. A measure of muscular endurance is
    A) One-repetition maximum.
    B) Three-repetition maximum.
    C) Number of sit-ups in 1 minute.
    D) Treadmill testing.

74. If an exerciser starts to exercise too much and either does not take a rest day at all and/or develops a minor injury and does not stop and rest so that the injury might heal, what can occur?
    A) An overuse injury.
    B) A fatal or near fatal automobile accident.
    C) Sleep deprivation.
    D) Decreased physical conditioning.

75. The ACSM recommends that exercise intensity be prescribed within what percentage of maximal heart rate?
    A) 40% and 50%.
    B) 50% and 70%.
    C) 60% and 90%.
    D) 70% and 100%.

76. The ACSM recommends how many repetitions of each exercise for muscular strength and endurance?
    A) 5 to 6.
    B) 8 to 12.
    C) 12 to 20.
    D) More than 20.

77. For higher intensity activities,
    A) The benefit outweighs any potential risk.
    B) The risk of orthopedic and cardiovascular complications are increased.

C) The risk of orthopedic and cardiovascular complications are minimal.

D) There is no increased risk of orthopedic and cardiovascular complications.

78. Auscultation of the heart rate refers to
   A) Feeling the pulse at the radial artery.
   B) Listening to the sounds of the heart through the chest.
   C) Counting the pulse rate at the carotid artery.
   D) Counting the pulse rate at the carotid, radial, or femoral arteries.

79. Which of the following are changes seen as a result of regular, chronic exercise?
   A) Decreased heart rate at rest.
   B) Increased stroke volume at rest.
   C) No change in cardiac output at rest.
   D) All of the above.

80. The heart (unlike skeletal muscle) has its own capability to produce an action potential. If an electrical impulse is not received from higher-level brain centers, cardiac muscle will stimulate itself. This is called
   A) Tetany.
   B) Simulated contraction.
   C) Diastole.
   D) Autorhythmicity.

81. Maximal exercise testing has been labeled by some medical experts as a dangerous situation for most people. Actually, the death rate during maximal exercise testing is approximately
   A) 0.01%.
   B) 1%.
   C) 10%.
   D) 5%.

82. Which of the following is an example of a cognitive process in the Transtheoretical Model?
   A) Counterconditioning.
   B) Reinforcement management.
   C) Dramatic relief.
   D) Self-liberation.

83. The purpose of the fitness assessment is to
   A) Develop the exercise prescription.
   B) Evaluate progress.
   C) Motivate.
   D) All of the above.

84. RICES means
   A) Dietary supplements.
   B) *Rest* and *ICE* are the best treatment for injury.
   C) *Rest, Ice, Compression, Elevation,* and *Stabilization.*
   D) None of the above.

85. Resistance exercises performed either in an ascending (increasing the resistance within a set of repetitions from one set to the next) or descending (decreasing the resistance within a set of repetitions from one set to the next) order are called
   A) Circuit weight training.
   B) Super-sets.
   C) Split routines.
   D) Pyramids.

86. The ACSM recommendation for the maximal rate of weight loss is
   A) 10 to 15 pounds per week (4.5–7 kg).
   B) 8 to 10 pounds per week (4–4.5 kg).
   C) 5 to 8 pounds per week (2.3–4 kg).
   D) 1 to 2 pounds per week (0.5–1 kg).

87. Which of the following is NOT an abnormal curvature of the spine?
   A) Kyphosis.
   B) Scoliosis.
   C) Chondrosis.
   D) Lordosis.

88. Which of the following assumes that an overall complex behavior arises from many small simple behaviors?
   A) Learning theories.
   B) Health Belief Model.
   C) Transtheoretical Model.
   D) Stages of Motivational Readiness.

89. Individuals who choose to begin a self-directed exercise program (on their own) should be advised to complete, at minimum, a quick screening of their health status using something like the
   A) Minnesota Multiphasic Personality Inventory (MMPI).
   B) Borg scale.
   C) PAR-Q.
   D) All of the above.

90. When a test battery of fitness assessments is administered to a client in a single session, the following order of tests is recommended.
   A) Resting measurements, flexibility, cardiorespiratory fitness, body composition, and muscular fitness.
   B) Flexibility, resting measurements, body composition, muscular fitness, and cardiorespiratory fitness.
   C) Resting measurements, body composition, cardiorespiratory fitness, muscular fitness, and flexibility.
   D) The order makes no difference, only that all the tests are done.

91. Implementing emergency procedures must include the fitness center
    A) Management.
    B) Staff.
    C) Clients.
    D) Management and staff.

92. Which of the following is a possible medical emergency that a client can experience during an exercise session?
    A) Hypoglycemia.
    B) Hypotension.
    C) Hypertension.
    D) All of the above.

93. During a graded exercise test, blood pressure must be taken at least
    A) Twice.
    B) Twice during each stage.
    C) Once during each stage.
    D) Every minute.

94. Which of the following muscle actions occurs when the length of the muscle does not change, but muscle tension is increased through enhanced neuromuscular recruitment patterns?
    A) Concentric isotonic.
    B) Eccentric isotonic.
    C) Isokinetic.
    D) Isometric.

95. Which of the following is the only nutrient that contains nitrogen?
    A) Fats.
    B) Proteins.
    C) Simple carbohydrates.
    D) Complex carbohydrates.

96. Which of the following activities provides the greatest improvement in aerobic fitness for someone who is beginning an exercise program?
    A) Weight training.
    B) Downhill snow skiing.
    C) Dieting.
    D) Walking.

97. In commercial settings, clients should be more extensively screened for potential health risks. The information solicited should include which of the following?
    A) Personal medical history.
    B) Present medical status.
    C) Medication.
    D) All of the above.

98. Generally, persons of poor fitness may benefit from
    A) Longer duration, higher intensity, and lower frequency of exercise.
    B) Longer duration, lower intensity, and lower frequency of exercise.
    C) Shorter duration, lower intensity, and higher frequency of exercise.
    D) Shorter duration, higher intensity, and higher frequency of exercise.

99. A document that details the marketing plan and justification for each action in the program as well as an analysis of each aspect of the research plus projections for success is called a
    A) Public relations plan.
    B) Marketing plan.
    C) Market research.
    D) Business plan.

ANSWERS AND EXPLANATIONS

1–D. Water exercise has gained in popularity, because the buoyancy properties of water help to reduce the potential for musculoskeletal injury and may even allow injured people an opportunity to exercise without further injury. A variety of activities may be offered in a water-exercise class. Walking, jogging, and dance activity all may be adapted for water. Water-exercise classes typically should combine the benefits of the buoyancy properties of water with the resistive properties of water. In this regard, both an aerobic stimulus as well as activity to enhance muscular strength and endurance may be provided.

[Chapter 8]

2–A. Because the number of reactions is small (basically two), the ATP-PC system can provide ATP at a very fast rate. The ATP-PC system is ranked number one in power. Enough PC is stored in skeletal muscle for approximately 25 seconds of high-intensity work. Therefore, the ATP-PC system will last for approximately 30 seconds (5 seconds for stored ATP, and 25 seconds for PC).

[Chapter 2]

3–C. Nitrates and nitroglycerine are antianginals (used to reduce chest pain associated with angina pectoris). α-Blockers are antihypertensives (used to reduce blood pressure by inhibiting the action of adrenergic neurotransmitters at the α-receptor, thereby promoting peripheral vasodilation). β-Blockers also are designed to reduce blood pressure by inhibiting the action of adrenergic neurotransmitters at the β-receptors, thereby decreasing cardiac output. Antihyperlipidemics control blood lipids, especially cholesterol and LDL.

[Chapter 4]

4–C. Dietary fats include triglycerides, cholesterol, and phospholipids. Triglycerides represent more than 90% of the fat stored in the body. A triglyceride is a glycerol molecule connected to three fatty acid molecules. The fatty acids are identified by the amount of "saturation" or the number of single or double bonds that link the carbon atoms. Saturated fatty acids only have single bonds. Monounsaturated fatty acids have one double bond, and polyunsaturated fatty acids have two or more double bonds.

[Chapter 9]

5–B. An adequate range of motion or joint mobility is requisite for optimal musculoskeletal health. Specifically, limited flexibility of the low back and hamstring regions may relate to an increased risk for development of chronic low back pain and disability. Activities that will enhance or maintain musculoskeletal flexibility should be included as a part of a comprehensive preventive or rehabilitative exercise program.

6–A. Minerals are inorganic substances that perform a variety of functions in the body. Many play an important role in assisting enzymes (or coenzymes) that are necessary for the proper functioning of body systems. They also are found in cell membranes, hormones, muscles, and connective tissues as well as electrolytes in body fluids. Minerals are considered to be either macrominerals (needed in relatively large doses), such as calcium, phosphorus, magnesium, potassium, sulfur, sodium, and chloride, or microminerals (needed in very small amounts), such as iron, zinc, selenium, manganese, molybdenum, iodine, copper, chromium, and fluoride.

[Chapter 9]

7–C. The body has three cardinal planes, and each plane is perpendicular to each of the other two. Movement occurs along these planes. The sagittal plane divides the body into right and left parts, and the midsagittal plane is represented by an imaginary vertical plane passing through the midline of the body, dividing it into right and left halves. The frontal plane is represented by an imaginary vertical plane passing through the body, dividing it into front and back halves. The transverse plane represents an imaginary horizontal plane passing through the midsection of the body and dividing it into upper and lower portions.

[Chapter 1]

8–D. The bones of the skeletal system perform five functions: They provide structural support for the entire body, serve as levers that can change the magnitude and direction of forces generated by skeletal muscles, protect organs and tissues, provide storage (calcium salts of bone serve as mineral reservoirs for maintaining concentrations of calcium and phosphate ions in body fluids, and fat cells in yellow bone marrow store lipids as energy reserve), and produce red blood cells and other elements within the bone marrow.

[Chapter 1]

9–D. To be classified as hypertensive, the systolic blood pressure must exceed 140/90 mm Hg as measured on two separate occasions, preferably days apart. An elevation of either the systolic or diastolic pressure is classified as hypertension.

[Chapter 4]

10–C. The purpose of risk stratification is to identify high-risk individuals (persons with contraindications leading to potential exclusion from testing or exercise, individuals with disease symptoms or risk factors that require medical evaluation before testing or exercise, individuals with clinically significant disease that requires medical supervision during testing or exercise, or individuals with special testing or exercise needs) and to select the appropriate activities for those persons. Risk categories include apparently healthy, low risk, moderate risk, and high risk.

[Chapter 6]

11–C. Heat exhaustion and heat stroke are serious conditions that result from a combination of the metabolic heat generated from exercise accompanied by dehydration and electrolyte loss from sweating. Signs and symptoms include uncoordinated gait, headache, dizziness, vomiting, and elevated body temperature. If these conditions are present, exercise must be stopped. Attempts to rehydrate, perhaps intravenously, should be attempted, and the body must be cooled by any means possible. The person should be placed in the supine position, with the feet elevated.

12–A. Angular movements decrease or increase the joint angle produced by the articulating bones. There are four types of angular movements: flexion (a movement that decreases the joint angle, bringing the bones closer together), extension (the movement opposite to flexion decreasing the joint angle between two bones), abduction (the movement of a body part away from the midline in a lateral direction), and adduction (the opposite of abduction, the movement toward the midline of the body).

[Chapter 1]

13–D. The oxygen system is capable of using all three fuels (carbohydrate, fat, and protein). Significant amounts of protein, however, are not used as a source of ATP energy during most types of exercise. Although all three fuels can be used, the two most important are carbohydrate and fat. When fat is used as a fuel, significantly more energy is released; however, this requires that more oxygen be supplied to produce this energy. If proteins are used, the amount of energy is comparable to that of carbohydrate. The carbohydrate, fat, and small amount of protein used by this energy system during exercise are metabolized completely, leaving only carbon dioxide (which is exhaled) and water. The nitrogen found in the protein is excreted as urea.

[Chapter 2]

14–B. The steps are as follows:

a. Choose the ACSM leg cycling formula.

b. Write down your knowns, and convert the values to the appropriate units:

$$116.6 \text{ pounds} \div 2.2 = 53 \text{ kg}$$
$$50 \text{ rpm} \times 6 \text{ m} = 300 \text{ m} \cdot \text{min}^{-1}$$
$$2.5 \text{ kp} = 2.5 \text{ kg}$$
$$30 \text{ minutes of cycling}$$

c. Write down the ACSM formula:

$$\text{Leg cycling} = (1.8 \times \text{work rate} \div \text{body weight}) + (3.5) + (3.5) \, (\text{mL} \cdot \text{kg}^{-1} \cdot \text{min}^{-1})$$

d. Calculate the work rate:

$$\text{Work rate} = (\text{kg} \cdot \text{m})/\text{min}$$
$$= 2.5 \text{ kg} \cdot 300 \text{ m} \cdot \text{min}^{-1}$$
$$= 750 \text{ kg} \cdot \text{min}^{-1}$$

e. Substitute the known values for the variable name:

$$\text{mL} \cdot \text{kg}^{-1} \cdot \text{min}^{-1} = (1.8 \times 750 \div 53) + (3.5) + (3.5)$$

f. Solve for the unknown:

$$\text{mL} \cdot \text{kg}^{-1} \cdot \text{min}^{-1} = 25.47 + 3.5 + 3.5$$
$$\text{gross leg cycling } \dot{V}o_2 = 32.47 \text{ mL} \cdot \text{kg}^{-1} \cdot \text{min}^{-1}$$

g. To find out how many calories she expends, we must first convert her oxygen consumption ($\dot{V}o_2$) to absolute terms:

$$\text{absolute } \dot{V}o_2 = \text{relative } \dot{V}o_2 \times \text{body weight}$$
$$= 32.47 \text{ mL} \cdot \text{kg}^{-1} \cdot \text{min}^{-1} \times 53 \text{ kg}$$
$$= 1,721 \text{ mL} \cdot \text{min}^{-1}$$

h. Convert $\text{mL} \cdot \text{min}^{-1}$ to $\text{L} \cdot \text{min}^{-1}$ by dividing by 1,000:

$$1,721 \text{ mL} \cdot \text{min}^{-1} \div 1,000 = 1.721 \text{ L} \cdot \text{min}^{-1}$$

i. Next, we must see how many calories she expends in 1 minute by multiplying her absolute $\dot{V}o_2$ (in $\text{L} \cdot \text{min}^{-1}$) by the constant 5.0:

$$1.721 \text{ L} \cdot \text{min}^{-1} \times 5.0 = 8.61 \text{ kcal} \cdot \text{min}^{-1}$$

j. Finally, multiply the number of calories she expends in 1 minute by the number of minutes she cycles:

$$8.61 \text{ kcal} \cdot \text{min}^{-1} \times 30 \text{ min} = 258.3 \text{ cal}$$

[Chapter 11]

15–B. Body composition refers to the relative proportions of fat and fat-free (lean) tissue in the body. It is commonly reported as "percent body fat," thereby identifying the proportion of the total body mass composed of fat. Fat-free mass is then determined as the balance of the total body mass. Hydrodensitometry and near-infrared interactance are ways to measure body composition.

[Chapter 6]

16–D. Exercise leadership is a skill that requires an understanding of the scientific concepts of exercise, the ability to interpret and teach these concepts effectively, and the ability to motivate individuals toward continued exercise participation. The ability to identify the level of supervision required for individuals based on their health/fitness status also is a key to safe and effective exercise leadership. It is incumbent on the health/fitness instructor to stay abreast of current information regarding exercise. He or she should be a resource for up-to-date and accurate information regarding health and fitness and should dispel myths and quackery. The health/fitness instructor also should be able to create an atmosphere and opportunity for learning by presenting a clear set of goals. Communication skills are fundamental to effective teaching as well.

17–D. Surrounding each myofibril is the sarcoplasmic reticulum, specialized endoplasmic reticulum consisting of a series of interconnected sacs and tubes. Calcium is stored in portions of the sarcoplasmic reticulum called **terminal cisternae**. Myofibrils contain the myofilaments, which are contractile proteins consisting primarily of actin and myosin.

[Chapter 1]

18–C. Anaerobic glycolysis also is known as the lactic acid system. A human stores carbohydrate in the body as muscle (or liver) glycogen. Glycogen is simply a long string of glucose molecules hooked end-to-end. Anaerobic glycolysis can use only carbohydrate, not fat or protein, as fuel. This system will use muscle glycogen, which is broken down to glucose and then enters anaerobic glycolysis. Only a small amount of ATP is produced, and the end-product is lactic acid (or lactate). If lactate is allowed to accumulate significantly in the muscle, it eventually will cause fatigue. Because no oxygen is required, this system is anaerobic.

[Chapter 2]

19–C. Cardiac output does not change significantly, primarily because the person is performing the same amount of work and, thus, responds with the same cardiac output. It should be noted, however, that the same cardiac output is now being generated with a lower heart rate and higher stroke volume compared with when the person was untrained.

[Chapter 2]

20–D. Every population that has been studied exhibits a decline in bone mass with aging. Therefore, bone loss is considered by most clinicians to be an inevitable consequence of aging. Osteoporosis refers to a condition that is characterized by a decrease in bone mass and density, producing bone porosity and fragility, and it refers to the clinical condition of low bone mass and the accompanying increase in susceptibility to fracture from minor trauma. The age at which bone loss begins and the rate at which it occurs vary greatly between males and females. Risk factors for age-related bone loss and development of clinical osteoporosis include being a white or Asian female, being thin-boned or petite, having a low peak bone mass at maturity, having a family history of osteoporosis, premature or surgically induced menopause, alcohol abuse and/or cigarette smoking, sedentary lifestyle, and inadequate dietary calcium intake.

[Chapter 3]

21–B. Outcomes are designed to measure the success of a program based on the outcome for a patient or client. Outcome studies require quantifiable data that can be analyzed, data that study the success of a program in terms of quantifiable measures (e.g., change in body composition). Measuring client satisfaction, level of change, length of time for change to occur, or percentage of clients who reach their goals are other examples of outcomes. Outcomes can be very helpful in marketing programs as well as in comparing one facility to another.

22–B. Although some learning is required on the part of the participant, the RPE should be considered an adjunct to heart rate measures. The RPE can be used as a reliable barometer of exercise intensity. The RPE is particularly useful when participants are incapable of monitoring their pulse accurately or when medications such as β-blockers alter the heart rate response to exercise. The ACSM recommends an exercise intensity that will elicit an RPE within a range of 12 to 16 on the original Borg scale of 6 to 20.

23–B. Fast-twitch (type II) muscle fibers can be subdivided into fast-twitch aerobic (type IIa) and fast-twitch glycolytic (type IIb). Although classified as a fast-twitch fiber, the type IIa fiber has the capability to perform some amounts of aerobic work. The motor nerve supplying fast-twitch fibers is larger than slow-twitch muscle fibers. Fast-twitch fibers are recruited when performing high-intensity, short-duration activities. Examples include weight lifting, sprints, jumping, and other similar activities. These fibers can produce large amounts of tension in a very short period; however, they fatigue quickly.

[Chapter 2]

24–A. Rotation is the turning of a bone around its own longitudinal axis or around another bone. Rotation of the anterior surface of the bone toward the midline of the body is medial rotation, whereas rotation of the same bone away from the midline is lateral rotation. Supination is a specialized rotation of the forearm that results in the palm of the hand being turned forward (anteriorly). Pronation (the opposite of supination) is the rotation of the forearm that results in the palm of the hand being directed backward (posteriorly).

[Chapter 1]

25–C. The trachea branches within the mediastinum to form the right and left primary bronchi. As each primary bronchus enters the lung, secondary bronchi branch off, with smaller and smaller branches continuing to branch until the smallest narrow passage is formed, which is called the bronchiole. Terminal bronchioles are the smallest-diameter bronchioles and supply air to the lobules of the lung. Varying the diameter of the bronchioles gives control over the resistance to airflow and distribution of air to the lungs.

[Chapter 1]

26–A. Cardiac output is calculated by multiplying heart rate and stroke volume. During dynamic exercise, cardiac output increases with increasing exercise intensity. Stroke volume increases only until approximately 40% to 50% of $\dot{V}O_2$max. Above this point, increases in cardiac output are accounted for only by an increase in heart rate. During static exercise, cardiac output may fall as a result of a drop in venous return. When the contraction is released, a rapid increase in cardiac output occurs as the venous return increases.

[Chapter 2]

27–D. Initial causes of coronary artery disease are thought to be an irritation of, or an injury to, the tunica intima (the innermost of the three layers in the wall) of the blood vessel. Sources of this initial injury are thought to be caused by dyslipidemia (elevated total blood cholesterol), hypertension (chronic high blood pressure, either an elevation of systolic blood pressure or diastolic blood pressure measured on two different days), immune responses, smoking, tumultuous and nonlaminar blood flow in the lumen of the coronary artery (turbulence), vasoconstrictor substances (chemicals that cause the smooth muscle cells in the walls of the vessel to contract, resulting in a reduction in the diameter of the lumen), and viral infections.

[Chapter 4]

28–C. Risk factors that contribute to the development of coronary artery disease include age (men, >45 years; women, >55 years), a family history of myocardial infarction or sudden death (male first-degree relatives < 55 years and female first-degree relatives < 65 years), cigarette smoking, hypertension (arterial blood pressure > 140/90 mm Hg measured on two separate occasions), hypercholesterolemia (total cholesterol > 200 mg/dL or 5.2 mmol/L, or high-density lipoprotein < 35 mg/dL or 0.9 mmol/L), diabetes mellitus in individuals older than 30 years or in individuals who have had type I diabetes more than 15 years or type II diabetes in individuals older than 35 years. Other risk factors contribute to the development of coronary artery disease but are not primary risk factors.

[Chapter 4]

29–B. The low-risk category is asymptomatic and has one or no major risk factor for coronary artery disease. A person is placed in the moderate-risk category if he or she has two or more major risk factors for coronary artery disease. A person in the high-risk category is someone with signs, symptoms of, or known cardiac disease, pulmonary disease, and metabolic disease.

[Chapter 6]

30–A. Lateral neck stretches are a safe alternative to full neck rolls. Full squats place high forces on the patellar tendon. The recommended alternative exercise is a half-squat. The hurdler's stretch also can place high stress on the medial collateral ligament and menisci. The recommended alternative is a seated hamstring stretch. Full sit-ups require recruitment of the hip flexors, which places stress on the lower back. Crunches are a good alternative.

[Chapter 7]

31–B. Vitamin A promotes healthy skin, resists infection, and improves night vision. Vitamin D helps to build strong bones and teeth. Sources of vitamin D include fortified milk, fish oils, and egg yolk. Vitamin K improves normal blood clotting. Thiamine is important in energy-releasing reactions.

[Chapter 9]

32–B. Each atrium communicates with the ventricle on the same side via an AV valve, which allows one-way flow of blood from the atrium to the ventricle. The right AV valve also is known as the tricuspid valve because of the three cusps, or flaps, of fibrous tissue that constitute the valve. The left AV valve is called the bicuspid valve (or mitral valve), because it contains a pair of cusps rather than a trio. Each cusp is braced by tendinous fibers called chordae tendinae, which, in turn, are connected to papillary muscles on the inner surface of the ventricle.

[Chapter 1]

33–B. The oxygen system is complicated and involves many reactions. The oxygen system takes 2 to 3 minutes to adjust to a new exercise intensity. This system is ranked third in power. An individual's $\dot{V}O_2$max is a measure of the power of the aerobic energy system. This value generally is regarded as the best indicator of aerobic fitness. The average $\dot{V}O_2$max of college-age males is approximately 45 mL $\cdot$ kg^{-1} $\cdot$ min^{-1}. The average $\dot{V}O_2$max of college-age females is 35 mL $\cdot$ kg^{-1} $\cdot$ min^{-1}.

[Chapter 2]

34–B. The action potential in cardiac muscle is much longer in duration compared with that in skeletal muscle. This prevents the cardiac muscle from being tetanized. If cardiac muscle were tetanized, no relaxation (diastole) of heart muscle would occur, preventing ventricular filling from occurring for the next contraction.

[Chapter 2]

35–C. Older people who exercise regularly report greater life satisfaction (older people who exercise regularly have a more positive attitude toward their work and generally are in better health than sedentary persons), greater happiness (strong correlations have been reported between the activity level of older adults and self-reported happiness), higher self-efficacy (older persons taking part in exercise programs commonly report that they can do everyday tasks more easily than before they began exercising), improved self-concept and self-esteem (older adults improve their score on self-concept questionnaires following participation in an exercise program), and reduced psychological stress (exercise is effective in reducing psychological stress without unwanted side effects).

[Chapter 3]

36–B. Angina pectoris is a heart-related chest pain caused by ischemia, which is insufficient blood flow that results from a temporary or permanent reduction of blood flow in one or more coronary arteries. Angina-like symptoms often are felt in the chest area, neck, shoulder, or arm.

[Chapter 4]

37–D. Psychological theories are the foundation for effective use of strategies and techniques of effective counseling and motivational skill-building for exercise adoption and maintenance. Theories provide a conceptual framework for assessment, development of programs or interventions, application of cognitive-behavioral or motivational principles, and evaluation of program effectiveness. Within the field of behavioral change, a theory is a set of assumptions that accounts for the relationships between certain variables and the behavior of interest.

[Chapter 5]

38–A. A-well designed health screening provides the exercise leader or health/fitness instructor with information that can lead to identification of those individuals for whom exercise is contraindicated. From that information, a proper exercise prescription also can be developed. A graded exercise test can be useful to measure heart rate and blood pressure responses.

[Chapter 6]

39–B. Regularly scheduled practices of responses to emergency situations, including a minimum of one announced and one unannounced drill, should take place. Emergency plans should include written, posted emergency plans and posted emergency numbers. The equipment and floor space should be arranged to allow safe egress from the facility in an emergency situation and to prevent accidental upsetting of equipment. A written maintenance procedures document that includes all daily, weekly, and monthly activities associated with each piece of equipment should be developed.

[Chapter 6]

40–B. Some externally applied forces do not act in a vertical direction, as do weights attached to the body. The forces exert effects that vary according to their particular angle of application. In the case of exercise pulleys, the angle of application changes in different parts of the range of motion. Each change in angle or force causes a change in magnitude of the rotary component of the force and, thus, the torque. In addition to the rotary component, weights applied to the extremities frequently exert traction on joint structures. This is known as a distractive force.

[Chapter 1]

41–A. If a motor unit is continuously stimulated without adequate time for relaxation to occur, tetanus will occur. When a motor unit is in tetany, there is sustained tension until the stimulus is removed or fatigue occurs.

[Chapter 2]

42–C. Heart rate is simply the total number of times the heart contracts in 1 minute. Normal resting heart rate is approximately 70 to 80 bpm. Heart rates during maximal exercise can exceed 200 bpm, depending on the age of the participant. Heart rate can be measured by counting the number of pulses in a specified time period at one of several locations. These locations commonly include the radial, femoral, and carotid arteries. The number of pulses is counted for 1 minute. If heart rate is taken at the carotid artery, take care not to press too hard, or a reflex slowing of the heart may occur and cause dizziness.

[Chapter 2]

43–C. Maximal heart rate does not change significantly with exercise training. Maximal heart rate does, however, decline with age. Maximal stroke volume increases after training as a result of an increase in contractility and/or an increase in the size of the heart. Because maximal heart rate is unchanged and maximal stroke volume increases, maximal cardiac output must increase.

[Chapter 2]

44–A. Because of the relatively underdeveloped musculature of the legs and difficulty following the pace of a metronome, the treadmill generally is preferred over cycle ergometers and step tests. However, ergometers used in adult exercise testing also can be used for children. Protocols to measure maximal aerobic power should last between 6 and 10 minutes, consisting of a progressively increasing load. Testing protocols developed for adults can be modified easily for children by lowering the initial power output and subsequent incremental increases. Protocols designed to predict maximal aerobic capacity from submaximal exercise should be interpreted cautiously, because several congenital conditions and diseases can cause peak heart rate to be reduced.

[Chapter 3]

45–D. Exercise has no effect on age and family history of heart disease and no direct effect on cigarette smoking. Regular endurance exercise does increase high-density lipoprotein, but it has limited influence on total cholesterol. Exercise has no direct effect on type I diabetes, but it can improve glucose tolerance for those with type II diabetes. Regular exercise will decrease systolic and diastolic blood pressure.

[Chapter 4]

46–A. At minimum, professionals performing fitness assessments on others should possess CPR and ACSM health/fitness instructor certification. Other certifications are available for other responsibilities.

[Chapter 6]

47–A. Intensity and duration of exercise must be considered together and are inversely related. Similar improvements in aerobic fitness may be realized if a person exercises at a low intensity for a longer duration or at a higher intensity for less time.

48–C. Three different stretching techniques typically are practiced and have associated risks and benefits. Static stretching is the most commonly recommended approach to stretching. It involves slowly stretching a muscle to the point of individual discomfort and holding that position for a period of 10 to 30 seconds. Minimal risk of injury exists and it has been shown to be effective. Ballistic stretching uses repetitive bouncing-type movements to produce muscle stretch. These movements may produce residual muscle soreness or acute injury. Proprioceptive neuromuscular facilitation stretching alternates contraction

and relaxation of both agonist and antagonist muscle groups. This technique is effective, but it may cause residual muscle soreness and is time-consuming. Additionally, a partner typically is required, and the potential for injury exists when the partner-assisted stretching is applied too vigorously.

49–C. Carbohydrates are compounds made of carbon, hydrogen, and oxygen. They are commonly known as simple carbohydrates (sugars) or complex carbohydrates (starch). Glucose, fructose, and sucrose are examples of sugars or simple carbohydrates. Some sources are refined sugar (white or brown) and fruits. Food sources for complex carbohydrates are grains, breads, cereals, pastas, potatoes, beans, and legumes. Proteins have nitrogen in them as well as carbon, hydrogen, and oxygen and may be found in such food sources as meats and nuts. Fats are found in foods such as butter and oils.

[Chapter 9]

50–C. Legal issues abound for fitness professionals involved in exercise testing, exercise prescription, and program administration. Legal concerns can develop with the instructor-client relationship, the exercises involved, the exercise setting, the purpose of the programs and exercises used, and the procedures used by the staff. A tort law is simply a type of civil wrong. Negligence is the failure to perform on the level of a generally accepted standard. Fitness professionals have certain documented and understood responsibilities to ensure the client's safety and to succeed in reaching predetermined goals. If these responsibilities are not followed, it is possible that one could be considered negligent.

51–A. All energy for muscular contraction must come from the breakdown of ATP. The energy is stored in the bonds between the last two phosphates. When work is performed (e.g., a biceps curl), the last phosphate is split (forming ADP), releasing heat energy. Some (but not all) of this heat energy is converted to mechanical energy to perform the curl. Because we are not 100% efficient at converting this heat energy to mechanical energy, the rest of the heat is released to the environment.

[Chapter 2]

52–C. A muscle is composed of muscle fibers (or cells). Each muscle fiber is composed of many myofibrils. Each myofibril is composed of sarcomeres. The sarcomere is the smallest part of muscle that can contract. The contractile (or muscle) proteins are contained in the sarcomere. Actin is a muscle protein (sometimes called the thin filament) that can be visualized as a twisted strand of beads. Actin also contains two other proteins, troponin and tropomyosin. Tropomyosin is a long, string-like molecule that wraps around the actin filament. Troponin is a specialized protein found at the ends of the tropomyosin filament.

[Chapter 2]

53–A. Systolic blood pressure is an indicator of cardiac output (the amount of blood pumped out of the heart in 1 minute) in a healthy vascular system. Cardiac output normally increases as workload increases, because the peripheral and central stimuli that control cardiac output normally increase with an increase in workload. Thus, systolic blood pressure should increase with an increase in workload. Failure of the systolic blood pressure to increase as workload increases indicates that cardiac output is not increasing, which, in turn, indicates an abnormal response to increasing workload. Additionally, an abnormally elevated systolic blood pressure response to aerobic exercise indicates an unhealthy vascular system.

[Chapter 4]

54–D. The majority of sedentary people are not motivated to initiate exercise programs and, if exercise is initiated, they are likely to stop within 3 to 6 months. In general, participants in earlier stages benefit most from cognitive strategies, such as listening to lectures and reading books without the expectation of actually engaging in exercise, whereas individuals in later stages depend more on behavioral techniques, such as reminders to exercise and developing social support to help them establish a regular exercise habit and be able to maintain it.

[Chapter 5]

55–D. Fitness testing is conducted in older adults for the same reasons as in younger adults, including exercise prescription, evaluation of progress, motivation, and education.

[Chapter 6]

56–C. Disordered eating covers a continuum from the preoccupation with food and body image to the syndromes of anorexia nervosa and bulimia. Anorexia nervosa is defined by symptoms that include a body weight that is 15% less than expected, a morbid fear of being or becoming fat, a preoccupation with food, and an abnormal body image (the thin person feels "fat"). Bulimia nervosa is defined by symptoms that include

binge eating twice a week for at least 3 months, loss of control over eating, purging behavior, and being overly concerned with body weight. Although specific psychiatric criteria must be met for a diagnosis to be made by a specialist, any degree of disordered eating may affect the eating pattern of the exerciser and place her or him at risk for nutritional deficiencies.

[Chapter 9]

57–C. A motor unit consists of the efferent (motor) nerve and all muscle fibers supplied (or innervated) by that nerve. The total number of motor units varies between different muscles. In addition, the total number of fibers in each motor unit varies between and within muscles. Different degrees of contraction can be achieved by varying the total number of motor units stimulated (or recruited) in a particular muscle. The major determinants of how much force is produced when a muscle contracts are the number of motor units that are recruited and the number of muscle fibers in each motor unit. When a motor unit is stimulated by a single nerve impulse, it responds by contracting one time and then relaxing. This is called a twitch. If a motor unit is continuously stimulated without adequate time for relaxation to occur, tetanus occurs. If a motor unit receives a second stimulation before it is allowed to relax, the two impulses are added (or summated), and the tension developed is greater.

[Chapter 2]

58–A. The steps are as follows:

a. Write out the running equation (accurate for speeds in excess of 5 mph):

$$\dot{V}O_2 \text{ (mL} \cdot \text{kg}^{-1} \cdot \text{min}^{-1}) = \text{horizontal} + \text{vertical} + \text{resting}$$

$$\dot{V}O_2 \text{ (mL} \cdot \text{kg}^{-1} \cdot \text{min}^{-1}) = \text{(speed} \times 0.2) + \text{(speed} \times \text{grade} \times 0.9) + 3.5$$

b. Convert speed (6.5 mph) to meters per minute:

$$6.5 \times 26.8 = 174.2 \text{ m} \cdot \text{min}^{-1}$$

c. Solve for the unknown:

$$\dot{V}O_2 \text{ (mL} \cdot \text{kg}^{-1} \cdot \text{min}^{-1}) = (174.2 \times 0.2) + (174.2 \times 0.05 \times 0.9) + 3.5$$

$$\dot{V}O_2 \text{ (mL} \cdot \text{kg}^{-1} \cdot \text{min}^{-1}) = 46.18 \text{ mL} \cdot \text{kg}^{-1} \cdot \text{min}^{-1}$$

d. Convert 46.18 mL $\cdot$ kg^{-1} $\cdot$ min^{-1} to MET:

$$1 \text{ MET} = 3.5 \text{ mL} \cdot \text{kg}^{-1} \cdot \text{min}^{-1}$$
$$46.18 \div 3.5 = 13.2 \text{ MET}$$

[Chapter 11]

59–B. Reinforcement is the positive or negative consequence for performing or not performing a behavior. Positive consequences are rewards that motivate behavior. This can include both intrinsic and extrinsic rewards. Intrinsic rewards are the benefits gained because of the rewarding nature of the activity. Extrinsic or external rewards are the positive outcomes received from others, which may include encouragement and praise or material reinforcements such as T-shirts and money.

[Chapter 5]

60–C. Exercise-induced asthma is a reversible airway obstruction that results directly from the ventilatory response to exercise. Hyperventilation causes an individual to breathe more through the mouth than through the nose and actually inhale deconditioned (cool, dirty, dry) air. The nose serves to warm, clean, and humidify the air. Deconditioned air triggers an immune or allergic response primarily in the small- and medium-sized airways in some individuals and may manifest in bronchoconstriction or bronchospasm. Medications are available that may prevent or reverse asthma attacks. These usually are administered in a tablet or aerosol form. Albuterol, terbutaline, glucocorticosteroids, cromolyn sodium, and theophylline are effective drugs to prevent or reverse asthma.

61–A. Creating a safe environment in which to exercise is a primary responsibility for any fitness facility. In developing and operating facilities and equipment for use by exercisers, the managers and staff are obligated to meet a standard of care for exerciser safety. The equipment to be used not only includes testing, cardiovascular, strength, and flexibility pieces, but also rehabilitation, pool, locker room, and emergency equipment. You must evaluate a number of criteria when selecting equipment. These criteria include correct anatomic positioning, ability to adjust to different body sizes, quality of design and materials, durability, repair records, and then price.

[Chapter 7]

62–A. The ability to take in and to utilize oxygen is dependent on the health and integrity of the heart, lungs, and circulatory systems. Efficiency of the aerobic metabolic pathways also is necessary to optimize cardiorespiratory fitness. The degree of improvement that may be expected in cardiorespiratory fitness relates directly to the frequency, intensity, duration, and mode or type of exercise. Maximal oxygen uptake may improve

between 5% and 30% with training. The exercise prescription may be altered for different populations to achieve the same results. However, for an apparently healthy person, the ACSM recommends an intensity of 60% to 90% maximal heart rate, duration of 20 to 60 minutes, and frequency of 3 to 5 days a week.

63–A. Plyometrics is a method of strength and power training that involves an eccentric loading of muscles and tendons followed immediately by an explosive concentric contraction. This stretch-shortening cycle may allow an enhanced generation of force during the concentric (shortening) phase. Most well-controlled studies have shown no significant difference in power improvement when comparing plyometrics with high-intensity strength training. The explosive nature of this type of activity may increase the risk for musculoskeletal injury. Plyometrics should not be considered a practical resistance exercise alternative for health/fitness applications but may be appropriate for select athletic/performance needs.

64–D. The characteristics of a good manager include designing programs and monitoring the implementation of programs. He or she also guides the staff or clients through the program. He or she is a good communicator who also purchases equipment and supplies. A good manager monitors the safety of the program or facility and surveys clients and staff to assess the success and value of the program.

65–A. Agreements, releases, and consents are documents that clearly describe what the client is participating in, the risks that are involved, and the rights of the client and the facility. If signed by the client, he or she is accepting some of the responsibility and risk by participating in this program. All fitness facilities are strongly encouraged to have program/service agreements and informed consents drafted by a lawyer for their protection.

66–B. The stores of ATP energy in skeletal muscle are very limited (5–10 seconds of high-intensity work). After this time, another high-energy source, PC, which has only one high-energy phosphate band, begins to break down. The energy from the breakdown of PC is used to re-form ATP, which then breaks down to provide energy for exercise. Only energy released from the breakdown of ATP, however, can provide energy for biologic work such as exercise.

[Chapter 2]

67–D. The sliding filament theory defines how skeletal muscles are believed to contract. These steps can best be described as what occurs during rest, stimulation, contraction, and then relaxation of the muscle. At rest, no nerve activity (except normal resting tone) occurs. Calcium is stored in a network of tubes in the muscle called the sarcoplasmic reticulum. If no calcium is present, the active sites (where the myosin cross-bridges can attach) are kept covered. If the active sites are uncovered, the enzyme that causes ATP to break down and release energy is kept inactive. During conditions when a nerve impulse is present, this impulse causes calcium to be released. The calcium binds to the troponin on the actin filament. When this occurs, the active sites are uncovered. Now, the myosin cross-bridges bind the active sites and form actomyosin (a connection between the actin and myosin proteins), and contraction occurs.

[Chapter 2]

68–C. After 30 years of age, skeletal muscle strength begins to decline. However, the loss of strength is not linear, with most of the decline occurring after 50 years of age. By 80 years of age, strength loss usually is in the range of 30% to 40%. The loss of strength with aging results primarily from a loss of muscle mass, which, in turn, is caused by both the loss of muscle fibers and the atrophy of the remaining fibers.

[Chapter 3]

69–C. Specific risks are associated with exercise for men and for women (although the statistics for women are not yet known). The rate of acute cardiovascular events is 1 in 187,500 hours of exercise. The rate of death during exercise for men is 1 in 396,000 hours. In addition, deaths during exercise are more common among men who have more than one risk factor for coronary artery disease. The risk of cardiovascular events or death is lower among men who are habitually active.

[Chapter 4]

70–D. Fiber is a type of complex carbohydrate that is indigestible by the body. This means that it will pass straight through the digestive system and is commonly referred to as "adding bulk to the diet." Fiber can be either water-soluble (pectin or gums) or water-insoluble (cellulose, hemicellulose, and lignin). Dietary fiber has been linked to the prevention of certain diseases.

[Chapter 9]

71–D. The Health Belief Model assumes that people will engage in a behavior (e.g., exercise) when there is a perceived threat of disease, there is a belief of susceptibility to disease, and the threat of disease is severe. This model also incorporates cues to action as critical to adopting and maintaining behavior. The concept of self-efficacy (confidence) is also added to this model.

[Chapter 5]

72–C. Informed consent is not a legal document. It does not provide legal immunity to a facility or individual in the event of injury to a client. It simply provides evidence that the client was made aware of the purposes, procedures, and risks associated with the test or exercise program. The consent form does not relieve the facility/individual of the responsibility to do everything possible to ensure the safety of the client. Negligence, improper test administration, inadequate personnel qualifications, and insufficient safety procedures all are items that are not expressly covered by informed consent. Because of the limitations associated with informed consent documents, legal counsel should be sought during the development of the document.

[Chapter 6]

73–C. Three common assessments for muscular endurance include the bench press, for upper body endurance (a weight is lifted in cadence with a metronome or other timing device; the total number of lifts performed correctly and in time with the cadence is counted); the push-up, for upper body endurance (the client assumes a standardized beginning position with the body held rigid and supported by the hands and toes for men and the hands and knees for women; the body is lowered to the floor, then pushed back up to the starting position; the score is the total number of properly performed push-ups completed without a pause by the client with no time limit); and the sit-up, for abdominal muscular endurance (the client begins in the bent-knee sit-up starting position with the hands resting on the floor and no foot restraint; the client then curls the upper body upward so that the hands slide along the floor a distance of 12.3 centimeters, with sit-ups performed at a cadence of 25 per minute until the client is no longer able to complete the action at the prescribed cadence).

[Chapter 6]

74–A. Overuse injuries become more common when people participate in more cardiovascular exercise. An exerciser starts to exercise too much and either does not take a rest day at all and/or develops a minor injury and does not stop and rest so that the injury might heal.

[Chapter 7]

75–C. Several methods are available to define exercise intensity objectively. The ACSM recommends that exercise intensity be prescribed within a range of 60% to 90% of maximum heart rate or between 50% and 85% of $\dot{V}O_2$max, maximum MET, or heart rate reserve. Lower intensities will elicit a favorable response in individuals with very low fitness levels. Because of the variability in estimating maximal heart rate from age, it is recommended that whenever possible, an actual maximal heart rate from a graded exercise test be used. Factors to consider when determining appropriate exercise intensity include age, fitness level, medications, overall health status, and individual goals.

76–B. The ACSM recommends that one set of 8 to 12 repetitions of each exercise should be performed to volitional fatigue. A 5- to 10-minute warm-up of aerobic activity or a light set (50–75% of the training weight) of the specific resistance exercise should precede the resistance exercise program. The ACSM recommends that these exercises be performed at least 2 days per week. Training two times per week will yield approximately 80% of the strength improvement seen with training three times per week, provided that the intensity is the same.

77–B. The risk of orthopedic and, perhaps, cardiovascular complications may be increased with high-intensity activity. Factors to consider when determining intensity include the individual's level of fitness, presence of medications that may influence exercise performance, risk of cardiovascular or orthopedic injury, and individual preference for exercise and individual program objectives.

78–B. During auscultation, a stethoscope is placed over the left aspect of the midsternum, or just under the pectoralis major. Take care to avoid placing the stethoscope bell over fat or muscle tissue, because this may interfere with the clarity of the sound. When measuring heart rate by auscultation, the initial sound is counted as zero. The longer the time for which heart sounds are counted, the less the error introduced by inadvertently missing a single beat yet the greater the risk of miscounting.

[Chapter 6]

79–D. The effects of regular (chronic) exercise can be classified or grouped into those that occur at rest, during moderate (or submaximal) exercise, and during maximal effort work. For example, you can measure an untrained individual's resting heart rate, train the person for several weeks or months, and then measure resting heart rate again to see what change has occurred. Resting heart rate declines with regular exercise, probably because of a combination of decreased sympathetic tone, increased parasympathetic tone, and decreased intrinsic firing rate of the sinoatrial node. Stroke volume increases at rest as a result of increased myocardial contractility. Little or no change occurs in cardiac output at rest, because the decline in heart rate is compensated for by the increase in stroke volume.

[Chapter 2]

80–D. Heart muscle has the capability of producing its own action potential (autorhythmicity). In other words, if an impulse is not received from higher-level brain centers, cardiac muscle will stimulate itself.

[Chapter 2]

81–A. The rate of death, either during or immediately after exercise testing, is 0.5 in 10,000 (~0.01%). The rate of myocardial infarction during or immediately after exercise testing is 3.6 in 10,000 (~0.04%). Complications during testing that require hospitalization are approximately 0.1%.

[Chapter 4]

82–C. Key components of the Transtheoretical Model are the Processes of Behavioral Change. These processes include five cognitive processes (consciousness raising, dramatic relief, environmental reevaluation, self-reevaluation, and social liberation) and five behavioral processes (counterconditioning, helping relationships, reinforcement management, self-liberation, and stimulus control).

[Chapter 5]

83–D. The purpose of the fitness assessment is to develop a proper exercise prescription (the data collected through appropriate fitness assessments assist the health/fitness instructor in developing safe, effective programs of exercise based on the individual client's current fitness status), to evaluate the rate of progress (baseline and follow-up testing indicate progression toward fitness goals), and to motivate (fitness assessments provide information needed to develop reasonable, attainable goals). Progress toward or attainment of a goal is a strong motivator for continued participation in an exercise program.

[Chapter 6]

84–C. Basic principles of care for musculoskeletal injuries include the objectives for care of exercise-related injuries, which are to decrease pain, reduce swelling, and prevent further injury. These objectives can be met in most cases by RICES (rest, ice, compression, elevation, and stabilization). Rest will prevent further injury and ensure that the healing process will begin. Ice is used to reduce swelling, bleeding, inflammation, and pain. Compression also helps to reduce swelling and bleeding. Compression is achieved by the use of elastic wraps or tape. Elevation helps to decrease the blood flow and excessive pressure to the injured area. Stabilization reduces muscle spasm by assisting in relaxation of associated muscles.

[Chapter 7]

85–D. Various systems of resistance training exist that differ in their combinations of sets, repetitions, and resistance applied, all in an effort to overload the muscle. Circuit weight training uses a series of exercises performed in succession with minimal rest between exercises. Various health benefits as well as modest improvements in aerobic capacity have been demonstrated as a result of circuit weight training. Super-sets refer to consecutive sets for antagonistic muscle groups with no rest between sets or multiple exercises for a specific muscle group with little or no rest. Split routines entail exercising different body parts on different days or during different sessions. Pyramids are performed either in ascending (increasing the resistance within a set of repetitions or from one set to the next) or descending (decreasing the resistance within a set of repetitions or from one set to the next) fashion.

86–D. The goal of the exercise component of a weight reduction program should be to maximize caloric expenditure. Frequency, intensity, and duration must be manipulated in conjunction with a dietary regimen in an attempt to create a caloric deficit of 500 to 1,000 calories per day. The recommended maximal rate for weight loss is 1 to 2 pounds per week.

87–C. Kyphosis is a posterior thoracic curvature. Scoliosis is a lateral deviation in the alignment of the vertebrae. Lordosis is an anterior lumbar curvature.

[Chapter 1]

88–A. Learning theories assume that an overall complex behavior arises from many small simple behaviors. By reinforcing partial behaviors and modifying cues in the environment, it is possible to shape the desired behavior.

[Chapter 5]

89–C. The PAR-Q is a screening tool for self-directed exercise programming. The MMPI is a psychological scale. The Borg scale is used to measure or to rate perceived exertion during exercise or during an exercise test.

[Chapter 6]

90–C. To get the best and most accurate information, the following order of testing is recommended: resting measurements (e.g., heart rate, blood pressure, blood analysis), body composition, cardiorespiratory fitness, muscular fitness and flexibility. Some methods of body composition assessment are sensitive to hydration status and some tests of cardiorespiratory and muscular fitness may affect hydration, so it is inappropriate to administer those prior to the body composition assessment. Assessing cardiorespiratory fitness often utilizes measures of heart rate. Some tests of muscular fitness and flexibility affect heart rate, so they are inappropriate to administer prior to cardiorespiratory fitness testing, since the elevated heart rate from those assessments may, in turn, affect the cardiorespiratory fitness testing results.

[Chapter 6]

91–D. When an emergency or injury occurs, the safe and effective management of the situation will assure the best care for the member. Implementing emergency procedures is an important part of the training of the staff. In-services, safety plans, and emergency procedures should be a part of the staff training. In addition, all exercise staff should be CPR certified and trained in first aid. Therefore, the fitness center management, staff, and clients all are included in the implementation of an emergency plan.

[Chapter 7]

92–D. Possible medical emergencies during exercise include heat exhaustion or heat stroke, fainting, hypoglycemia, hyperglycemia, simple or compound fractures, bronchospasm, hypotension or shock, seizures, bleeding, and other cardiac symptoms.

[Chapter 7]

93–C. During most graded exercise tests, the following measurements are taken: heart rate (during a 2-

minute stage, every minute; during a 3-minute stage, at minutes 2 and 3 and additionally at every subsequent minute until steady state is achieved), blood pressure (once during each stage, toward the end of the stage), and RPE (once during each stage, toward the end of the stage). In most graded exercise tests for which the stages are 3 minutes in length, it is practical to take the measurements according to the following schedule: minute 2:00, heart rate; minute 2:15, RPE; minute 2:30, blood pressure; minute 3, heart rate.

[Chapter 6]

94–D. Resistance exercise may be performed by incorporating exercises requiring different muscle actions. Isometric muscle action occurs when the length of the muscle does not change but the muscle tension is increased through enhanced neuromuscular recruitment patterns. These actions occur when we attempt to push or pull against an immovable object. Although isometric activities have been shown to elicit improvements in muscular strength, these improvements seem to be limited to the joint angle(s) at which the action is applied. Therefore, it would require many isometric contractions at many joint angles for isometrics to be considered effective. Additionally, exaggerated increases in blood pressure may accompany isometric muscle actions. This type of exercise has some application in the management of select musculoskeletal injury.

95–B. Protein is made of carbon, hydrogen, and oxygen, but it also uniquely includes nitrogen. The building blocks of protein are the more than 20 amino acids. The amino acids make specific, long-sequenced chains of proteins. Eight essential amino acids cannot be manufactured by the human body; these are necessary for protein production and must be obtained in the dietary intake.

[Chapter 9]

96–D. Large muscle group activity performed in rhythmic fashion over prolonged periods facilitates the greatest improvements in aerobic fitness. Walking, running, cycling, swimming, stair climbing, aerobic dance, rowing, and cross-country skiing are examples of these types of activities. Weight training should not be consid-

ered an appropriate activity for enhancing aerobic fitness, but it should be employed in a comprehensive exercise program to improve muscular strength and anaerobic muscular endurance. The mode(s) of activity should be selected based on the principle of specificity—that is, with attention to the desired outcomes and to maintain the participation and enjoyment of the individual.

97–D. Different types of health screenings are used for various purposes. In commercial settings, clients should be screened more extensively for potential health risks. At minimum, a personal medical history should be taken. In addition, present medical status should be examined and questions asked regarding the use of medications (both prescription and over-the-counter), family history of heart disease and other medical conditions, and other lifestyle health habits (nutritional habits, exercise history, stress, and smoking).

[Chapter 6]

98–C. The number of times per day or per week that a person exercises is interrelated with both the intensity and the duration of activity. Generally, persons with poor fitness may benefit from multiple short-duration, low-intensity exercise sessions per day. Individual goals, preferences, limitations, and time constraints also will determine frequency and the relationship between duration, frequency, and intensity.

99–D. Marketing and promoting a program is one of the significant functions of a manager. Promotions can be internal (within the facility to generate member interest) or external (bringing new members into the club). Developing ideas is a key component of a marketing plan. Idea development requires preparation, research, and an understanding of your audience. Ideas for marketing strategies often come from studying the market (research). A business plan is the next step; this plan describes in detail the marketing plan and justification for each action and program. Analysis of each aspect of the research is made, as are projections of the success of the plan, including a cost/benefit analysis. The decision to accept the marketing plan by management is made by the information found in the business plan.

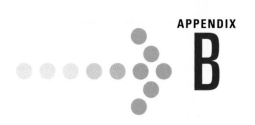
Clinical Comprehensive Exam

DIRECTIONS: Each of the numbered items or incomplete statements in this section is followed by answers or by completions of the statement. Select the ONE lettered answer or completion that is BEST in each case.

1. Which of the following medications is an endogenous catecholamine that optimizes blood flow to the heart and brain by increasing aortic diastolic pressure and preferentially shunts blood to the internal carotid artery, thus enhancing cerebral blood flow?
   A) Lidocaine.
   B) Oxygen.
   C) Atropine.
   D) Epinephrine.

2. If a healthy young man exercises at an intensity of $45 \text{ mL} \cdot \text{kg}^{-1} \cdot \text{min}^{-1}$ three times per week for 45 minutes each session, how long would it take him to lose 10 pounds of fat? Assume that he weighs 70.0 kg.
   A) 4 weeks.
   B) 7.14 weeks.
   C) 16.5 weeks.
   D) 19 weeks.

3. All of the following techniques are commonly used in the diagnosis of coronary artery disease EXCEPT
   A) Electrocardiography.
   B) Radionuclide imaging.
   C) Echocardiography.
   D) Cardiac spirometry.

4. During mild to moderate exercise, minute ventilation increases primarily through an increase in
   A) Tidal volume.
   B) Respiratory rate.
   C) Forced expiratory volume.
   D) Forced inspiratory volume.

5. Which of the following would be an adequate exercise prescription for a patient who has undergone a heart transplant?
   A) High intensity, short duration, small muscle groups, and high frequency.
   B) High intensity, long duration, small muscle groups, and high frequency.
   C) Low to moderate intensity, 6 days per week, large muscle groups, and moderate duration.
   D) Low intensity, three days per week, large muscle groups, and moderate duration.

6. Recommendations for exercise in patients with diabetes include all of the following EXCEPT
   A) Avoiding injection of insulin into an exercising muscle.
   B) Exercising with a partner.
   C) Exercising only when temperature and humidity are moderate.
   D) Avoiding exercise during peak insulin activity.

7. Which of the following is a reversible pulmonary condition caused by some type of irritant (e.g., dust, pollen) and characterized by obvious narrowing of the bronchial airways, dyspnea and, possibly, hypoxia and hypercapnia?
   A) Emphysema.
   B) Bronchitis.
   C) Asthma.
   D) Pulmonary vascular disease.

8. Atrial flutter and atrial fibrillation are examples of
   A) Ventricular arrhythmias.
   B) Supraventricular arrhythmias.
   C) Atrioventricular conduction delays.
   D) Preexcitation syndromes.

9. Which of the following statements regarding contraindications to graded exercise testing is NOT accurate?
   A) Some individuals have risk factors that outweigh the potential benefits from exercise testing and the information that may be obtained.
   B) Absolute contraindications refer to individuals for whom exercise testing should not be performed until the situation or condition has stabilized.
   C) Relative contraindications include patients who might be tested if the potential benefit from exercise testing outweighs the relative risk.
   D) All of the above statements are true.

10. An impulse originating in the sinoatrial node and then spreading to both atria, causing atrial depolarization, appears on the electrocardiogram as a
   A) P wave.
   B) QRS complex.
   C) ST segment.
   D) T wave.

11. Whole-body and segmental movement occurs in three spatial dimensions. Which plane divides the body into symmetrical right and left halves?
   A) Frontal.
   B) Transverse.
   C) Sagittal.
   D) Medial.

12. To reduce the risk for certain diseases and to gain health benefits, the recommended daily energy expenditure from physical activity is
   A) 50–80 kcal/day.
   B) 80–100 kcal/day.
   C) 150–400 kcal/day.
   D) >400 kcal/day.

13. Exercise has a beneficial effect on reducing the mortality rate in patients with coronary artery disease. The mechanisms responsible for this include
   A) Its effect on other risk factors.
   B) Reduced myocardial oxygen demand at rest and at submaximal workloads.
   C) Reduced platelet aggregation.
   D) All of the above.

14. The degradation of carbohydrate to pyruvate or lactate occurs through
   A) The adenosine triphosphate system.
   B) Anaerobic glycolysis.
   C) Aerobic glycolysis.
   D) Fat metabolism.

15. Which of the following is LEAST likely to be an effective means of permanent weight loss?
   A) Dietary changes.
   B) Increased exercise.
   C) Rapid weight loss.
   D) Diet and exercise.

16. Which of the following strategies is most commonly used in patients with multiple-vessel coronary artery disease who are not responding to other treatments?
   A) Percutaneous transluminal coronary angioplasty.
   B) Coronary artery stent.
   C) Coronary artery bypass graft surgery.
   D) Pharmacologic therapy.

17. Which of the following statements BEST describes the precautions for exercise taken in patients with an automatic implantable cardioverter defibrillator (AICD)?
   A) Heart rate must be monitored closely during exercise to ensure that it does not reach the level of the activation rate and trigger a shock to the patient.
   B) Most AICDs are set to deliver a shock to the patient only when the heart rate nears 300 bpm.
   C) The patient should avoid exercise-related increases in heart rate.
   D) The intensity of exercise should be kept very low for this patient.

18. Oxidative phosphorylation uses oxygen as the final acceptor of hydrogen to form adenosine triphosphate (ATP) and
   A) Phosphocreatine.
   B) Lactate.
   C) Carbon monoxide.
   D) Water.

19. Healthy, untrained subjects have an anaerobic threshold at approximately what percentage of maximal oxygen consumption?
   A) 25%.
   B) 55%.
   C) 75%.
   D) 95%.

20. Which of the following medications reduces myocardial ischemia by lowering myocardial oxygen demand, with some increase in oxygen supply, and is used to treat typical and variant angina?
   A) β-Adrenergic blockers.
   B) Calcium-channel blockers.
   C) Aspirin.
   D) Nitrates.

21. Which of the following structures is located in the posterior wall of the right atrium, just inferior to the opening of the superior vena cava?
   A) Sinoatrial node.
   B) Atrioventricular node.
   C) Bundle of His.
   D) Purkinje fibers.

22. How many calories will a 110-pound woman expend if she pedals on a Monark cycle ergometer at 50 rpm against a resistance of 2.5 kp for 60 minutes?
   A) 12.87 calories.
   B) 31.28 calories.
   C) 510 calories.
   D) 3500 calories.

23. Electrocardiographic precordial lead V_4 is placed at the
    A) Fourth intercostal space, left sternal border.
    B) Fourth intercostal space, right sternal border.
    C) Midaxillary line, fifth intercostal space.
    D) Midclavicular line, fifth intercostal space.

24. Which of the following increases curvilinearly with the work rate until it reaches near maximum at a level equivalent to approximately 50% of aerobic capacity, increasing only slightly thereafter?
    A) Stroke volume.
    B) End-diastolic volume.
    C) Cardiac output.
    D) Oxygen consumption.

25. Exposure to which of the following environments causes vasoconstriction (higher blood pressure response), lowering the anginal threshold and, possibly, provoking angina at rest (variant or Prinzmetal's angina), and can induce asthma, general dehydration, and dryness or burning of the mouth and throat?
    A) Extreme cold.
    B) Extreme heat.
    C) High altitude.
    D) High humidity.

26. What is the equivalent total caloric content of 3.0 pounds (1.36 kg) of fat?
    A) 1,000 kcal.
    B) 5,500 kcal.
    C) 10,500 kcal.
    D) 15,000 kcal.

27. Which of the following is NOT a major symptom or sign that is suggestive of cardiopulmonary or metabolic disease?
    A) Ankle edema.
    B) Claudication.
    C) Orthopnea.
    D) Bronchitis.

28. Irreversible necrosis of the heart muscle resulting from prolonged ischemia describes
    A) Thrombosis.
    B) Aneurysm.
    C) Infarction.
    D) Thrombolysis.

29. Which of the following medications used to treat heart failure and some arrhythmias can produce electrocardiographic changes of QT-interval shortening and ST-segment depression (often known as "scooping")?
    A) β-Blockers.
    B) Calcium-channel blockers.
    C) Potassium.
    D) Digitalis.

30. The energy to perform physical work comes from the breakdown of
    A) Testosterone.
    B) Oxygen.
    C) ATP.
    D) Phosphocreatine.

31. For a patient who has had coronary artery bypass graft surgery or valve replacement surgery, which of the following care measures is NOT indicated?
    A) The patient should avoid extreme tension on the upper body because of sternal and leg wounds for 2 to 4 months.
    B) The clinician should observe for infection or discomfort along the incision.
    C) The patient should be monitored for chest pain, dizziness, and dysrhythmias.
    D) The patient should avoid high-intensity exercise early in the rehabilitation period.

32. Which of the following is a MODIFIABLE risk factor for the development of coronary artery disease?
    A) Increasing age.
    B) Male gender.
    C) Family history.
    D) Tobacco smoking.

33. Regular aerobic exercise 5 days/week at 50–85% of maximal oxygen consumption ($\dot{V}O_{2max}$) for 45 minutes will most favorably affect
    A) Homocysteine levels.
    B) Triglycerides.
    C) Lipoprotein (a).
    D) Low-density lipoprotein cholesterol.

34. Which of the following redistributes blood flow from the trunk to peripheral areas, decreases resistance in the tissues for movement, and increases the tissue temperature and energy production?
    A) Training effect.
    B) Cool-down.
    C) Warm-up.
    D) Orthostatic response.

35. Regarding risk stratification for exercise testing, individuals with signs or symptoms suggesting cardiopulmonary or metabolic disease and/or two or more risk factors are considered to be at
    A) No risk.
    B) Low risk.
    C) Moderate risk.
    D) High risk.

36. Which of the following conditions is marked by progressively more difficult conduction of an electrical impulse through the atrioventricular (AV) junction, producing a progressively longer PR interval until a P wave is not conducted (with the

electrocardiogram showing a P wave not followed by a QRS complex)?
A)   First-degree AV block.
B)   Second-degree AV block, Mobitz type I.
C)   Second-degree AV block, Mobitz type II.
D)   Third-degree AV block.

37. Heart rate increases in a linear fashion with work rate and oxygen uptake during dynamic exercise. The magnitude of the heart rate response is related to
A)   Age.
B)   Body position.
C)   Medication use.
D)   All of the above.

38. Regular exercise can have a positive effect on all of the following conditions EXCEPT
A)   Obesity.
B)   Dyslipidemia.
C)   Hypertension.
D)   Cirrhosis.

39. On the electrocardiogram, which of the following is considered to be a sensitive indicator of myocardial ischemia or injury?
A)   Q wave.
B)   PR interval.
C)   ST segment.
D)   T wave.

40. Which of the following evaluation techniques provides the LEAST accurate measurement of obesity?
A)   Body mass index.
B)   Waist-to-hip ratio.
C)   Body composition analysis.
D)   Height/weight tables.

41. A balance between the energy required by the working muscles and the rate of ATP production through aerobic metabolism is referred to as
A)   Oxygen debt.
B)   Oxygen deficit.
C)   Steady state.
D)   Adaptation.

42. On the electrocardiogram, various combinations of ST-segment abnormalities, the presence of Q waves, or the absence of R waves may suggest
A)   Cerebrovascular accident.
B)   Acute myocardial infarction.
C)   Ventricular aneurysm.
D)   Mitral valve prolapse.

43. What is the relative oxygen consumption of walking on a treadmill at 3.5 mph up a 10% grade?
A) $181.72 \text{ mL} \cdot \text{kg}^{-1} \cdot \text{min}^{-1}$.
B) $18.17 \text{ mL} \cdot \text{kg}^{-1} \cdot \text{min}^{-1}$.

C) $29.76 \text{ mL} \cdot \text{kg}^{-1} \cdot \text{min}^{-1}$.
D) $27.96 \text{ mL} \cdot \text{kg}^{-1} \cdot \text{min}^{-1}$.

44. Which of the following axes lies perpendicular to the frontal plane?
A)   Longitudinal.
B)   Mediolateral.
C)   Anteroposterior.
D)   Transverse.

45. Expected benefits of regular exercise in patients with peripheral vascular disease include all of the following EXCEPT
A)   Redistribution and increased blood flow to the legs.
B)   Increased tolerance for walking (improved claudication pain tolerance).
C)   Increased blood viscosity.
D)   Improved muscle cell metabolism.

46. Which of the following patients do NOT need a physician's evaluation before initiating a vigorous exercise program?
A)   Men over age 50 and women over age 50 with fewer than two risk factors.
B)   Men under age 40 and women under age 50 with fewer than two risk factors.
C)   Men under age 40 and women under age 50 with two risk factors.
D)   Men under age 50 and women under age 50 with known disease.

47. All of the following are types of intraventricular conduction disturbances EXCEPT
A)   Left bundle branch block.
B)   Right bundle branch block.
C)   AV nodal reentrant tachycardia.
D)   All of the above are types of intraventricular conduction disturbances.

48. For persons free of absolute contraindications to exercise, the health and medical benefits of exercise clearly outweigh any associated risks. To ensure as safe an environment as possible during exercise testing and training, the clinical exercise specialist must be prepared to do all of the following EXCEPT
A)   Understand the risks associated with exercise and exercise testing.
B)   Be able to perform emergency medical procedures.
C)   Have knowledge regarding the care of an injury or medical emergency.
D)   Be able to implement preventive measures.

49. What is defined as a surplus of adipose tissue, resulting from excess energy intake relative to energy expenditure?
A)   Overweight.
B)   Android obesity.

C)   Obesity.

D)   Gynoid obesity.

50.   Although certification of clinical exercise rehabilitation programs is a relatively new concept, it involves many already established components of the exercise program. Which of the following is NOT a important component of clinical exercise rehabilitation program certification?

A)   Staff certification and/or licensure.

B)   Program outcomes measures.

C)   The policy and procedures manual.

D)   Adherence to insurance codes for billing.

51.   Preload of the left ventricle refers to

A)   Contractility.

B)   Diastolic filling.

C)   Ventricular outflow.

D)   Ejection fraction.

52.   A constricting, squeezing, burning, or heavy feeling in the chest area, neck, cheeks, shoulder, or arms, provoked by physical work or stress, is characteristic of

A)   Angina.

B)   Asthma.

C)   Atherosclerosis.

D)   Arteriosclerosis.

53.   Health screening before participation in a graded exercise test is indicated for all of the following reasons EXCEPT

A)   To determine the presence of disease.

B)   To consider contraindications for exercise testing or training.

C)   To determine the need for referral to a medically supervised exercise program.

D)   To evaluate aerobic capacity.

54.   The proper emergency response for a patient who has experienced a cardiac arrest but now is breathing and has a palpable pulse includes

A)   Continuing the exercise test to determine why the patient had this response.

B)   Placing the patient in the recovery position with the head to the side to prevent an airway obstruction.

C)   Placing the patient in a comfortable seated position.

D)   Beginning Phase I cardiac rehabilitation.

55.   A patient weighing 200 pounds sets the treadmill at a speed of 4.0 mph and a grade of 5%. During exercise, his blood pressure rises to 150/90 mm Hg, and his heart rate increases to 150 bpm. What is his estimated energy expenditure in terms of L/min?

A)   1.07 L/min.

B)   2.17 L/min.

C)   4.28 L/min

D)   8.56 L/min

56.   Advancing age brings a progressive decline in bone

A)   Mineral density and calcium content.

B)   Distensibility.

C)   Fractures.

D)   None of the above.

57.   Which of the following procedures provides the LEAST sensitivity and specificity in the diagnosis of coronary artery disease?

A)   Coronary angiography.

B)   Echocardiography.

C)   Radionuclide imaging.

D)   Electrocardiography.

58.   When an electrical impulse is generated in a particular area in the heart, the outside of the cells in this area become negatively charged, and the inside of the cells become positively charged, in a process known as

A)   Polarization.

B)   Repolarization.

C)   Depolarization.

D)   Excitation.

59.   Cardiac output increases linearly with increased work rate. At exercise intensities up to 50% of maximal oxygen consumption, increased cardiac output is facilitated by an increase in

A)   Heart rate and stroke volume.

B)   Heart rate only.

C)   Stroke volume only.

D)   Neither heart rate nor stroke volume.

60.   Which of the following is TRUE of flow-resistive training (a type of breathing retraining for patients with pulmonary disease)?

A)   It helps to coordinate breathing with activities of daily living.

B)   It increases respiratory muscle strength and endurance.

C)   It uses a preset inspiratory pressure, usually at a consistent fraction of the maximal inspiratory pressure.

D)   It consists of breathing through a progressively smaller opening.

61.   A sustained muscle contraction against a fixed load or resistance with no change in the joint angle describes

A)   Isometric contraction.

B)   Isotonic contraction.

C)   Eccentric contraction.

D)   Isokinetic contraction.

62.   Which of the following is a NONMODIFIABLE risk factor for the development of coronary artery disease?

A)   Tobacco smoking.

B)   Dyslipidemia.

C) Family history.

D) Hypertension.

63. All of the following are examples of capital expenses EXCEPT

A) Tangible assets.

B) Staff salaries

C) Equipment purchases.

D) Construction.

64. A push or a pull that produces or has the capacity to produce a change in motion of a body is known as

A) Force.

B) Torque.

C) Newton's law of gravity.

D) Inertia.

65. The thickest, middle layer of the artery wall, which is composed predominantly of smooth muscle cells and is responsible for vasoconstriction and vasodilation, is known as the

A) Endothelium.

B) Intima.

C) Media.

D) Adventitia.

66. What electrocardiographic electrode is positioned at the fourth intercostal space, left sternal border?

A) V_1.

B) V_2.

C) V_3.

D) V_6.

67. An exercise program for a man weighing 154 pounds (70 kg) includes 5 minutes of warm-up at 2.0 MET, 20 minutes of treadmill running at 9 MET, 20 minutes of leg cycling at 8 MET, and 5 minutes of cool-down at 2.5 MET. What is this patient's total energy expenditure for an exercise session?

A) 162 kcal.

B) 868 kcal.

C) 444 kcal.

D) 1256 kcal.

68. The "average" cardiac output at maximal exercise is

A) 5 L/min

B) 10 L/min

C) 20 L/min

D) 20 mL/min

69. For a patient exercising in the heat or in a humid environment, the exercise prescription should be altered by

A) Increasing the intensity and decreasing the duration.

B) Decreasing the intensity and increasing the duration.

C) Decreasing the intensity and decreasing the duration.

D) Increasing the intensity and varying the duration.

70. Which of the following statements regarding an emergency plan is accurate?

A) The emergency plan does not need to be written down as long as everyone understands it.

B) As long as everyone knows his or her individual responsibilities during an emergency, a list of each staff member's responsibilities is not needed.

C) All emergency situations must be documented with dates, times, actions, people involved, and outcomes.

D) There is no need to practice emergencies as long as the staff members fully understand their responsibilities.

71. Which of the following is NOT considered to be an orthopedic condition that can lead to limitation of regular exercise (physical conditioning)?

A) Osteoarthritis.

B) Rheumatoid arthritis.

C) Osteoporosis.

D) Multiple sclerosis.

72. What disorder is characterized by an inflammation and edema of the trachea and bronchial tubes; hypertrophy of the mucous glands, which narrows the airway; arterial hypoxemia, leading to vasoconstriction of smooth muscle in the pulmonary arterioles and venules; and in the presence of continued vasoconstriction, pulmonary hypertension?

A) Emphysema.

B) Bronchitis.

C) Atherosclerosis.

D) Asthma.

73. For any high-risk patient, it is prudent to

A) Skip both the warm-up and the cool-down entirely.

B) Increase the intensity of the warm-up, and decrease the intensity of the cool-down.

C) Decrease the intensity of the warm-up, and increase the intensity of the cool-down.

D) Prolong both the warm-up and the cool-down.

74. Oxygen consumption can be measured by all of the following methods EXCEPT

A) Direct calorimetry.

B) Indirect calorimetry.

C) Estimation from workload.

D) Chest radiography.

75. Which of the following is NOT a symptom of transient ischemic attacks?
    A) Fatigue.
    B) Burning or tingling sensation in extremities.
    C) Ventricular fibrillation.
    D) Pain in jaw or neck.

76. The sum of the oxygen cost of physical activity and the resting energy expenditure is known as the
    A) Relative oxygen consumption.
    B) Absolute oxygen consumption.
    C) Net oxygen consumption.
    D) Gross oxygen consumption.

77. Ventricular tachycardia is marked by
    A) Two premature ventricular contractions (PVCs) in a row.
    B) One PVC on every other beat repeatedly.
    C) Two PVCs on every other beat repeatedly.
    D) Three PVCs in a row.

78. In which of the following conditions do necrotic heart muscle fibers degenerate, causing the muscle wall to become very thin and, thus, increasing the risk of thrombus, arrhythmias, and heart failure?
    A) Papillary dysfunction.
    B) Ventricular dilation.
    C) Myocardial infarction.
    D) Ventricular aneurysm.

79. The exercise prescription for muscular fitness (endurance) when using resistance training is
    A) 10–40% of one repetition maximum.
    B) 20–40% of one repetition maximum.
    C) 40–60% of one repetition maximum.
    D) 60–80% of one repetition maximum.

80. A slotted, stainless-steel tube that acts as a scaffold to hold the walls of a coronary artery open, thereby improving blood flow and relieving the symptoms of coronary artery disease, is known as a
    A) Balloon angioplasty.
    B) Stent.
    C) Lysing device.
    D) Coronary artery graft.

81. Which of the following conditions is indicated by a PR interval prolonged beyond 0.20 seconds, with all P waves conducted and all PR intervals the same?
    A) First-degree AV block.
    B) Second-degree AV block, Mobitz type I.
    C) Second-degree AV block, Mobitz type II.
    D) Third-degree AV block

82. Q waves detected by electrocardiogram leads V_1, V_2, V_3, and V_4 are an indication of
    A) Left anterior hemiblock.
    B) Left posterior hemiblock.
    C) Anterior infarction.
    D) Posterior infarction.

83. Atherosclerosis is thought to begin
    A) At birth.
    B) During adolescence.
    C) During middle age.
    D) Only after significant exposure to risk factors.

84. What graded exercise test protocol includes a momentary stoppage while measures are obtained?
    A) Step test.
    B) Continuous protocol.
    C) Discontinuous protocol.
    D) Field test.

85. For patients with congestive heart failure, which of the following statements about the efficacy of regular exercise is ACCURATE?
    A) Most of the improvement resulting from regular exercise is within the myocardium.
    B) These patients can never expect improved physical fitness.
    C) Exercise capacity is improved because of peripheral adaptations.
    D) Complete bed rest is prescribed for these patients.

86. In which of the following conditions would regular resistance training generally provide the MOST benefit?
    A) Osteoporosis.
    B) Rheumatoid arthritis.
    C) Stroke.
    D) Hypertension.

87. Above 1,500 m (4,921 feet) in altitude, what percentage reduction in maximal oxygen consumption can be expected for each subsequent 1,000 m (3,280 feet) in altitude?
    A) 2%.
    B) 10%.
    C) 25%.
    D) 50%.

88. The QRS complex on an electrocardiogram is measured from the beginning of the first wave to the end of the last wave of the complex. A QRS complex duration exceeding 0.20 second may point to
    A) AV conduction delay.
    B) Normal cardiac function.
    C) Intraventricular conduction delay.
    D) Acute myocardial infarction.

89. The incidence of cardiac arrest during clinical exercise testing is
    A) 1 in 10,000.
    B) 1 in 2,500.
    C) 1.4 in 10,000.
    D) 1 in 1 million.

90. A regular exercise program will primarily affect which lipid value?
    A) Total cholesterol level.
    B) Very-low-density and high-density lipoprotein cholesterol levels.
    C) Low-density lipoprotein cholesterol level.
    D) Total cholesterol:low-density cholesterol ratio.

91. In the terminology of the health behavior change model, which of the following refers to early phases of making a change in a health behavior or the intention to make a change?
    A) Antecedents.
    B) Adoption.
    C) Maintenance.
    D) Instruction.

92. An effective strategy in limiting the progression and promoting regression of atherosclerosis is to lower
    A) Low-density lipoprotein cholesterol.
    B) High-density lipoprotein cholesterol.
    C) Triglycerides.
    D) Glucose.

93. Which of the following is NOT a common type of "field test"?
    A) Cooper 12-minute test.
    B) 1.5-mile run test.
    C) Rockport walking test.
    D) Treadmill test.

94. A transmural myocardial infarction, marked by tissue necrosis in a full-thickness portion of the left ventricular wall, typically produces what changes on the electrocardiogram?
    A) T-wave inversion.
    B) U-wave inversion.
    C) ST-segment depression.
    D) ST-segment elevation.

95. Slow, safe activation of the body's responses to exercise and increased range of motion to prepare joints and muscles for vigorous activity occurs during
    A) Stimulus phase.
    B) Cool-down.

    C) Warm-up.
    D) Resistance training.

96. Which of the following statements is TRUE?
    A) For certain individuals, the risks of testing and exercise outweigh the potential benefits.
    B) For all patients, the risks of testing and exercise outweigh the benefits.
    C) Only a small percentage of patients should undergo exercise testing, because it is too dangerous.
    D) The potential benefits of testing and exercise always outweigh the risks.

97. Which of the following has a risk ratio in the development of coronary artery disease similar to that of hypertension, hypercholesterolemia, and cigarette smoking?
    A) Physical inactivity.
    B) Obesity.
    C) Diabetes mellitus.
    D) Psychological stress.

98. Which of the following is the best example of physical activity requiring anaerobic glycolysis to produce energy in the form of ATP?
    A) 40-yard dash.
    B) 400-m sprint.
    C) 5,000-m run.
    D) Marathon run.

99. A mean electrical axis (as measured on the electrocardiogram) of $-45°$ is considered to be
    A) Normal.
    B) Right-axis deviation.
    C) Left-axis deviation.
    D) Extreme left-axis deviation.

100. Which of the following medications significantly reduces first-year mortality rates in postmyocardial infarction patients by 20% to 35%?
    A) Aspirin.
    B) Calcium-channel blockers.
    C) β-Adrenergic blockers.
    D) Nitrates.

ANSWERS AND EXPLANATIONS

1–D. Epinephrine is an endogenous catecholamine that optimizes blood flow to the heart and brain by increasing aortic diastolic pressure and preferentially shunting blood to the internal carotid artery. Lidocaine is an antiarrhythmic agent that can decrease automaticity in the ventricular myocardium as well as raise the fibrillation threshold. Supplemental oxygen ensures adequate arterial oxygen content and greatly enhances tissue oxygenation. Atropine is a parasympathetic blocking agent used to treat bradyarrhythmias.

[Chapter 7]

2–C. The steps are as follows:

    a. Convert relative $\dot{V}O_2$ to absolute $\dot{V}O_2$ by multiplying relative $\dot{V}O_2$ (mL $\cdot$ kg^{-1} $\cdot$ min^{-1}) by his body weight.

    b. Assuming that the young man weight 70 kg:

$$\text{absolute } \dot{V}O_2 = \text{relative } \dot{V}O_2 \times \text{body weight}$$
$$= 45 \text{ mL} \cdot \text{kg}^{-1} \cdot \text{min}^{-1} \times 70 \text{ kg}$$
$$= 3{,}150 \text{ mL} \cdot \text{min}^{-1}$$

    c. To get L $\cdot$ min^{-1}, divide mL $\cdot$ min^{-1} by 1,000:

$$3{,}150 \text{ mL} \cdot \text{min}^{-1} \div 1{,}000 = 3.15 \text{ L} \cdot \text{min}^{-1}$$

    d. Multiply 3.15 L $\cdot$ min^{-1} by the constant 5.0 to get kcal $\cdot$ min^{-1}:

$$3.15 \text{ L} \cdot \text{min}^{-1} \times 5.0 = 15.75 \text{ kcal} \cdot \text{min}^{-1}$$

    e. Multiply 15.75 kcal $\cdot$ min^{-1} by the total number of minutes that he exercises (45 minutes $\times$ 3 times per week = 135 total minutes) to get the total caloric expenditure:

$$15.75 \text{ kcal} \cdot \text{min}^{-1} \times 135 \text{ minutes}$$
$$= 2126.25 \text{ kcal per week}$$

    f. Divide by 3,500 to get pounds of fat:

$$2{,}126.25 \text{ kcal} \div 3{,}500$$
$$= 0.6075 \text{ pounds of fat per week}$$

    g. Divide 10 pounds by 0.6075 pounds of fat per week to get how many weeks it will take him to lose 10 pounds of fat:

$$10 \div 0.6075 = 16.46 \text{ weeks}$$

    or approximately 16.5 weeks.

[Chapter 11]

3–D. In the diagnosis of coronary artery disease, electrocardiography, radionuclide imaging, and echocardiography are commonly used by themselves or with other tests. Other important diagnostic studies for coronary artery disease include coronary angiography.

[Chapter 4]

4–A. During mild to moderate exercise, minute ventilation increases primarily through tidal volume. During vigorous exercise, respiratory rate also increases. The increase in minute ventilation is directly proportional to oxygen consumption and carbon dioxide production during low-intensity exercise.

[Chapter 2]

5–C. Patients who have had heart transplant should exercise at a rating of perceived exertion of between 11 and 15 (moderate), between 60% and 70% of maximum metabolic capacity (MET), or 40% to 75% of maximal oxygen consumption. Frequency should be 4 to 6 days per week. Duration should include a prolonged warm-up. In addition, resistance training can be used in moderation.

[Chapter 8, ACSM's Guidelines for Exercise Testing and Prescription, 7th ed., pg. 197]

6–C. Recommended precautions for the exercising patient with diabetes include wearing proper footwear, maintaining adequate hydration, monitoring blood glucose level regularly, always wearing a medical identification bracelet or other form of identification, avoiding injecting insulin into exercising muscles, always exercising with a partner, and avoiding exercise during peak insulin activity. There is no reason why a patient with diabetes cannot exercise at any time if proper precautions are followed.

[Chapter 8]

7–C. The only reversible pulmonary disease, asthma is triggered by a mediator (e.g., dust, pollen) that increases calcium influx into mast cells, resulting in the release of chemical mediators (e.g., histamine). These mediators trigger bronchoconstriction (an increase in smooth muscle contraction of the bronchial tubes) and an inflammatory response. During asthma attacks, the individual becomes dyspneic and is likely to be hypoxic and hypercapnic. Attacks can last for hours or even days if they are not self-reversing or responsive to drug therapy.

[Chapter 4]

8–B. In the presence of atrial flutter and atrial fibrillation, the atria are not stimulated from the sinoatrial node but from some ectopic atrial focus or foci. The rate of atrial depolarization varies between 250 and 350 bpm for atrial flutter and between 400 and 600 bpm for atrial fibrillation. In either atrial flutter or atrial fibrillation, the rate of ventricular depolarization depends on the rate at which the AV node conducts the supraventricular stimuli.

[Chapter 12]

9–D. All of these statements are true regarding contraindications to exercise testing.

[Chapter 6]

10–A. The cardiac impulse originating in the sinoatrial node that spreads to both atria causing atrial depolarization is indicated on the electrocardiogram as a P wave. Atrial repolarization usually is not seen on the electrocardiogram, because it is obscured by the ventricular electrical potentials. Ventricular depolarization is represented on the electrocardiogram by the QRS complex. Ventricular repolarization is represented on the electrocardiogram by the ST segment, the T wave, and at times, the U wave.

[Chapter 12]

11–C. The sagittal plane divides the body into symmetric right and left halves. The frontal plane divides the body into front and back halves. The transverse plane divides the body in half superiorly and inferiorly. There is no medial plane.

[Chapter 1]

12–C. The principles of exercise prescription for health and physical fitness dictate that the average physical activity caloric expenditure needed to gain health benefits to reduce the risk for certain chronic diseases is between 150 and 400 kcal per day.

[Chapter 8, ACSM's Guidelines for Exercise Testing and Prescription, 7th ed., pg. 148]

13–D. The mechanisms responsible for a reduction in deaths from coronary artery disease include its effect on other risk factors, reduced myocardial oxygen demand both at rest and at submaximal workloads (resulting in an increased ischemic and angina threshold), reduced platelet aggregation, and improved endothelial-mediated vasomotor tone.

[Chapter 4]

14–B. The degradation of carbohydrate (glucose or glycogen) to pyruvate or lactate occurs in a process termed **anaerobic glycolysis**. Because pyruvate can participate in the aerobic production of ATP, glycolysis also can be considered as the first step in the aerobic production of ATP. Anaerobic metabolism results in the accumulation of lactic acid in the blood, which can contribute to fatigue; lactic acid also can be used as a fuel both during and after exercise.

[Chapter 2]

15–C. Rapid weight loss is considered to be 3 pounds per week for women and 3 to 5 pounds per week for men after the first 2 weeks of the diet. Long-term maintenance usually is a problem with rapid weight loss; one study reported total recidivism within 3 to 5 years. Modifications in diet and exercise generally are associated with more permanent weight loss.

[ChaptFer 9]

16–C. Coronary artery bypass graft surgery usually is reserved for patients who have a poor prognosis for survival or are unresponsive to pharmacologic treatment, stents, or percutaneous transluminal coronary angioplasty. Such patients include those with angina, left main coronary artery stenosis, multiple-vessel disease, and left ventricular dysfunction.

[Chapter 4]

17–A. There are many benefits of chronic exercise for a patient with an AICD. Several precautions need to be taken, however, including monitoring the heart rate and knowing the rate at which the AICD is set to shock the patient. The rate for activation is preset and varies for each patient. Depending on the exercise prescription, it generally is safe to exercise a patient up to that heart rate.

[Chapter 8, ACSM's Guidelines for Exercise Testing and Prescription, 7th ed., pg. 197]

18–D. The metabolic end products of oxidative phosphorylation include ATP and water. Other byproducts include carbon dioxide. Lactate is the metabolic end product of anaerobic glycolysis.

[Chapter 2]

19–B. A normal, unconditioned person has an anaerobic threshold of approximately 55% of maximal oxygen consumption. A conditioned person can have an anaerobic threshold as high as 70% to 90% of maximal oxygen consumption. The onset of metabolic acidosis or anaerobic metabolism can be measured through serial measurements of blood lactate level or assessment of expired gases, specifically pulmonary ventilation and carbon dioxide production.

[Chapter 2]

20–D. Nitrates reduce ischemia by reducing myocardial oxygen demand, with some increase in oxygen supply, and are used in the treatment of typical and variant angina. β-Adrenergic blockers reduce myocardial ischemia by lowering myocardial oxygen demand. These agents lower blood pressure, control ventricular arrhythmias, and significantly reduce first-year mortality rates in patients after myocardial infarction by 20% to 35%. Calcium-channel blockers reduce ischemia by altering the major determinants of myocardial oxygen supply and demand, but these agents have not been shown to reduce mortality rates after myocardial infarction. Aspirin is a platelet inhibitor.

[Chapter 4]

21–A. Cardiac impulses normally arise in the sinoatrial or sinus node of the heart. The sinoatrial node is located in the right atrium (posterior wall), near the opening of the superior vena cava. From the sinoatrial node, impulses travel to the left atrium and to the AV node, through the bundle of His, and then to Purkinje fibers in the ventricles.

[Chapter 12]

22–C. The steps are as follows:

a. Choose the ACSM leg cycling formula.

b. Write down your knowns, and convert the values to the appropriate units:

110 pounds ÷ 2.2 = 50 kg
50 rpm × 6 m = 300 m · min⁻¹
2.5 kp = 2.5 kg
60 minutes of cycling

c. Write down the ACSM formula:

$$\text{Leg cycling (mL · kg}^{-1} \cdot \text{min}^{-1}) = (1.8 \times \text{work rate} \div \text{body weight}) + 3.5 + 3.5 \text{ (mL · kg}^{-1} \cdot \text{min}^{-1})$$

d. Calculate the work rate:

$$\text{Work rate} = \text{kg · m · min}^{-1}$$
$$= 2.5 \text{ kg · } 300 \text{ m · min}^{-1}$$
$$= 750 \text{ kg · m · min}^{-1}$$

e. Substitute the known values for the variable name:

$$\text{mL · kg}^{-1} \cdot \text{min}^{-1} = (1.8 \times 750 \div 50) + 3.5 + 3.5$$

f. Solve for the unknown:

$$\text{mL · kg}^{-1} \cdot \text{min}^{-1} = 27 + 3.5 + 3.5$$
Gross leg cycling $\dot{V}_{O_2}$ = 34 mL · kg⁻¹ · min⁻¹

g. To find out how many calories she expends, we must first convert her oxygen consumption to absolute terms:

$$\text{absolute } \dot{V}_{O_2} = \text{relative } \dot{V}_{O_2} \times \text{body weight}$$
$$= 34 \text{ mL · kg}^{-1} \cdot \text{min}^{-1} \times 50 \text{ kg}$$
$$= 1,700 \text{ mL · min}^{-1}$$

h. Convert mL · min⁻¹ to L · min⁻¹ by dividing by 1,000:

$$1,700 \text{ mL · min}^{-1} \div 1,000 = 1.7 \text{ L · min}^{-1}$$

i. Next, we must see how many calories she expends in 1 minute by multiplying her absolute $\dot{V}_{O_2}$ (in L · min⁻¹) by the constant 5.0:

$$1.7 \text{ L · min}^{-1} \times 5.0 = 8.5 \text{ kcal · min}^{-1}$$

j. Finally, multiply the number of calories she expends in 1 minute by the number of minutes that she cycles:

$$8.5 \text{ kcal · min}^{-1} \times 60 \text{ minutes} = 510 \text{ total calories}$$

[Chapter 11]

23–D. The proper anatomical location of V_4 is the midclavicular line, fifth intercostal space. Precordial leads V_1 and V_2 are located at the fourth intercostal space, right and left sternal borders. There is no precordial lead site at the midaxillary line, fifth intercostal space.

[Chapter 12]

24–A. During exercise, stroke volume increases curvilinearly with work rate until it reaches near maximum at a level equivalent to approximately 50% of aerobic capacity, increasing only slightly thereafter. The left ventricle is able to contract with greater force during exercise because of a greater end-diastolic volume and enhanced mechanical ability of muscle fibers to produce force.

[Chapter 2]

25–A. Exposure to the cold causes vasoconstriction (higher blood pressure response), lowers the anginal threshold in patients with angina, can provoke angina at rest (variant or Prinzmetal's angina), and can induce asthma, general dehydration, and dryness or burning of the mouth and throat.

[Chapter 4]

26–C. To convert from pounds of fat to total kilocalories, multiply the fat weight (in pounds) by 3,500. The correct answer is 3 × 3,500 = 10,500 kcal.

[Chapter 11]

27–D. Bilateral ankle edema is a characteristic sign of heart failure, whereas unilateral edema of a limb often results from venous thrombosis or lymphatic blockage in the limb. Intermittent claudication, a condition caused by an inadequate blood supply, is an aching, crampy, tired, and sometimes burning pain in the legs that typically occurs with exercise and disappears with rest. Orthopnea is characterized by the inability to breathe easily unless one is sitting up straight or standing erect and is a symptom of heart failure. Bronchitis, a pulmonary disorder, is characterized by inflammation and edema of the trachea and bronchial tubes. Classic symptoms of bronchitis include chronic cough, sputum production, and dyspnea.

[Chapter 4]

28–C. A thrombosis is a specific clot that may cause a myocardial infarction. An aneurysm is a condition caused by necrotic muscle fibers of the heart that degenerate, causing the myocardial wall to become very thin. During systole, these non-functional muscle fibers do not contract but, rather, bulge outward, increasing the risk of thrombus, ventricular arrhythmia, and heart failure. Thrombolysis (thrombolytic therapy) uses a specific clot-dissolving agent administered during acute myocardial infarction to restore blood flow and to limit myocardial necrosis. Myocardial infarction is irreversible necrosis of the heart muscle resulting from prolonged ischemia.

[Chapter 4]

29–D. Digitalis is used to treat heart failure and certain arrhythmias. Shortening of the QT interval and a "scooping" of the ST–T complex characterize the effects of digitalis on the electrocardiogram.

[Chapter 12]

30–C. The energy to perform physical work comes from the breakdown of ATP. The amount of directly available ATP is small, with action lasting only 5 to 10 seconds; thus, ATP must be resynthesized constantly.

[Chapter 2]

31–A. Avoiding tension on the upper body typically is recommended for 4 to 8 weeks, not for 2 to 4 months. All of the other precautions are accurate.

[Chapter 8]

32–D. Aging, male gender, and family history of coronary artery disease are risk factors that cannot be controlled. Tobacco smoking can be modified or eliminated.

[Chapter 4]

33–B. Triglycerides are the only substance listed that has been proven to be directly affected by exercise. Homocysteine and lipoprotein (a) have not been shown to change favorably with exercise. Low-density lipoprotein cholesterol is affected by diet and may be lowered indirectly from weight loss associated with exercise.

[Chapter 9]

34–C. Warm-up exercises tend to redistribute blood flow from the trunk to peripheral areas, to decrease resistance in the tissues for movement, and to increase tissue temperature and energy production. Cool-down has an opposite effect.

[Chapter 2]

35–D. Low-risk individuals are those men younger than 45 years and women younger than 55 years who are asymptomatic and meet no more than one risk factor. Moderate-risk individuals are those men ≥45 years and women ≥55 years of age or those who meet the threshold for two or more risk factors. High-risk individuals are those with one or more signs and symptoms or known cardiovascular, pulmonary, or metabolic disease.

[Chapter 6, ACSM's Guidelines for Exercise Testing and Prescription, 7th ed., Table 2-4, pg 280]

36–B. Second-degree AV block is subdivided into two types: Mobitz type I, and Mobitz type II. Mobitz type I also is known as the Wenckebach phenomenon. In this condition, the conduction of the impulse through the AV junction becomes increasingly more difficult, resulting in a progressively longer PR interval, until a QRS complex is dropped following a P-wave. This indicates that the AV junction failed to conduct the impulse from the atria to the ventricles. This pause allows the AV node to recover, and the following P-wave is conducted with a normal or slightly shorter PR interval.

[Chapter 12]

37–D. The magnitude of heart rate response is related to age, body position, fitness, type of activity, presence of heart disease, medications, blood volume, and the environment. In unconditioned persons, a proportionally greater increase in heart rate is observed at any fixed submaximal work rate compared with that seen in conditioned persons.

[Chapter 2]

38–D. Regular exercise increases caloric expenditure in an effort to reduce body weight for those who are obese; increases the activity of lipoprotein lipase, which alters blood fats (e.g., triglycerides); and lowers blood pressure. In addition to helping to reduce these risk factors for the development of coronary artery disease, exercise also can have positive benefits for those with diabetes mellitus, peripheral arterial disease, osteoporosis, and pulmonary disease.

[Chapter 4]

39–C. ST segments are considered to be sensitive indicators of myocardial ischemia or injury. A Q wave is a negative deflection of a QRS complex preceding an R wave. A "pathological" Q wave is an indication of a old transmural myocardial infarction. The PR interval is the time that it takes from the initiation of an electrical impulse in the sinoatrial node to the initiation of electrical activity in the ventricles. The T wave indicates ventricular repolarization.

[Chapter 12]

40–D. The identification and classification of obesity has been somewhat discretionary, with a multitude of available techniques. It appears that height/weight tables provide the least accurate technique, because they do not include any variance for body composition (i.e., amount of fat vs. amount of lean tissue).

[Chapter 8]

41–C. A steady-state condition occurs when a balance exists between the energy required by the working muscles and the rate of ATP production through aerobic metabolism. Oxygen debt is the oxygen consumption in excess of the resting oxygen consumption at the end of an exercise session. Oxygen deficit is the difference between total oxygen actually consumed and the amount that would have been consumed in a steady state. Adaptation is a result of long-term, sustained exercise training.

[Chapter 2]

42–B. The electrocardiogram is an excellent tool for detecting rhythm and conduction abnormalities, chamber enlargements, ischemia, and infarction. ST-segment elevation is a sign of acute myocardial infarction, with resulting loss of R waves that are replaced by Q waves.

[Chapter 4]

43–C. The steps are as follows:

a. Choose the ACSM walking formula.

b. Write down your knowns, and convert the values to the appropriate units:

$$3.5 \text{ mph} \times 26.8 = 93.8 \text{ m} \cdot \text{min}^{-1}$$
$$10\% \text{ grade} = 0.10$$

c. Write down the ACSM walking formula:

$$\text{walking} = (0.1 \times \text{speed}) + (1.8 \times \text{speed} \times \text{fractional grade}) + 3.5 \ (\text{mL} \cdot \text{kg}^{-1} \cdot \text{min}^{-1})$$

d. Substitute the known values for the variable name:

$$\text{mL} \cdot \text{kg}^{-1} \cdot \text{min}^{-1} = (0.1 \times 93.8) + (1.8 \times 93.8 \times 0.1) + 3.5$$
$$\text{mL} \cdot \text{kg}^{-1} \cdot \text{min}^{-1} = 9.38 + 16.884 + 3.5$$

e. Solve for the unknown:

$$\text{mL} \cdot \text{kg}^{-1} \cdot \text{min}^{-1} = 9.38 + 16.884 + 3.5$$
$$\text{gross walking } \dot{V}O_2 = 29.76 \text{ mL} \cdot \text{kg}^{-1} \cdot \text{min}^{-1}$$

[Chapter 11]

44–C. Segmental movements occur around an axis and in a plane. Each of the planes has an associated axis that is perpendicular to it. The mediolateral axis is perpendicular to the sagittal plane, and the anteroposterior axis is perpendicular to the frontal plane. There is no transverse axis.

[Chapter 1]

45–C. The benefits of regular (endurance) exercise for patients with peripheral vascular disease include redistribution of and increased blood flow to the legs, increased tolerance for walking and improved claudication pain tolerance, decreased blood viscosity, and improved muscle cell metabolism.

[Chapter 8]

46–B. The purpose of health screening before engaging in vigorous exercise is to identify clients who require additional medical testing to determine the presence of disease, contraindications for exercise testing or training, or referral to a medically supervised exercise program. Men younger than 40 years and women younger than 50 years with fewer than two coronary artery disease risk factors do not require a physician's evaluation before initiating vigorous exercise.

[Chapter 6]

47–C. An intraventricular conduction disturbance is an abnormal conduction of an electrical impulse below the bundle of His. Intraventricular conduction disturbances include right and left bundle branch block as well as right and left anterior hemiblock.

[Chapter 12]

48–B. Emergency plans must be created, practiced, and implemented in the event of a medical emergency. Clinical personnel must understand the risks associated with exercise and exercise testing, be able to implement preventive measures, and have knowledge regarding the care of an injury or medical emergency.

[Chapter 7]

49–C. Obesity is defined as a surplus of adipose tissue, resulting from excess energy intake relative to energy expenditure. Overweight is defined as a deviation in body weight from some standard or "ideal" weight related to height. Android obesity describes fat accumulation over the chest and arms rather than the lower trunk, which is gynoid obesity.

[Chapter 9]

50–D. Program certification of clinical exercise rehabilitation programs, although a new concept, involves many components that have already been established as part of the exercise program, such as a clearly articulated mission statement, a defined organizational chart, a method of measuring client outcomes, a well-used policy and procedures manual, and so forth. Certification of a program is about the quality of the program, not the financial operations of a program (e.g., billing practices, use of insurance codes).

[Chapter 10]

51–B. Preload refers to diastolic filling (i.e., the amount of blood in the left ventricular prior to ejection). Contractility is the vigor of contraction and may be influenced by ventricular outflow (afterload). Ejection fraction is the ratio of stroke volume to end-diastolic volume.

[Chapter 2]

52–A. Angina pectoris is the pain associated with myocardial ischemia. The pain often is felt in the chest, neck, cheeks, shoulder, or arms. It can be brought on by physical or psychological stress and is relieved when the stressor is removed. Angina can be either classic (typical) or vasospastic (variant or Prinzmetal's).

[Chapter 4]

53–D. The overall goal of health screening before participation in a graded exercise testing or an exercise program is to obtain essential information that will ensure the safety of the participant. Thus, health screening helps to determine the presence of disease, enables one to consider possible contraindications to exercise testing and training, and helps to determine whether referral to a medically supervised exercise program is needed.

[Chapter 6]

54–B. The proper response to a patient who has experienced a cardiac arrest yet is breathing and has a pulse is to call to the emergency medical system immediately; place the patient in the recovery position, with the head to the side to avoid an airway obstruction; and then stay with the patient and continue to monitor his or her vital signs.

[Chapter 7]

55–B. Use the walking metabolic equation to determine the relative oxygen consumption $[(0.1 \times \text{speed}) + (1.8 \times \text{speed} \times \text{grade}) + 3.5]$. Then, convert $\text{mL} \cdot \text{kg}^{-1} \cdot \text{min}^{-1}$ to $\text{L} \cdot \text{min}^{-1}$, and then $\text{L} \cdot \text{min}^{-1}$ to $\text{kcal} \cdot \text{min}^{-1}$:

5% grade = 0.05

4.0 mph = 107.2 m · min^{-1}

200 pounds = 90.91 kg

$\dot{V}\text{O}_2 = (0.1 \times 107.2) + (1.8 \times 107.2 \times 0.05) + 3.5$

$\dot{V}\text{O}_2 = 23.87$ mL · kg^{-1} · min^{-1}

$\dot{V}\text{O}_2 = 23.83$ mL · kg^{-1} · min^{-1} × 90.01 kg/1,000

$\dot{V}\text{O}_2 = 2.17$ L · min^{-1}

[Chapter 11]

56–A. Advancing age brings a progressive decline in bone mineral density and calcium content. This loss accelerates in women immediately after menopause. As a result, older women are at increased risk for bone fractures, which are a significant cause of morbidity and mortality in the elderly. Hip fractures are the most common type and account for a large share of the disability, death, and high medical costs associated with falls.

[Chapter 3]

57–D. Electrocardiography is the least sensitive and least specific of all these tests. Directly visualizing the coronary arteries using coronary angiography provides the highest sensitivity and specificity. Radionuclide imaging and echocardiography have about the same sensitivity and specificity.

[Chapter 4]

58–C. In the resting period of the myocardial cell, the inside of the cell membrane is negatively charged, and the outside of the cell membrane is positively charged. As such, the term **polarized cell** is reserved for the normal "resting myocardial cell" and describes the presence of electrical potential across the cell membrane caused by the separation of electrical charges. When an electrical impulse is generated in a particular area in the heart, the outside of the cell in this area becomes negative, whereas the inside of the cell in this same area becomes positive. This state of cell excitation (caused by a change in polarity) is called **depolarization**. The simulated myocardial cells return to their resting state in a process called **repolarization**.

[Chapter 12]

59–A. At exercise intensities up to 50% of maximal oxygen consumption, the increase in cardiac output is facilitated by increases in heart rate and stroke volume. Thereafter, the increase results almost solely from the continued rise in heart rate.

[Chapter 2]

60–D. Flow-resistive training involves breathing through a progressively smaller opening. Paced breathing helps to coordinate breathing with activities of daily living. Respiratory muscle training increases respiratory muscle strength and endurance. A preset inspiratory pressure, usually at the same fraction of maximal inspiratory pressure, is known as **threshold loading training**.

[ACSM's Guidelines for Exercise Testing and Prescription, 7th ed., pg. 229]

61–A. Isometric contractions occur when the muscle group contracts against a fixed load with no apparent movement and no change in joint angle. In isotonic contractions, the joint angle decreases or increases with production of muscle force. Isokinetic contractions can refer to either a concentric or an eccentric contraction. An isokinetic contraction occurs at a fixed speed of movement and usually involves use of an isokinetic device that can control the speed of rotation along a joint's entire range of motion.

[Chapter 6]

62–C. Family history of coronary artery disease cannot be changed. The other factors listed can, with some intervention, can be changed or modified.

[Chapter 4]

63–B. Staff salaries are not capital expenses; capital expenses are used to procure something tangible for the program. Rather, staff salaries are an example of a variable expense. The purchase of equipment and the cost associated with construction are excellent examples of capital expenses.

[Chapter 10]

64–A. Torque is the product of a force and the perpendicular distance from the line of action of the force, whereas force can be seen as a push or a pull that produces or has the capacity to produce a change in motion of a body. Multiple forces from multiple directions may act on a body; however, it is the sum of the forces, or the **net force**, that determines the resulting change in motion. Newton's laws describe the relationship between forces, torques, and the resulting movements.

[Chapter 1]

65–C. The endothelium comprises a single layer of cells that form a tight barrier between blood and the arterial wall to resist thrombosis, promote vasodilation, and inhibit smooth muscle cells from migration and proliferation into the intima. The intima is the very thin, innermost layer of the artery wall and is composed mainly of connective tissue with some smooth muscle cells. The media, the thickest layer, comprises predominantly smooth muscle cells and is responsible for arterial vasoconstriction and vasodilation. The adventitia is the outermost layer of the artery wall and provides the media and intima with oxygen and other nutrients.

[Chapter 4]

66–B. The electrode position for V_1 is the right sternal border, fourth intercostal space. Electrode V_2 is located in the fourth intercostal space, left sternal border. The position of V_3 is at the midpoint of a straight line between V_2 and V_4, and electrode V_6 is located on the midaxillary line and horizontal to V_4 and V_5.

[Chapter 12]

67–C. The energy expenditure for the warm-up is 2.0 MET × 5 minutes = 10 MET.

The energy expenditure for the treadmill is 9.0 MET × 20 minutes = 180 MET.

The energy expenditure for the cycle is 8.0 MET × 20 minutes = 160 MET.

The energy expenditure for the cool-down is 2.50 MET × 5 minutes = 12.5 MET.

The total energy expenditure is 10 + 180 + 160 + 12.5 = 362.5 MET. Multiply 362.5 MET by 3.5 (because 1 MET = 3.5 mL · kg^{-1} · min^{-1}), which equals 1,268.75 mL · kg^{-1}. Multiply 1,268.75 mL · kg^{-1} by body weight (70 kg), which equals 88,812.5 mL. Divide that number by 1,000 (because 1,000 mL = 1 L), which equals 88.81 L. Multiply 88.81 L by 5 (because 5 kcal equals 1 L of oxygen consumed), which equals 444 kcal.

[Chapter 11]

68–C. Average maximal heart rate is 200 bpm, and average maximal stroke volume is 100 mL/stroke. Average maximal cardiac output is the product of these two values, or 20 L · min^{-1}.

[Chapter 2]

69–C. High ambient temperature or relative humidity increases the risk of heat-related disorders, including heat cramps, heat syncope, dehydration, heat exhaustion, and heat stroke. Exercise will increase heart rate responses at submaximal workloads and lower oxygen consumption at maximal workloads. In this type of environment, the exercise prescription should be altered by lowering the intensity and, possibly, also the duration and, if necessary, by including intermittent rest periods.

[Chapter 4]

70–C. The emergency plan must be written down and available in all testing and exercise areas. The plan should list the specific responsibilities of each staff member, required equipment, and predetermined contacts for an emergency response. All emergencies must be documented with dates, times, actions, people involved, and results. The plan should be practiced with both announced and unannounced drills on a quarterly basis. All staff members, including nonclinical staff members, should be trained in the emergency plan.

[Chapter 7]

71–D. Osteoarthritis is a degenerative joint disease that generally is localized first on an articular cartilage. Rheumatoid arthritis is an inflammatory disease affecting joints as well as organs. Osteoporosis involve the loss of bone density. Multiple sclerosis is a neuromuscular disease.

[Chapter 8]

72–B. Classic symptoms of bronchitis include sputum production, chronic cough, and dyspnea associated with the characteristics listed. The clinical symptom of emphysema is dyspnea associated with hypoxia and hypercapnia, resulting from hypoventilation of the alveoli; minute ventilation also is very high. Asthma is a reversible condition that is characterized by an obvious narrowing of the bronchial airways, causing dyspnea. Atherosclerosis is a progressive disease of the systemic arterial system.

[Chapter 4]

73–D. Exercise training can counteract the harmful physiological effects of inactivity that often are associated with chronic diseases. A number of precautions and contraindications to exercise exist. However, one such precaution is to ensure adequate warm-up and cool-down periods.

[Chapter 8]

74–D. Direct measurement of oxygen consumption requires an extensive laboratory and specialized equipment. Oxygen consumption can be meas-

ured in the laboratory using techniques of direct and indirect calorimetry, or it can be estimated from the workload.

[Chapter 2]

75–C. Transient ischemic attacks are sudden, brief ischemic attacks usually involving the carotid or vertebral arteries in the neck. They do not affect the heart directly. Other common symptoms are slight paralysis on one side (hemiparesis) and difficulty speaking (transient ischemic attacks).

[Chapter 7]

76–D. Physical activity elevates oxygen consumption above resting levels. This additional oxygen uptake by the body is known as the **net oxygen consumption**. Total oxygen consumption (the resting energy expenditure and the oxygen consumption of physical activity) is the gross energy expenditure (i.e., gross oxygen consumption). Net and gross oxygen consumption can be expressed in relative or absolute terms.

[Chapter 11]

77–D. Two PVCs in a row is known as a **PVC couplet**. Ventricular tachycardia is when three PVCs (or more) occur in a row without any normal beats.

[Chapter 12]

78–D. A complication of an extensive myocardial infarction is a ventricular aneurysm. Characteristics of a ventricular aneurysm include a degeneration of the myocardial wall, which becomes very thin and often bulges out during systole. These fibers do not contract during systole.

[Chapter 4]

79–C. The amount of weight or resistance and repetitions will vary for strength versus endurance. Rapid strength gains will be realized at higher resistance or weight (80–100% of one repetition maximum) and lower repetitions (six to eight). For muscular endurance, a lower weight is used (40–60% of one repetition maximum) and higher repetitions (8–15).

[Chapter 8]

80–B. Mounted on a balloon catheter that is inflated or expanded at the site of a coronary artery blockage, a stent is a slotted, stainless-steel tube that is permanently implanted in the artery, where it acts as a scaffold to hold the walls of a coronary artery open.

[Chapter 4]

81–A. The PR interval is measured from the beginning of the P wave to the beginning of the QRS complex. It represents the time that is required for the impulse to spread through the atria and to pass through the AV junction. A normal PR interval is 0.12 to 0.20 second; a PR interval prolonged beyond 0.20 second with all P waves conducted and all PR intervals the same indicates first-degree AV block.

[Chapter 12]

82–C. Myocardial infarction can be determined and localized by careful inspection of certain electrocardiographic leads. Pathological Q waves on the anterior leads indicate a transmural myocardial infarction of the anterior wall of the left ventricle.

[Chapter 12]

83–A. Atherosclerosis is thought to begin at an early age—at birth, according to some. The disease process is related to the presence of risk factors. Progression does not necessarily occur in a stable, linear manner. Some lesions may develop slowly and are relatively stable, whereas other lesions progress very quickly as a result of frequent plaque rupture, formation of thrombi, and changes in the intima.

[Chapter 4]

84–C. Various graded exercise test protocols are available. Some are continuous (with measurements taken without interruption), and others are discontinuous (involving a momentary stop while measurements are obtained). Some test protocols are taken during a step test, whereas others are taken in the field.

[Chapter 6]

85–C. Exercise has various benefits for patients with congestive heart failure. It appears as though most of the physical improvements are peripheral (i.e., within the skeletal muscle) and not central. Other benefits of regular exercise for patients with congestive heart failure are a decrease in symptoms and an enhanced quality of life.

[Chapter 8]

86–A. Although strength training (resistance training) may be beneficial in all of these special populations, regular resistance training helps to conserve bone mass, thus decreasing the progression of osteoporosis.

[Chapter 8]

87–B. Even after exposure and training, an approximately 10% reduction in maximal oxygen consumption occurs per every 1,000 m of altitude above 1,500 m. After acclimatization, expect a continued increase in pulmonary ventilation and heart rate response at submaximal workloads but a reduced cardiac output, stroke volume, and heart rate at maximal exercise.

[Chapter 4]

88–C. A QRS duration exceeding 0.20 second indicates an intraventricular conduction delay. Examples of intraventricular conduction delays include PVCs and left bundle branch block.

[Chapter 12]

89–B. With the physical demands of exercise, emergency situations can occur, especially in a clinical setting where patients with disease are exercising. The incidence of a cardiac arrest during exercise testing is 0.4 in 10,000 (1/2,500).

[Chapter 6]

90–B. Very-low-density lipoprotein cholesterol is composed almost entirely of triglycerides, which are converted to a fuel source by the enzyme lipoprotein lipase (which increases with exercise). High-density lipoprotein cholesterol also is increased by regular exercise: The very-low-density lipoprotein remnants serve as precursors to high-density lipoprotein cholesterol.

[Chapter 4]

91–B. The health behavior change model comprises three phases: antecedents, adoption, and maintenance. Antecedents refers to all conditions that exist that can support, initiate, or hinder changes in health behavior, including information, instruction, role models, and previous experience. Adoption is the early phase of making a change in a health behavior or the intention to make a change (often a difficult decision). This phase involves any environmental and physical prerequisites, self-efficiency and outcome efficiency, cues to action, goal setting, and behavioral intention. The maintenance phase is one of continued response and includes relapse prevention, reinforcement, monitoring, and contracting.

[Chapter 5]

92–A. Lowering total cholesterol and low-density lipoprotein cholesterol has proven to be effective in reducing and even reversing atherosclerosis. The goal is to reduce the availability of lipids to the injured endothelium. In primary-prevention trials, lowering total cholesterol and low-density lipoprotein cholesterol has been shown to reduce the incidence and mortality of coronary artery disease.

[Chapter 9]

93–D. Field tests are those that can be administered with minimal equipment and in varying conditions. In the Cooper 12-minute test, the subject covers the greatest distance possible during the 12-minute test period. Maximal oxygen consumption is estimated from the distance covered in meters. The 1.5-mile test is an estimate of maximal oxygen consumption taken as a result of the time needed to cover the distance. The Rockport walking test is a submaximal test that requires the patient to walk 1 mile as fast as possible. Immediate postexercise heart rate is measured, and maximal oxygen consumption is predicted based on gender, time, and heart rate. Treadmill testing is a complicated procedure that normally is performed in a laboratory setting.

[Chapter 6]

94–D. Transmural myocardial infarction produces changes in both the QRS complex and the ST segment. ST-segment elevation or tall, upright T waves are the earliest signs associated with transmural myocardial infarction. ST-segment elevation may persist for a few hours to a few days.

[Chapter 12]

95–C. The purpose of the warm-up is to slowly and safely activate the body's responses to exercise and to increase the range of motion to prepare joints and muscles for vigorous activity. Beneficial physiological responses include increased heart rate and stroke volume, increased body temperature and muscle temperature, and increased metabolic activity.

[Chapter 8]

96–A. It is essential that clinicians be familiar with contraindications to exercise and exercise testing. For certain groups of patients, the risks of exercise testing (and of exercise in general) outweigh the benefits.

[Chapter 7]

97–A. Physical inactivity (sedentary life style) has been determined to have a similar risk in the development of atherosclerosis as the other major risk factors (smoking, hypertension, and elevated cholesterol). Obesity, diabetes mellitus, and stress are important risk factors but are not thought to be as significant as smoking, high blood pressure, or high cholesterol.

[Chapter 4]

98–B. The 400-m sprint is an example of physical activity requiring anaerobic glycolysis to produce energy in the form of ATP. Shorter sprints rely on ready stores of ATP and phosphocreatine. Longer runs require aerobic metabolism to produce ATP.

[Chapter 2]

99–C. A mean electrical axis between $-30°$ and $+100°$ is considered to be normal. An axis that is more negative than $-30°$ is considered to be left-axis deviation; an axis greater than $+100°$ is considered to be right-axis deviation until it reaches $-180°$ and then is considered to be extreme right- or extreme left-axis deviation.

[Chapter 12]

100–C. β-Adrenergic blockers significantly reduce first-year mortality rates in patients after myocardial infarction. Aspirin is a platelet inhibitor. Calcium-channel blockers reduce ischemia by altering the major determinants of myocardial oxygen supply and demand but have not been shown to reduce mortality rates in patients after myocardial infarction. Nitrates reduce ischemia by reducing myocardial oxygen demand, with some increase in oxygen supply, and are used in the treatment of typical and variant angina.

[Chapter 4]

Recommended Readings

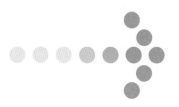

General Recommendations

American College of Sports Medicine. ACSM's Exercise Management for Persons with Chronic Diseases and Disabilities. Champaign, IL: Human Kinetics, 2003.

American College of Sports Medicine. ACSM's Guidelines for Exercise Testing and Prescription. 7th Ed. Baltimore: Lippincott Williams & Wilkins, 2005.

American College of Sports Medicine. ACSM's Resource Manual for Guidelines for Exercise Testing and Prescription. 5th Ed. Baltimore: Lippincott Williams & Wilkins, 2005.

American College of Sports Medicine. ACSM's Resources for Clinical Exercise Physiology: Musculoskeletal, Neuromuscular, Neoplastic, Immunologic, and Hematologic Conditions. Baltimore: Lippincott Williams & Wilkins, 2002.

American College of Sports Medicine. ACSM's Resources for the Personal Trainer. Baltimore: Lippincott Williams & Wilkins, 2005.

Selected List of ACSM Position Stands

Physical Activity and Bone Health, November 1, 2004.

Exercise and Hypertension, March 1, 2004.

Automated External Defibrillators in Health/Fitness Facilities, March 1, 2002.

Progression Models in Resistance Training for Healthy Adults, February 1, 2002.

Appropriate Intervention Strategies for Weight Loss and Prevention of Weight Regain for Adults, December 1, 2001.

Nutrition and Athletic Performance, December 1, 2000.

Exercise and Type 2 Diabetes, July 1, 2000.

Recommended Quantity and Quality of Exercise for Developing and Maintaining Cardiorespiratory and Muscular Fitness and Flexibility in Healthy Adults, June 1, 1998.

Exercise and Physical Activity for Older Adults, June 1, 1998.

The Female Athlete Triad, May 1, 1997.

www.acsm-msse.org

Current Comments

The ACSM has developed Current Comments on many topics. For more information, see http://www.acsm.org/health%2Bfitness/comments.htm.

CHAPTER 1: ANATOMY AND BIOMECHANICS

Hamil J, Knutzen KM. Biomechanical Basis of Human Movement. Baltimore: Lippincott Williams & Wilkins, 2003.

Nordin M, Frankel VH. Basic Biomechanics of the Musculoskeletal System. 2nd Ed. Philadelphia: Lea & Febiger, 1989.

CHAPTER 2: EXERCISE PHYSIOLOGY

McArdle W, Katch F, Katch V. Exercise Physiology. Energy, Nutrition, and Human Performance. 5th Ed. Baltimore: Lippincott Williams & Wilkins, 2001.

CHAPTER 3: HUMAN DEVELOPMENT AND AGING

Skinner JS, ed. Exercise Testing and Exercise Prescription for Special Cases: Theoretical Basis and Clinical Application. Philadelphia: Lippincott Williams & Wilkins, 2005.

CHAPTER 4: PATHOPHYSIOLOGY/RISK FACTORS

Campaigne BN, Lampman RI. Exercise in the Clinical Management of Diabetes Mellitus. Champaign, IL: Human Kinetics, 1994.

Grundy SM, et al. Implications of recent clinical trials for the National Cholesterol Education Program Adult Treatment Panel III Guidelines. Circulation 2004;110:227–239.

Fuster V, et al. Atherothrombosis and Coronary Artery Disease. Baltimore: Lippincott Williams & Wilkins, 2004.

Chobanian AV, et al. Seventh Report of the Joint National Commission on Prevention, Detection, Evaluation, and Treatment of High Blood Pressure. JAMA 2003:289:2560–2572

Lazarus SL, et al. Third Report of the National Cholesterol Education Program (NCEP) Expert Panel on Detection, Evaluation, and Treatment of High Blood Cholesterol in Adults (Adult Treatment Panel II.) JAMA 2001;285:2486–2497.

CHAPTER 5: HUMAN BEHAVIOR AND PSYCHOLOGY

Prochaska JO, Norcross JC, DiClemente CC. Changing for Good: A Revolutionary Six-Stage Program for Overcoming Bad Habits and Moving Your Life Positively Forward. New York: Avon Books, 1994.

Sallis J, Owen N. Physical Activity and Behavioral Medicine. Thousand Oaks, CA: Sage Publications, 1999.

U.S. Department of Health and Human Services, Public Health Service, Centers for Disease Control and Prevention, National Center for Chronic Disease Prevention and Health Promotion, Division of Nutrition and Physical Activity. Physical Activity: A Guide for Community Action. Champaign, IL: Human Kinetics, 1999.

CHAPTER 6: HEALTH APPRAISAL AND FITNESS TESTING

Heyward VH. Advanced Fitness Assessment and Exercise Prescription. 3rd Ed. Champaign, IL: Human Kinetics, 1998.

Howley ET, Franks BD. Health Fitness Instructor's Handbook. 4th Ed. Champaign, IL: Human Kinetics, 2003.

Skinner JS. Exercise Testing and Prescription for Special Cases. 3rd Ed. Baltimore: Lippincott Williams & Wilkins, 2005.

Wasserman K. Principles of Exercise Testing and Interpretation. Baltimore: Lippincott Williams and Wilkins, 2004.

CHAPTER 7: SAFETY, INJURY PREVENTION, AND EMERGENCY CARE

Lieber R. Skeletal Muscle Structure and Function: The Physiological Basis of Rehabilitation. Baltimore: Lippincott Williams & Wilkins, 2002.

Tharrett SJ, Peterson JA, eds. ACSM's Health/Fitness Facility Standards and Guidelines. 2nd Ed. Champaign, IL: Human Kinetics, 1997.

CHAPTER 8: EXERCISE PROGRAMMING

Ehrman JK, Gordon PM, Visich PS, Keteyian SJ. Clinical Exercise Physiology. Champaign, IL: Human Kinetics, 2003.

Pollock ML, Wilmore JH. Exercise in Health and Disease: Evaluation and Prescription for Prevention and Rehabilitation. 2nd Ed. Philadelphia: WB Saunders, 1990.

CHAPTER 9: NUTRITION AND WEIGHT MANAGEMENT

Grundy SM, et al. Implications of recent clinical trials for the National Cholesterol Education Program Adult Treatment Panel III Guidelines. Circulation 2004;110:227–239.

Fuster V. Atherothrombosis and Coronary Artery Disease. Baltimore: Lippincott Williams & Wilkins, 2004.

Shape Up America, American Obesity Association. Guidance for Treatment of Adult Obesity. Bethesda, MD: Shape Up America, 1996.

Lazarus SL. Third Report of the National Cholesterol Education Program (NCEP) Expert Panel on Detection, Evaluation, and Treatment of High Blood Cholesterol in Adults (Adult Treatment Panel II). JAMA 2001;285:2486–2497.

CHAPTER 10: PROGRAM ADMINISTRATION/MANAGEMENT

Cleverly WO. Essentials of Health Care Finance. Gaithersburg, MD: Aspen Publishers, 1997.

Grantham WC, Patton RW, York TD, Winick ML. Health Fitness Management. Champaign, IL: Human Kinetics, 1998.

Langley TD, Hawkins JD. Administration for Exercise Related Professions. Englewood, CO: Morton Publishing, 1999.

Patton RW, Grantham WC, Gerson RF, Gettman LR. Developing and Managing Health/Fitness Facilities. Champaign, IL: Human Kinetics, 1989.

Tharrett SJ, Peterson JA, eds. ACSM's Health/Fitness Facility Standards and Guidelines. 2nd Ed. Champaign, IL: Human Kinetics, 1997.

CHAPTER 11: METABOLIC CALCULATIONS

Kaminsky L. Metabolic Calculations Tutorial. CD-ROM, version 1.00.

CHAPTER 12: ELECTROCARDIOGRAPHY

Huff J. ECG Workout: Exercises in Arrhythmia Interpretation. Baltimore: Lippincott Williams & Wilkins, 2001.

Wagner GS. Marriot's Practical Electrocardiography. 10th Ed. Baltimore: Lippincott Williams & Wilkins, 2000.

Index

Page numbers in *italics* denote figures; those followed by "t" denote tables